# NURSING ACTIONS
# FOR
# HEALTH PROMOTION

M. Heath

# NURSING ACTIONS FOR HEALTH PROMOTION

## COLLEEN SMITHERMAN, M.Ed., R.N.

**FORMERLY, ASSISTANT PROFESSOR OF NURSING
DEPAUW UNIVERSITY SCHOOL OF NURSING
GREENCASTLE, INDIANA**

 **F. A. DAVIS COMPANY • Philadelphia**

**Library of Congress Cataloging in Publication Data**

Smitherman, Colleen.
  Nursing actions for health promotion.
  Includes bibliographies and index.
    1. Nursing—Psychological aspects.   2. Nursing—
Social aspects.   I. Title. [DNLM: Nursing care.
2. Sick role.   3. Crisis intervention. WY100 S664i]
RT86.S64      610.73        80-17464
ISBN 0-8036-7941-6

*To Marvin,*
*who provided unfailing support and*
*encouragement.*
*To Todd and Teri,*
*who provided welcome diversion.*

# PREFACE

This book explores areas of nursing practice which are usually independent from medically related nursing activities. It assumes that nurses are involved in providing health care which goes beyond medical care and in promoting wellness which goes beyond medical wellness.

Part 1 discusses processes which the nurse uses as she works with individuals and families to improve or maintain their level of wellness. An attempt is made to thoroughly explain each process, provide evaluative criteria, and provide examples of the use of the process. It is hoped that this knowledge, when combined with practice and experience, can lead to expertise in the use of each process.

The second and third parts explore common situations which are appropriate for nursing diagnosis and nursing management. Part 2 describes common responses that individuals or families may make to actual or threatened changes in their level of wellness. Part 3 explores selected situations which may potentially promote growth for the individuals involved if the situation is resolved optimally. For each response and situation, background theory, management suggestions, assessment criteria, and examples of intervention are given.

This book has been designed to be useful for nurses who work in any setting and with individuals at any stage in the life cycle. Therefore, the material presented concentrates on similarities among individuals rather than on dissimilarities such as the presence of a specific medical diagnosis or their presence in a specific health care facility. A consistent attempt has been made throughout the text to portray the individual or family being served as active and responsible for their wellness and not as passive recipients of nursing care. Therefore, the nurse is encouraged throughout the book to "work with" rather than to "do to" the individual or family. The term "client" has not been used. Client is defined as a person under the protection of another—a vassal or dependent. This is definitely not the relationship of the nurse to those she works with that is promoted here.

It is believed that the consumer must be understood and helped within the social constellation of his primary reference group, most often the family in the broadest sense of the term. Rarely is an individual's problem solely his own. What affects him affects his immediate social contacts. For this reason, the family is considered an important focus in the book.

Consistent emphasis is placed in the book on the importance of the nurse's understanding of herself and her reactions to those she serves. She must be in touch with her own feelings, attitudes, and values, and must explore her responses to others. Self-knowledge will enable her to recognize her own strengths and weaknesses, to deal with her own problems, and to avoid imposing her biases and needs on others. Therefore, consideration is given to relating each topic explored to the nurse personally.

The aim of this text is not primarily to present new knowledge. Rather the intent has been to analyze and synthesize existing information into concise commentaries on a number of subjects. Unfortunately, the information presented is not always based on statistical research, but often represents the theories and concepts of recognized authorities. Therefore, it remains for the reader to validate the usefulness of this material in her practice situation. Numerous examples have been given to show how the material has been applied. The examples presented are based on the actual experiences of the author and of other nurses or students. They are not "perfect" interventions because they represent for the most part the actions and accomplishments of nurses working in real settings under the real pressures nurses experience.

Throughout the text, the nurse has usually been referred to as "she." This has been done in order to avoid clumsy and distracting circumlocutions. No slight is intended to the growing number of men active in nursing. Physicians and patients have generally been referred to as "he" for the same reasons.

This book should be useful to the student of nursing and to the graduate nurse whose basic education did not include the topics presented. Readers should consider this text as a point of departure from which they must exert time and effort to reach competence in the use of the processes discussed and in intervention in the situations described.

*Colleen Smitherman*

# ACKNOWLEDGMENTS

I am indebted to Marjorie Fine Mead and Corinne Hudson Reutebuch, who collaborated with me initially in determining the contents of this book. Margie deserves special thanks for writing the first drafts of the preface and the chapter on the helping process.

I wish to thank the faculty of the Department of Nursing of the College of St. Catherine, in St. Paul, Minnesota, who have influenced my thinking on nursing processes and on independent nursing practice situations.

I would also like to thank Judith M. Kim and Karen R. Emilson of F. A. Davis Company, who encouraged the publication of this book. I am especially thankful for the secretarial skills of Janice E. Coleman, who turned my scribbled and sometimes unpolished thoughts into a crisp, legible manuscript.

C.S.

# CONTENTS

# PART 1

## NURSING PROCESSES

This section provides an introduction to five basic processes: the communication process, the helping process, the problem solving process, the teaching process, and the leadership process. The processes discussed can be used in any setting and with any individual or family to assist them to attain optimal wellness.

These processes do not stand alone but the use of each one requires the concomitant application of nursing knowledges appropriate to the situation. In addition, conscientious practice and experience are required to develop skill in the use of each process. While each process is presented separately in order to facilitate comprehension, it is to be expected that in practice the nurse may find that these processes overlap and may merge into one unique nursing process.

The nurse may find that use of these processes is helpful in contacts with coworkers and in her personal life as well as in her professional work with the consumers of her services.

# CHAPTER 1

# THE COMMUNICATION PROCESS

Nursing is a profession which involves in all settings communicating with people such as patients, families, and others in the health care system. When one enters the profession of nursing one has been communicating with others since shortly after birth and has had considerable experience in interacting with others. However, there is still more which can be learned about the communication process.

Communication is basic to all of the processes that a nurse uses. For example, through communication the nurse forms helping relationships, identifies and solves problems, and performs health teaching. Indeed, the nurse might be described as a communication specialist because of the central nature of communication to her practice. The nurse is frequently the person who has the greatest potential contact with patients and families so that she may be able to use her time with others to promote meaningful communication.

At first glance, communication is usually assumed to be synonymous with conversation, but broadly defined, communication includes all messages, verbal or otherwise, conscious or unconscious, which two or more individuals send through any channel of communication between themselves.

## FORMS OF COMMUNICATION

There are many forms of communication which can occur. *Social communication* is probably one of the most common and most familiar to all individuals. Social communication is primarily engaged in for its time filling or entertainment value. There is usually a free give-and-take among those involved and topics are covered at levels which usually exclude discussion of feelings or personal significance. The following is an example of the verbal portion of a social conversation.

Jane: Hi, Jill. How are you doing?
Jill:    Just fine. Have you been busy this week?
Jane: Not too bad. How about you?
Jill:    It's been really slow this week actually.

Jane: Do you work this weekend?
Jill:   No. Betty and I are going to . . .

There is another common form of communication called *formal communication*. The man or woman reading the evening news on the radio or television, a panel discussion of a school problem, an entertainer performing on stage, and the individual presenting a lecture to a class are engaging in formal communication. This type of communication is usually characterized by much less give-and-take with one individual primarily sending a message and the rest receiving even though some forms allow for audience interaction. Most individuals have experienced formal communications as the receiver but have much less experience as the sender of formal communication. Written information such as this book is also an example of formal communication as are works of art in which an artist communicates a message through a painting or a piece of music.

*Therapeutic communication* involves another dimension. In therapeutic communication, a situation occurs in which one individual experiences attention to his concerns and needs so that he has been helped by the interaction toward wellness. Social conversations may at times be nearly therapeutic. Many individuals can recall feeling better after a good chat which was purely social with a friend. A formal communication situation may also be nearly therapeutic at times. Individuals often report being helped by a meaningful sermon or article, for example. Although these situations may be therapeutic on occasion, therapeutic communication which is deliberately planned and contains specific characteristics is believed to be most likely to be consistently helpful. Therapeutic communicaiton can be identified when an interaction occurs which involves an individual who is focusing on helping another and has temporarily put aside his own needs and concerns.

A nurse may use all three forms of communication in her practices. For example, a nurse who works in a hospital may use patient focused social communication as she orients a new patient and his family to the room. By the use of patient focused social communication she might convey to the patient useful information and her interest, availability, and friend-liness. Formal communication might be used by a nurse when she speaks to a group of parents in a rehabilitation center about helping their preschool children prepare for school entry. But it is through the use of therapeutic individualized communication that a nurse has the greatest potential for influencing the health and well-being of patients.

Unfortunately, individuals beginning their professional nursing education are usually unfamiliar with therapeutic communication. Many of the goals and methods of therapeutic communication may seem very contrary to their previous experiences in formal and especially social communication. Underlying the process of therapeutic communication is the assumption that an individual desires to and is helped by having someone actively guide him to discover and express his problems, his feelings about the problems, and hopefully to facilitate his efforts at resolving his problems. The unwritten rules of social conversation, however, discourage one from bringing up or dwelling on problems, concerns, or difficulties. If one conversant in a conversation does mention a problem, other conversants usually act promptly to dismiss the problem. Therefore, learners usually enter nursing with a mental set appropriate for social communication but contrary to therapeutic communication. Some of the ideas which are often expressed by the learner beginning to study therapeutic communication are:

1. People are better off if you don't bring up their problems.
2. Talking about problems only makes them seem worse.
3. People would rather have someone divert their attention from their problems than have someone focus on them.

4. One shouldn't let people bring up questions or problems if one doesn't know the answers to them.
5. Allowing people to talk about their innermost fears and anxieties is actually prying into their private lives and not appropriate.
6. Learning therapeutic communication is confusing and one will never know what to say to people afterwards.
7. If therapeutic communication is so important, why does one never hear nurses or anyone else talking that way?
8. What's wrong with social communication? One sounds phoney if he tries to use therapeutic skills.
9. Do all nurses really need to learn this or only those going into psychiatric nursing?
10. What good does talking about problems do anyway?

Because of these beliefs which an individual often brings with her into nursing, learning therapeutic communication is one of the largest tasks many nurses face because it requires extensive attitude and behavior change. Some individuals seem to naturally adapt and some never do. There is no magic formula to help individuals accomplish this awesome task but hard work and practice are useful. Most individuals never truly accept the concept of therapeutic communication until they have had an experience in which they help another and begin to realize the powerfulness of their interaction. It is hoped that this chapter will help provide examples which demonstrate the value and usefulness of therapeutic communication as a sometimes appropriate addition to the other types of communication skills which an individual brings into nursing situations.

## COMMUNICATION DYNAMICS

### Components of Messages

A communication may be looked at from many perspectives. One such perspective is that of message components. Most obvious is the element of *verbal* message or the actual words spoken. Less obvious but of more importance is the *paraverbal* message, or how the words are spoken. This includes such elements as the tone of voice, rate of speech, pitch of voice, tempo, inflections, emphasis, and loudness. Whining and other vocal sounds such as sighs, groans, moans, and grunts are also paraverbal messages. These numerous infinitesimal characteristics imply messages such as uncertainty, excitement, hesitation, surprise, anger, disgust, love, joy, sarcasm, and so forth. The paraverbal message is more influential than the verbal message so that the listener usually gets the message sent accurately even if he was not able to distinguish the actual verbal message. The influence of the paraverbal message on the verbal message can be appreciated by performing this exercise. Say the phrase, "Come here" combined with the paraverbal messages of annoyance, anticipation, elation, regret, fear, or affection. The words stay the same but the message becomes vastly different in each situation. If the verbal and paraverbal messages are in opposition to each other, the receiver will be more influenced by the paraverbal message as in the communication, "I'm so glad to see you" combined with a paraverbal message of boredom and disinterest.[9]

In addition to the verbal and paraverbal messages contained in a communication, there is a third important message called the *nonverbal message*. The nonverbal message is conveyed in a large number of ways as will be explored.

## FACIAL EXPRESSION

The facial expression can communicate messages which agree with, distract from, or contradict the verbal and paraverbal message. Even while not speaking, an individual's facial expression communicates messages to the one who is speaking to that individual or one who might speak. The face has the greatest potential and usefulness for nonverbal communication,[10,11] and for this reason an individual usually learns at a young age to begin exercising control over his facial expression. For example, a child learns through trial and error that telling a fib with a "straight face" will more likely fool Mom or Dad. A nurse may be advised to carefully control her facial expression when changing an unpleasant dressing or seeing a deformed body part, for example.

One is not always able to completely control his facial expression in all situations and the facial expression may show traces of this lack of complete control if one looks closely.[10,11]

## EYE MOVEMENTS

Eye movements, while a part of facial expression, can communicate much to another.[2,9] They can be used as signals from one person to another. These signals indicate whether another individual should speak, continue, or stop. The speaker also may use eye movements to indicate his truthfulness, interest, seriousness, and so on. Status may be communicated by eye movements because the person in a group with the most status gives less eye contact than he receives. It has been suggested that eye movements can indicate who should talk in a group because the one speaking will usually indicate who is to be the next speaker before he finishes by looking at him.[9] The importance of eye movements is noted in the phrase, "Look me straight in the eye and say that." Also, the new mother is felt to be adjusting appropriately to her infant if she holds her infant so that their eyes can meet.

In formal communication situations, a speaker may watch the eye movements of his audience to determine their reaction to his message. Trying to avoid eye contact with another may indicate avoidance, shyness, deference, dishonesty, or fear. Eye contact may be used to signal interest, desire, or an invitation such as in, "She gave him the eye." A child being scolded lowers his eyes to the floor and his exasperated father raises his to the heavens. Eyes can shift, dance, roll, stare coldly, piercingly, or blankly, and cry. Eyelashes can be lowered, raised, batted, or winked. Eyebrows can be raised in surprise or lowered in consternation. It is believed that although one may control a facial expression to deny an emotion, the eyes are subject to less control and may betray the facial expression.

## LIP MOVEMENTS

Lip movements are another part of facial expression and have a significance all their own. There is the frozen smile, the plastic smile, the wicked smile, the friendly smile, and so on. Lips can be taut, pouting, quivering, or snarling. The person anxious to speak may wet his lips or partially open his mouth. The person hesitant to speak may "button" his lips or may bite his lip. Parents describe a tremendous increase in feeling for their infant when he bestows his first smile upon them.

## BODY MOVEMENTS

How people who talk together use their bodies can communicate their relationship. Hall has identified distances which adults use if possible to separate themselves from others according to the relationship.[16] From 0 to 18 inches is considered an intimate distance which can be violated by only those most close to the individual. From 18 inches to 4 feet is a personal distance which most people find acceptable for talking to friends. From 4 feet to 8 feet is a social distance which is comfortable for relating to acquaintances. Over 12 feet is described as a public distance which provides little possibility for personal involvement. Of course, many situations demand that these optimal distances be violated and not everyone shares the same ideas about acceptable distances.

Posture can present messages as to whether the conversants are relaxed—shown by extension of the body—or anxious—shown by contraction of the body.[9] Leaning forward at the waist toward another may communicate increasing interest.[1] Leaning away may signify rejection or withdrawal. Slow motion videotape recordings of behavior show that individuals who are talking with one another move in a synchronous dance with one another in time to the conversation.[9] This dancing phenomenon has been seen in studies of the interaction between an infant and an adult. Babbling babies will take turns speaking with an adult. This tends to indicate that infants are attuned to the role of body movements in communication from the beginning.[7,22]

The movements of body parts are highly significant in a communication. The individual may use his hands and arms to emphasize a point, give directions, and regulate the flow of the conversation. Hands and arms can be used to touch another affectionately or spank a child in anger. Hands and arms alone have communicative value as in signaling to a friend with a wave. One may use his hands to gain comfort as does the child holding his favorite blanket and the adult playing with a paper clip.

Feet may convey messages as in the incessant tapping foot of one who is impatient, the kick under the table to another to change topics, or the rhythmically kicking foot of one who is anxious.

Children stand or sit closer together and touch each other more than adults with a gradual decrease in closeness and touching developing as the child ages.[29] Adults touch children less as the child ages.[27]

The way one uses his body parts and the positions he puts them in are probably very reliable indicators of the person's internal state and are subject usually to very little conscious control. Thus, they can provide valuable, accurate, and authentic information. Consider the patient who is pretending to be relaxed but is betrayed by his hands clenched on the edges of his chair. There are several interesting books on body language which explore body movements and postures in detail.

## PHYSICAL APPEARANCE

Physical appearance has been described as of communicative value in an interaction.[9] Individuals who are close to the current appearance idealized by society are often favored in interpretations of situations. If an unkempt young man with long hair, an elderly lady with white hair, and a smartly dressed handsome middle-aged man were all speeding in identical automobiles in a residential zone, an observer might decide that the young man was a radical carelessly defying the law, the elderly lady was too old to drive, and the middle-aged man was a businessman who was en route to an important meeting but was driving carefully under the circumstances. If the individuals had been of different racial groups, the conclusions the average observer arrived at might have been different.

The hairstyle, clothes, jewelry, and makeup one wears may communicate social status, economic status, occupation, and personality characteristics. Thus, individual traits may be focused on or ignored by an observer because of physical appearance.

Nonverbal messages are believed to be more influential than verbal and paraverbal messages in a communication. When the nonverbal message contradicts the verbal and paraverbal message, the receiver will usually perceive the nonverbal message. This situation is demonstrated in the classic example of the nurse saying, "I would be glad to answer any of your questions" as she glances at her watch and edges towards the door. Thus the old saying, "Actions speak louder than words."

In summary, messages have three components. The least obvious or unconscious component is the most accurate and influential. Nurses need to learn to analyze the different components they use to send messages and analyze the verbal, paraverbal, and nonverbal components of the messages they send. It has been estimated that in any communication, the verbal message accounts for 7 percent of what is communicated, the paraverbal message accounts for 38 percent, and the nonverbal message communicates the remaining 55 percent of the content.[25]

## The Environment

In addition to the message sources described previously, aspects of the environment have communicative value. The use of *space* has significance.[9] The more important one is, the larger and more private one's space becomes. Thus, the director of nursing in an imaginary hospital has a large private office. The head nurse has a small office with a glass window which others use daily. Staff nurses have lockers in a room shared by many others. Patients have rooms, without door locks, which they are temporarily occupying.

The element of use of *time* has communicative value about the relationships.[9] The patient waits for the nurse and for quite long periods. The physician must never wait very long for the nurse. The most important speaker holds the floor longest and is interrupted less.

Objects in the environment communicate information about the prestige and personality of the user of the objects.[9] In the imaginary hospital the physician's lounge is furnished in much more opulence than the nurse's lounge. There may not even be a patient's lounge.

## Message Channels

Messages in most situations are sent on a variety of channels. In other words, when one sends a message such as, "Come here," it is sent on the *auditory* channel by the words one speaks. It is often accompanied with a gesture of summons on the *visual* channel. One could also reach out and pull someone towards them on the *tactile* channel. There are many situations in which only one channel is used. Use of the telephone presently limits one to only the auditory channel. It is interesting to speculate on why some individuals dislike talking to others on the telephone and others would prefer to conduct all business over the phone. A letter usually communicates only on the visual channel. Reaching out to another in the dark with a squeeze of the hand could be purely tactile.

The use of these three channels is most obvious, but the *olfactory* channel is also commonly used. The wife who applies perfume just before meeting her husband may be communicating a message with various connotations. A letter can be written on scented stationery. One who blows cigarette smoke in others' faces may be sending unconscious messages. The smell of food cooking may remind others that they are hungry. Communication between humans on the olfactory channel is probably better developed than we realize as recent studies with infants and their mothers are indicating.

Communications which use many channels are usually more accurately perceived and desirable than those using only one channel. Most of us are familiar with the uncomfortable frustration of watching a television when the auditory portion is missing or talking to someone who is not watching us. An individual can become more discerning about a message as he is exposed to more channels. Thus, one who watches someone as he speaks perceives the message more accurately than one who listens but is looking elsewhere and vice versa.

The messages sent on various channels may not agree. Usually, one selects the message on the visual channel as more reliable than the message on the aural-auditory channel if there is discrepancy. This is reflected by the old adage to believe half of what one sees and almost nothing of what one hears. Therefore, verbal and paraverbal messages, which are sent on the auditory channel, are less influential than nonverbal messages, which are sent on the visual channel. This leads again to the example of the visual message sent by the nurse backing from the room overshadowing the auditory message, "I'll be glad to answer any of your questions."

Individuals vary in how receptive they are to different channels. Increasing the perceptual abilities of various senses by practice and experience is one of the challenging tasks a nurse faces. One can learn to increase what he receives on the visual channel by conscious effort to look more carefully and more discriminatingly at what he is seeing. One can develop the auditory channel similarly until even slight paraverbal messages are heard. Developing the olfactory sense is important also. Some nurses report, for example, that they can distinguish an organism causing an infection by its particular odor. Nurses develop their tactile sense when they learn to differentiate a weak pulse from a strong pulse, palpate body structures, feel skin temperature, and so forth. Some individuals have physiologic limitation on how much of a channel may be developed such as a hearing impairment, for example. It is believed that other channels may be more fully developed to compensate for deficiencies in another channel.

Anything that is present on a channel besides the message being sent is called noise.[29,34] The presence of noise will decrease the reception of the message. One of the most common sources of noise is within the individual himself. Thinking about something else during the conversation is an example of interpersonal noise which decreases receptivity. Interpersonal noise also occurs when one lets preconceived perceptions of another distort the message being sent. Environmental noise such as distractions and interruptions can decrease communication. Noise can be controlled to a considerable extent through planning and mental effort as will be described later. Suggestions which relate to some of these will be given later.

Two necessary preconditions for communication have now been identified. There must be at least one component of a message—verbal, paraverbal, or nonverbal—and there must be at least one intact channel by which the message is sent. Thus, even the lowly grunt (paraverbal, aural-auditory channel) or the arched eyebrow (nonverbal, visual channel) can be considered an intact communication whether sent intentionally or not. It is, of course, useful to have a receiver who gets the message and interprets it accurately. However, each individual in an interaction, even if the interaction is without conversation, is usually sending and receiving messages at the same time although they may not be consciously aware of the fact. It is significant that even an unconscious patient is sending and receiving messages.

In a two person interaction, the individual who speaks first cannot be assumed to be the sender and the other the receiver, because both individuals probably responded to nonverbal cues about the possibility of a conversation before either spoke. Consider two individuals who are unacquainted with each other looking at the same display in a grocery store. If one speaks to the other, it is probably because he unconsciously reads the behavior of the other to indicate a receptivity to communication. And the one who did not speak may have read an earlier message that the other wished to talk to him and sent a message of permission. All of this was probably unnoticed by conscious attention. It is difficult to say which one actually initiated the conversation.

The interpretation of verbal and nonverbal messages is not always accurate, as demonstrated by two passengers in an airplane. One may continue to attempt a conversation with another despite a lack of continued messages and a preponderance of stop messages. Insensitivity to nonverbal messages may have been the cause for the mistaken interaction. Obviously, the potential for communication inaccuracy and failure is great.

Other factors which can influence communication include the preoccupations, needs, and motives of the sender and receiver, the relationship they have, the content of the message, the setting in which the interaction occurs, the method of transmission, past experience, perceptual abilities, and preparation.[27,33]

## Levels of Messages

Another helpful way of looking at communications involves analyzing the levels of the interactions which occur between two individuals when a conversation occurs. This was first described as transactional analysis by Eric Berne and popularized further by Thomas Harris.[4,17] The theory is based on the idea that at any given time an individual may be in one of three ego states: parent, adult, or child.

There are characteristic messages, verbal, paraverbal, and nonverbal, sent by individuals when in each of these states. Messages from the parent state are often demanding, authoritative, and evaluative such as, "That was a stupid thing to do" and "Bring me my pipe and slippers." They are accompanied by a stern voice, the pointing finger, and the authoritative stance. Messages from the child state are full of emotion and may appear argumentative, helpless, or submissive such as, "Why can't I go?" "You never come see me," and "I don't care." They are accompanied by whining, crying, or submissive or rebellious stances. The adult state, which is a mediator between the parent and child states, represents rational, mature thinking and behavior. Messages from the adult state reflect objective data processing such as, "What happened?" "How is this going to work?" and "Where can we find that?" It is assumed that they are accompanied by neutral paraverbal and nonverbal behavior.

Nurses and their patients will benefit most when their interactions are adult to adult because this is the state in which the most optimal cognitive abilities occur. However, because one can interact from any state, nurses and other health care professionals may develop the habit of always interacting from their parent state[13] with messages such as, "You must . . .," "You should . . .," and "You will feel better if . . . ." When the nurse initiates an interaction in the parent state, the patient is most likely to assume the child state and the following type of dialogue is likely:

> Nurse: Why haven't you been taking your medicine as you were told to do? You know that this will make you better.
> Patient: I guess I forgot.

Suppose that the nurse had initiated the interaction from an adult state. She might have obtained a more useful response from her patient's adult ego state:

> Nurse: I noticed that you haven't taken the medicine that the physician prescribed. Is there some reason?
> Patient: Yes. It caused me to have diarrhea so I quit taking it.

It is obvious that the second interaction could lead to a more productive discussion than the first.

A patient who initiates an interaction from a parent state may activate the nurse's child state. For example:

> Patient: Where have you been? I've been calling the agency for hours.
> Nurse: You're not the only patient I have, you know.

However, the nurse could have responded from an adult ego state instead of the child state and again a more profitable interaction might have ensued because the patient may move to his adult state.

> Patient: Where have you been? I've been calling the agency for hours.
> Nurse: I'm here now. What did you want to see me about?

A nurse and patient may interact as two parents or two children as shown below.

> Patient: Dr. Smith hasn't been in to see me. Where is he anyway? He should be here.
> Nurse: You know how those surgeons are—you can't depend on them.

> Nurse: Why weren't you home last week? I waited out here for 20 minutes in the cold.
> Patient: How did I know you were coming last week? I had other things to do anyway.

In order to promote therapeutic communications, the nurse will need to operate from her adult ego state with recognition of information from her parent and child states. This is not always easy. In addition to the temptation to stay in the parent state, there may also be reasons to stay in the child state. Physicians, educators, and supervisors sometimes relate to nurses only with parent-to-child interactions. The nurse may either stay perpetually in a child ego state or she may emulate her superiors and assume the parent state when she has a chance with subordinates and patients. Lange[21] has suggested that the nurse can strengthen her adult state by:

1. Becoming familiar with her child and parent states through reflection.
2. Allowing a slight pause before initiating a conversation or responding to others to give the adult a chance to determine parent input, child input, and reality.

When the nurse communicates with others from her adult state, it increases the possibilities that the conversation will move to or progress on an adult-to-adult level, the most useful level. More suggestions about reaching the adult level will be given later when discussing problematic interactions.

## The Role of Culture in Analyzing Communication Dynamics

Culture has an indelible influence, which cannot be lightly dismissed, on all the dynamics which have been discussed. The components of a message—verbal, paraverbal, and non-verbal—are all conditioned during development and heavily influenced by cultural over-lays. Thus, the words one speaks, the use and manipulation of voice sounds, and the accompanying nonverbal elements of facial expression, eye movements, lip movements, body movements, physical appearance, and the interpretation of the environment will vary within cultures and even within cultural subgroups. Such is also true for the channels one uses to send messages. For example, the use of touch varies extremely. American culture requires more judicious use of the tactile channel than many other cultures. Even the levels of communication one uses are culturally conditioned. For example, recent studies have suggested that individuals in lower socioeconomic groups engage in very little communi-cation on the adult-to-adult level. Marriage partners relate to each other alternately as parent-to-child and siblings relate to each other as parent-to-child with the older child using the parent state towards other younger children.

Therefore, the nurse will be most accurate in analyzing the communication dynamics of individuals whose background and experiences have been similar to her own. Her accu-racy will decrease progressively as the background and experiences of her patient increas-ingly vary from hers. This can be mediated by learning about others, however. The reverse applies in that others who share the cultural background of the nurse will understand her most accurately and others less accurately.

## Communication Impairment

We have assumed here that the individual has no impairments in his communication abilities. The nurse will encounter many individuals who lack the optimal communication abilities such as those with speech impairments, hearing impairments, visual impairments, receptive impairments, or combinations of these. In each of these situations, the nurse will need to consider which channels are affected and which types of messages may be possible and plan how to maximally use the abilities the patient has. More information on this area is available in specific nursing texts.

## THERAPEUTIC COMMUNICATION

Individuals who become nurses are usually sufficiently familiar with social communi-cation and can engage in it successfully with patients. Therefore, social communica-tion in particular will not be discussed. Some information on formal communication is provided in the chapter on the teaching process. What will be emphasized here is the more difficult art and skill of therapeutic communication. Facility in therapeutic communication can greatly improve one's social communication skill so that one who studies and practices therapeutic communication receives a frequently useful bonus.

Two types of therapeutic communication will be presented—nondirective and directive. These two types will be considered separately, although this is an artificial separation in some aspects as will be seen. There are vastly differing viewpoints on communication within and outside of the nursing literature. The material to be presented here has been selected because it is reportedly useful in general nursing situations given the usual time and access constraints under which nurses work, and because it is generally usable by nurses with differing backgrounds and orientations with commitment and practice. This discussion is not intended to provide the competence needed by a nurse who must communicate with individuals with extensive emotional or mental illnesses.

## Nondirective Therapeutic Communication

Nondirective communication is used when the patient can be instrumental in focusing the interaction on his own needs or concerns. It is most useful when the nurse does not need to collect any specific information from the patient.

### ANATOMY OF A NONDIRECTIVE THERAPEUTIC CONVERSATION

While a conversation is never based on an absolute pattern, there does seem to be a general pattern which occurs in a nondirective therapeutic conversation under optimal circumstances. An understanding of this pattern will enable the nurse to determine what action she can take to complement and facilitate this pattern. Most nondirective therapeutic conversations have certain phases. These often overlap each other.

1. *Beginning phase.* During this period the nurse and patient engage in patient focused social conversation about a few or several topics.
2. *Content phase.* At this time, the patient introduces and tells the nurse about one or more situations that are meaningful to him.
3. *Mood phase.* This period involves the patient as he describes his past and present emotional feelings about the situation he has previously described.
4. *Reflection and integration phase.* During this period, the patient looks back in review. He may return to earlier phases to add more content about the situation and present more emotional feelings. A certain summary of the situation begins to emerge. Attempts which have been made to cope with the situation will be described.
5. *Problem solving phase.* At this stage, the patient focuses on what can be done about the situation. The patient will present one or more methods of resolution and accept some of them.
6. *Ending phase.* During this phase, the patient and nurse return to topics of less meaningfulness to the patient.

The following is an example of an interaction between a nurse and a patient which demonstrates the progression of this pattern. Notice that phases are not always clear-cut.

## Beginning Phase

Mr. Brown and the nurse assigned to him for the evening are discussing his stay in the hospital.

## Content Phase

Mr. Brown begins to tell the nurse about his morning in the x-ray department where he had a barium enema. He talks about how physically uncomfortable the procedure was. He remarks on how no one there seemed to care about him at all except as a "colon." He describes how difficult it was to cooperate with everything he was asked to do. He remarks that he had felt cold the rest of the morning after being in the chilly x-ray room so lightly dressed.

## Mood Phase

Mr. Brown begins to become increasingly agitated as he talks more about his morning. He describes how embarrassed he was at having his body so casually exposed in front of so many people—especially the young female technicians. He next remarks about how surprised he was that his physician had not been there because he had assumed he would need to see the procedure to know the results. As he talks, he begins to describe increasing annoyance at his physician for even ordering the test. His voice grows louder as he describes having to wait in the cold room on the table because of an argument two of the personnel were having over a problem that did not concern him at all. He is now quite flushed in the face.

## Reflection and Integration Phase

After ventilation of his feelings, Mr. Brown sighs and remarks how glad he is that the procedure is over and how he hopes he never has to go to x-ray again. He comments that he knows the test was needed. He returns to periodically describe other incidents of the morning and how he feels about them. In particular, he tells how one technician had yelled at him for not cooperating with the test. He describes that he had lost his temper and yelled back at her. Becoming more quiet again, he mentions that he is not accustomed to being ill, and that being in the hospital is a real threat to his image of himself as vigorous and healthy. He also describes anxiety over his condition and what the potential diagnosis could mean. Again he mentions yelling at the technician and how surprised he was that he had lost his temper and behaved in such an uncharacteristic manner. His conversation begins to repeat the theme then that he is mostly upset and perplexed with himself for not being able to better control himself in spite of the complexity of the situation he was in.

## Problem Solving Phase

Mr. Brown grows calmer as he reiterates how unprepared he had been for the ordeal and how his behavior was caused by his complete surprise at the procedure. He comments that he had so many things on his mind. He remarks that he was sure the x-ray department was accustomed to the behavior of people who were "pushed to their limit." He states that if he ever had to have another barium enema, he would be more prepared. He comments that he was going to get more information from his physician from now on before he consented to tests. He remarks that he would like to apologize to the technician he yelled at but that he hopes she understands how patients feel under the circumstances he was going through. He concludes by remarking that he is glad he can get out of the hospital soon. Mr. Brown turns to discussing his possible discharge.

## Ending Phase

Mr. Brown and the nurse return to discussing other aspects of the day and his experiences in the hospital.

The pattern described could conceivably be completely covered in a few minutes as in the previous example or it may be a process lasting much longer with the patient moving from one stage to another slowly. Each phase might even occur in separate interactions with the nurse. Some stages may require more than one interaction period. When the entire pattern has not been covered in one interaction period, the level where the interaction was suspended may be returned to in the next interaction. This has been known to occur even though the interval of time separating the interactions has been as long as several years. Some patients may stall at a certain phase.

The following points about the pattern, usually followed by a nondirective therapeutic communication under optimal circumstances, must be considered:

1. It cannot be assumed that the interaction will inevitably follow this pattern. It is somewhat dependent on the interactions of the nurse.

2. The patient will usually learn a lot about his emotional reaction to the situation he is describing as he speaks. He may comment, "I didn't realize this was bothering me so much," or "I'm surprised at how much I'm talking about this." His true feelings about the situation may emerge with more intensity than he realized.

3. The theme which develops in the reflection and integration phase may be different from the theme which was introduced in the content phase or the mood phase. It may be of more personal significance and more difficult for the patient to express. For example, Mr. Brown initiated the interaction with the theme which might be stated as: "I had a terrible time in x-ray. The people there were inconsiderate and it was cold and uncomfortable." The theme which eventually developed was much different and more personal and might be stated as: "I guess what I really feel badly about is that I wasn't able to put up with it and I lost my temper. That isn't like me." The theme which develops may be a learning experience for the patient. The patient may say, "I didn't realize until now that this was really the problem." Mr. Brown might have said, "I thought I was just angry at the

x-ray department and Dr. Jones. Now I see that I am mostly angry at myself for how I reacted."

4. The resolution attempts that develop may be acceptable to the patient, but not necessarily the nurse. Patients will occasionally resolve a lot of their feelings with denials or rationalizations which the nurse may not feel are appropriate. Other resolution attempts which the nurse may not be pleased with are ones which accept the problem without proposed corrective action such as, "There is nothing I can do about this and I have to accept that." It may be helpful for the nurse to remind herself that everyone uses these approaches sometimes, even she herself, and that the solutions offered by the patient are the best ones he can make at the moment. The patient may not be ready to face more reality.

5. The pattern shows movement from a patient focused social communication to progressively more meaningful communication, sometimes with considerable emotional display, and a gradual return to patient focused social communication. This might be thought of as representing a slow spiral. The interaction circles into the essence of another human being as he shares a concern or problem and his feelings from his inner conscious or unconscious thoughts and then a slow circling outward. Individuals vary greatly in how close to their central core they are willing to allow another to come.

6. The pattern shows that a helpful interaction is usually one in which the patient learns about himself. This is one of the reasons that the nurse should facilitate therapeutic communications. In our example, Mr. Brown probably learned several useful pieces of information about his reaction to the hospital environment, his concern over his diagnosis, his reaction to illness, and his limits of coping while ill and in another environment.

7. A helpful interaction usually is one in which the patient gains some practice in problem solving. Resolution attempts are actually equal to problem solving attempts and the patient will discuss, reject, and accept them until he feels he has solved his problem. Mr. Brown's problem solving attempts included justifying his behavior because of his unpreparedness and by believing that the x-ray department must be accustomed to upset patients. He also rejected apologizing to the technician. He planned ahead to get more information from his physician and to get away from the hospital as soon as possible. It should be remembered that deciding one can do nothing is still a solution.

8. The patient may need to repeat his conversation more than once with different outcomes about any one particular situation. Mr. Brown told his x-ray story to his wife when she came later. If one assumes that their relationship is characterized by openness and acceptance, he may tell her even more details of his behavior and reactions than he was willing to share with the nurse and reach even more understanding of his behavior. A patient may have a need to relate some situations over and over, such as a labor and delivery experience or an operation. Each time the experience is related, he may reach a greater level of understanding about the events and their feeling. Man is presumed to think with language so that transforming vague events and emotional feelings into words allows for a greater ability to mentally think about them. Repeating a story may be necessary because each telling may lead to more precise and accurate verbal descriptions of what one actually felt and what actually occurred. The patient may become more willing to remember elements which he had been denying to himself before.

9. Patients will often express that they feel better during the reflection and integration phase. Several factors probably contribute to this. Ventilation of moderate or strong feelings which have been previously unexpressed appears by itself to be a psychological relief.[35]

10. Some patients may present the mood phase before the content phase. The nurse can easily adjust to this by helping the patient to express his feelings and then helping him to tell the story which has led to his feelings.

## NURSING ACTIONS TO FACILITATE NONDIRECTIVE THERAPEUTIC COMMUNICATION

There are specific goals during each phase of a nondirective therapeutic interaction.

### Beginning Phase

The goal of nursing action during this stage could be described as creating a climate where the patient is free to discuss whatever he wishes. The focus of the conversation is, therefore, on the patient. The nurse uses her interaction to demonstrate interest, concern, and understanding. This is sometimes referred to as establishing rapport. The nurse does not arbitrarily probe or pry into the patient's situation, but she provides the patient with an available listener should he desire to discuss a subject meaningful to him. She is especially sensitive to cues the patient may communicate which may indicate a willingness to discuss a particular subject. An example of a patient sending a cue to a nurse is described below.

Mrs. Jackson has brought her 18-month-old twins into the neighborhood clinic for well child care. The nurse has been talking to Mrs. Jackson, who has just moved to a new apartment, about the trials and tribulations of moving.

Mrs. Jackson: Well, I'm just glad the move is over. We sure do have a lot more space. It's funny though. My husband was the one who wanted to move to a larger place so we could have more room. It doesn't seem to have helped much though. (Voice becoming lower) Things seem to be getting worse. (Sighs, looks down at her hands)

Mrs. Jackson is in essence, consciously or unconsciously, sending a message to the nurse that she would like to discuss an area of importance to her. The patient is frequently very tentative, vague, and elusive about presenting the situation he wishes to discuss as was Mrs. Jackson. How the nurse responds to this cue is crucial for if the nurse misses the cue or disregards it, the patient will usually not bring it up again because he has found out that the nurse does not wish to engage in more meaningful discussion. The following is an example of a cue missed by a nurse.

Mr. Honeywell is recuperating after having a below-the-knee leg amputation.

Mr. Honeywell: I used to spend a lot of time at my daughter's helping her with the yard work. I guess I won't have to worry about getting her mower to start any more. It was the most stubborn thing I've ever seen.
Nurse: What kind of mower was it?
Mr. Honeywell: It was a Cutrite.

Another nurse could have responded by picking up on the cue.

Mr. Honeywell: I used to spend a lot of time at my daughter's helping her with the yard work. I guess I won't have to worry about getting her mower to start any more. It was the most stubborn thing I've ever seen.

Nurse:          You won't be mowing her yard any more?
Mr. Honeywell: I guess not. The doctor says I could learn to walk with an artificial leg but I'm not sure. I
                know people can learn to get around with them really well, but I don't know if I could . . . .

Notice that in the first interaction the nurse was listening and did follow up on
Mr. Honeywell's last remark. She was not listening for the subtle, almost hidden
meaning that the second nurse heard. The difference in responses the two nurses received
is striking.

The nurse who picks up on a cue is not probing into her patient's life. If the patient does
not wish to discuss a subject being approached, he probably would not have alluded to it
to begin with. The nurse can always allow the patient to change his mind after communicating a cue. He may decide he is not ready to discuss the subject after all.

Does a patient always have concerns to discuss with a nurse? Probably not. Some
people really do not like talking about their problems. Others may talk about their problems, but not with a stranger. In general situations, the nurse should not force patients to
discuss something they do not wish to discuss. She should only create the climate for
meaningful discussion and let the patient decide. An emotional catharsis is not the goal of
therapeutic communication as has been sometimes assumed.

The social communication which the nurse engages in has been referred to as patient
focused. This means that the topics discussed are of a social conversation nature, but that
the nurse does not participate in the conversation in the same manner she would with a
friend. She avoids focusing the conversation on herself and her interests or concerns. The
following represents a social conversation which is not patient focused.

Nurse:   Good morning, Mrs. Rosenbaum. How are you today?
Patient: Just fine. Isn't it a lovely day? Just look at that sunshine.
Nurse:   It sure is nice. I hope it doesn't rain tonight. I want to go on a picnic with my boyfriend.
Patient: Oh, where are you going?
Nurse:   We usually go over to Como Park . . .

The nurse started out by expressing interest in her patient but soon she showed that she
would rather talk about herself. The following illustrates how the focus could have been
kept on the patient.

Nurse:   Good morning, Mrs. Rosenbaum. How are you today?
Patient: Just fine. Isn't it a lovely day? Just look at that sunshine.
Nurse:   It sure is nice. Would you like to eat your breakfast over here by the window?
Patient: That would be nice. Can you help me out of bed? You know, I'm not as strong as I was before
         surgery.
Nurse:   Do you mean that you feel weaker?
Patient: Yes, but I think . . .

Some sources of information will suggest that the nurse should never engage in social
conversation with a patient. The approach of using deliberate patient focused social communication is being advocated because:

1.  A patient might be uncomfortable with a nurse who will not engage in some discussion on a social level
    when they first met. An opening phase of social communication may be more comfortable and normal.
2.  The beginning nurse can learn to engage in patient focused social communication rather easily. Then she
    can learn to use patient focused social communication as a beginning point from which to work towards
    therapeutic communication. This avoids the anxiety and resistance which might come from being told to
    completely abandon the only type of communication she is experienced in—social communication—for
    another type of communication which seems very difficult.

3. Experience with counselors and their patients has shown that the patient is aware of and responds to the person he talks with as a human being and is less concerned about or aware of any particular techniques the counselor uses or doesn't use.[12] If this is true, the nurse, through patient focused social communication, reveals herself as a real person with interests, ideas, and a unique personality. The patient may respond to and attempt to communicate with her because of what she has revealed about herself during the patient focused social communication phase. Hopefully, she has revealed that she is trustworthy, sensitive, and more interested in the patient than herself.

## Content Phase

During this phase, the nursing goal could be described as one of facilitating the patient's description of his situation. The nurse might be tempted to move prematurely toward trying to see how the patient felt about the situation or trying to offer him solutions. This could lead to an inadequate appreciation for the situation. The nurse should remember that she will not be able to understand fully how the patient feels until she understands the content. Nor will she be able to appreciate feasible solutions if she has not heard the entire problem. The following illustrates how the nurse could inappropriately introduce the mood theme too quickly.

Nurse:        Well, I see your physican just left. Do you get to go home today?
Mr. Nelson: No, he said I need to stay another day.
Nurse:        I'll bet you are really disappointed.
Mr. Nelson: Yeah, I guess so. Well, no need to pack.

Contrast that with another nurse who wanted to get the whole story first.

Nurse:        Well, I see your physician just left. Do you get to go home today?
Mr. Nelson: No, he said I need to stay another day.
Nurse:        Oh really.
Mr. Nelson: Yes. Some of the test results have raised the possibility of another problem he wants to check out. I'll be glad to get the needed tests done now without having to come back again . . .

The following is an example of the possible results when a nurse who is eager to offer solutions is paired with a patient who wants to just tell her story.

Mrs. Becker: I don't know what I am going to do. They just called me from the day care center. Tim has the chicken pox and I'll have to find someplace for him to stay tomorrow. This is going to be such a hectic week and now this!
Nurse:        Can't you stay home from work?
Mrs. Becker: Not this week. We are doing our inventory and I'm the only one who has done it before. Besides that, I have a night class I'm starting tonight and my car won't start.
Nurse:        Could your neighbors watch Tim tomorrow?
Mrs. Becker: I hate to bother them. They have their own problems. If I could just get my shopping done maybe I could figure this out.
Nurse:        Could your mother come?
Mrs. Becker: She stayed with Toni last week and she said she was going to be busy this week. My sister-in-law and her husband are coming for dinner tomorrow night so that means a fancy meal and cleaning the house between now and then too.
Nurse:        How about your mother-in-law?
Mrs. Becker: She hasn't been well. Sometimes my schedule gets too much. Toni needs refreshments tomorrow afternoon for a meeting. I don't know when I can get that done.
Nurse:        Does the day care center know of anyone who stays with children?

The nurse was trying to be helpful. Mrs. Becker was not ready for solutions yet. This conversation might have gone on forever with the nurse offering solutions and Mrs. Becker rejecting them, although Mrs. Becker is most likely to soon give up on trying to explain how things are. The nurse might have realized that there was much Mrs. Becker had to say if she had listened more carefully to the first statement and responded to the content.

> Mrs. Becker: I don't know what I am going to do. They just called me from the day care center. Tim has the chicken pox and I'll have to find someplace for him to stay tomorrow. This is going to be such a hectic week and now this!
> Nurse: It sounds like you have quite a problem.
> Mrs. Becker: Yes, and besides that I haven't done my shopping, Toni needs refreshments for her club meeting, I'm having company for dinner . . .

The nurse can remind herself that in order to help the patient she must first understand the situation and direct her actions toward helping the patient describe the situation.

## Mood Phase

The goal of nursing action during the mood phase of a nondirective therapeutic interaction is to facilitate the patient's expression of emotional feelings. It is important that the nurse not dismiss the patient's feelings as shown in this example.

> Jimmy: I don't want to go back to school. All of the kids will laugh at my arm and call me Captain Hook.
> Nurse: You mustn't feel that way. They are your friends. You can't let their comments bother you. They don't mean to be cruel.

By what she replied, the nurse has told the patient that the way he feels is wrong. She has communicated to him that she is not very interested in how he really feels. She would rather have him feel as she suggests he should feel. Jimmy probably won't tell her his true feelings again. The nurse could have encouraged him to express his feelings.

> Jimmy: I don't want to go back to school. All of the kids will laugh at my arm and call me Captain Hook.
> Nurse: You're afraid you will be made fun of.
> Jimmy: Yes, I'm embarrassed when people watch me. This thing looks hideous. I feel like a character in a pirate movie.

Listening to a patient express emotional feelings can be difficult. Patients may express anger or cry while talking. The nurse may be tempted to avoid a discussion of emotional feelings for her own comfort. It is equally difficult to facilitate a patient's expression of feelings if his feelings are expressions of dissatisfaction with the nurse herself or other aspects of the health care setting.

> Mrs. White: I wish that medical student would stay out of here. He acts like I'm not really trying to have this baby. He keeps telling me to relax. Relax! He's never had a baby. All of you treat me like I'm acting like a baby.
> Nurse: You feel we aren't being very understanding?
> Mrs. White: Yes. These contractions really hurt. I never dreamed it would be this bad.
> Nurse: You weren't prepared for this much pain?
> Mrs. White: Not this much . . .

If the nurse had become defensive, the interaction might have gone like this.

Mrs. White:   I wish that medical student would stay out of here. He acts like I'm not really trying to have this baby. He keeps telling me to relax. Relax! He's never had a baby. All of you treat me like I'm acting like a baby.

Nurse:   We're only trying to help. You aren't cooperating with us.

Mrs. White:   I'm trying but you keep . . .

## Reflection and Integration Phase

In this phase, the nurse uses her interaction to help clarify and summarize what has occurred previously. She will check her understanding of the situation with the patient and encourage the patient to elaborate about anything which is unclear. As this stage progresses, she is alert for any shifts in understanding of the situation which may occur as the patient grasps a more realistic view of his problems. She will help the patient identify and verbalize the theme which will eventually materialize. The nurse may be more verbally active during this stage than she was previously when the patient easily conversed with occasional input from her.

The following demonstrates an example of the nurse attempting to summarize and clarify a discussion which had occurred and the important realization that the mother makes as she reflects on the situation.

Nurse:   Let me see if I understand this now. You dislike going to the diabetic clinic with Julie because you feel the staff members are unfriendly and critical, and the doctors never are the same, and because it is difficult to get there.

Mrs. Nichols:   Yes. There's no place to park either.

Nurse:   Can you explain to me what you mean when you say the staff is critical?

Mrs. Nichols:   The dieticians always ask me how Julie's diet is going and if we are following it. I try so hard but I can't plan every meal that carefully. They want everything just perfect. I feel bad when they start in on the importance of her eating properly. (Pause) I guess I try to avoid the clinic mainly because they remind me that I'm not careful enough about her diet and I want to be. I know it is important but I need more help planning meals. Maybe I should tell the dietician I need more help.

An example of the nurse helping the patient to summarize a situation follows. Notice the insight the patient gained because of the summary.

Nicky:   So that's the story. I feel very confused about what to do.

Nurse:   Tell me if I've got this right. You need the surgery but your mother doesn't want you to have it.

Nicky:   No, she wants me to have it but she wants me to wait. My dad insists that I have the surgery now. He wants to borrow the money so I can go ahead. Mom says that Dad has enough problems without going more in debt.

Nurse:   So you are caught in the middle. Whichever decision you make will cause conflict between your parents.

Nicky:   Hey! That's just it. I didn't realize it until you said it that way. I couldn't figure out why I was having so much trouble deciding what to do.

The following example demonstrates a discussion between two nurses, one a supervisor and the other a staff nurse, that shows that much new content and emotional expression normally can arise during this stage as reflection and integration occur.

Jo:   All right, let's try to put this together. You are upset because the head nurse sent you to the other unit today. You are a pediatric nurse and you feel you shouldn't have to work with adult patients.

Ellen: Yes. I don't see why I have to go when some of the others don't care where they work. I never know what I'm doing there. No one is very helpful.

Jo: You feel uncertain and confused on the other unit.

Ellen: Yes. Things there are so different—the meds and the patients' conditions. And lifting all those obese women with hip fractures.

Jo: It is very different from this unit.

Ellen: Yes. There are so many older men. They are always wanting something all the time and they want to hold your hand. They bother me.

Jo: They bother you?

Ellen: You know. They sometimes try to grab you and stuff.

Jo: (Nodding)

Ellen: There is this one guy there who has to have irrigations and he has his hands all over you. It really gives me the creeps. I never did like taking care of older men. I don't know what to say when they start acting up. I just want to run out of the room. Do you know what I mean?

Jo: I'm not sure. Do you mean that you feel frightened?

Ellen: Yes. I don't know why it should bother me so much but I'm afraid some guy will attack me or something. I know most of them don't really know what they are doing, but it makes me angry to be used for their gratification.

Jo: You are upset by it and also frightened?

Ellen: I feel abused and I don't know what to do. I talked to some of the other nurses down there and they just laugh about it. It doesn't seem to bother them.

Jo: So you wonder why it should bother you so much?

Ellen: Right, but it sure does. In all honesty, I guess I really wouldn't mind having to go down to that unit at all if I could figure out how to cope with the older men. That's really the only part that bothers me now that I think about it.

This phase works best if the patient arrives at his own interpretations. It is seldom helpful for the nurse to offer her interpretations of the situation to the patient but she can state to the patient what he seems to be saying.

## Problem Solving Phase

The goal of nursing action during this phase could be described as helping the patient to work through his problems. This is not to be confused with telling the patient how to solve his problems. The nurse is most helpful who allows the patient to arrive at alternatives on his own. When the nurse offers advice, the patient may feel frustration because he was not able to think of the solution on his own or because the advice is not acceptable to him, but he feels he is obliged to accept it or at least pretend to accept it. Even if the patient asks for the nurse's advice, she should consider referring the question back to the patient. For example:

Mr. Rubin: What would you do if Jack was your son? Would you want him to do this?

Nurse: I would like to hear more of what you have been considering.

Mr. Rubin: I know I am old fashioned but I just can't see this . . .

This interaction demonstrates a point which is frequently overlooked. When people ask others for advice, they almost invariably have already decided what they want to do and are actually looking for confirmation of their decision. If the nurse offers advice in this situation, she runs the risk of assuming the responsibility which the patient should face himself. And if her advice differs from his decision, she increases his discomfort.

Although the nurse should not necessarily offer a solution to her patient, she can help him to evaluate solutions. The following example is intended to show how a nurse can help a patient explore alternatives.

Millie: So I have to decide soon what I am going to do about this pregnancy. The more I think about it, the more confused I get.
Nurse: As of now, what choices have you considered?
Millie: Well, I could terminate the pregnancy for one thing.
Nurse: How do you feel about that?
Millie: I really can't see myself going through with that. It sounds very scary to me. I don't think Joe wants me to do that either. But I can't plan my life based on what he wants. I have to please myself too.
Nurse: So you aren't really ready to decide one way or the other about termination of the pregnancy.
Millie: No. I don't want to do that but it is still a possibility.
Nurse: What else have you thought about doing?
Millie: I guess the only other alternative I can accept is going ahead with the pregnancy and keeping the baby. That would take so long and be so difficult.

This phase is frequently difficult for the nurse who has definite opinions on how others should lead their lives and a narrow range of acceptable variations. Also, not all problems can be neatly solved and the nurse must learn to tolerate interactions which end without resolution of the problem.

## Ending Phase

During this phase, the nurse has as her goal again the creation of a climate where the patient can focus the conversation as he wishes, as she did in the beginning stage. Patients usually appreciate a gradual, less emotionally charged ending to an interaction which is facilitated by concluding with some social conversation. This may not necessarily be true if the patient indicates instead that he has a lot of things to think about. Then it might not be best to disrupt his contemplation by introducing irrelevant topics at this time. In general, the nurse should let the patient signal the end of the interaction by introducing social conversation rather than changing the subject herself.

## *Directive Therapeutic Communication*

Directive communication has not always been seen as necessary or appropriate in nursing situations. A total reliance on nondirective communication would indicate that a nurse never needs to focus the interaction of the patient nor to direct the conversation to collect specific information. But sometimes a nurse does need to introduce problem areas and assist the patient in focusing on them and discussing them. Nurses are increasingly becoming aware of the need to increase their skills in information gathering. Nursing assessment based on structured outlines is becoming common in some health care settings. Therefore, directive communication has a legitimate place in nursing practice and there are ways to polish one's skill in directing patient interactions and collecting data.

It is sometimes suggested that directive communication is nontherapeutic and that could potentially be the case if improperly done. The directive communication approach to be presented here presumes that directive communication has the same potential as nondirective communication to be therapeutic because the interaction focuses on the patient and ultimately on helping him to identify and meet his needs. Like nondirective communication, directive communication does not focus on the needs and problems of the nurse. Directive communication is most useful when the patient should, but might not otherwise, focus on an important problem or situation, and when the nurse needs information which the patient has but may not know how to present to the nurse. As mentioned earlier, directive and nondirective communication approaches are being presented for the sake of clarity as two separate and distinct types of interactions. After this discussion, the ways in which the two types interrelate will be considered.

## ANATOMY OF A DIRECTIVE THERAPEUTIC CONVERSATION

The following outline is intended to describe the general pattern of a directive interaction under optimal circumstances. Variations are, of course, possible.

1. *Opening phase.* During this period, the nurse explains the purpose or introduces the topic of the interaction.
2. *Data collection phase.* During this period, the nurse guides the patient in presenting and discussing appropriate data.
3. *Problem solving phase.* At this stage, the data are analyzed and plans for any further necessary action are made.
4. *Closing phase.* At this time, the participants evaluate the achievement of the purposes of the interaction and the conversation returns to general topics.

An example of a directive therapeutic communication which involves guiding a patient in focusing on a specific topic follows.

Mr. Brown is to be discharged from the hospital in a few days. The nurse has planned to talk to Mr. Brown this morning to see what his needs are in relation to discharge teaching. The nurse enters Mr. Brown's room at a time when she believes he will be available to discuss the subject.

### Opening Phase

The nurse talks with Mr. Brown for a few minutes about his hospital stay. She then tells him that she would like to discuss the subject of his approaching release from the hospital if it is a good time to do so. Mr. Brown acknowledges that it is.

### Data Collection Phase

The nurse begins by asking Mr. Brown to discuss what questions he may have about going home. She brings up specific topics later to ascertain what information he has about them.

### Problem Solving Phase

As they discuss the approaching discharge, the nurse and Mr. Brown identify that he needs more information on what medications he might need to take at home, what activities he can engage in, how to know if he should call his physician, and if he will have any dietary restrictions. The nurse is aware of the special diet he will be placed on and she briefly describes it to him. They plan together for Mr. Brown to discuss his medications, activities, and followup with the physician when he next visits. The nurse offers to alert the dietician to Mr. Brown's need for dietary information and Mr. Brown plans to arrange with his wife a time when they both could meet with the dietician.

## Closing Phase

The nurse offers her services to Mr. Brown as he thinks of other concerns related to discharge. They talk for a few minutes more about general topics. The nurse leaves to follow up on contacting the dietician.

As was true with regard to nondirective therapeutic communication, the length of time for a directive interaction can vary considerably. The patient will usually learn about his situation and himself because of the interaction. The problems that are discovered may not have been obvious to the patient or nurse in the beginning. The nurse will need to accept the patient's resolution attempts of the moment. The interaction may show a spiraling inward and outward pattern. The patient will usually gain some practice in problem solving. The patient may express that he feels better because of the interaction.

## NURSING ACTIONS TO FACILITATE DIRECTIVE THERAPEUTIC COMMUNICATION

In order to facilitate each phase of a helpful directive interaction, the nurse must realize the goals of each phase.

## Opening Phase

The nurse has as her goal during this phase to establish rapport and to introduce the topic to be pursued. She is careful to first determine if her timing is appropriate. If the patient has other more pressing needs, she may wish to postpone the proposed topic and attend to the patient's other needs, although this may not always be possible.

## Data Collection Phase

During this phase, the goal of the nurse is to obtain accurate and complete data about the specific topic. One temptation to be resisted during this stage is to engage in other activities which will hamper data collection. For example, the nurse working with Mr. Brown might have disbanded attempts at data collection as soon as Mr. Brown identified a need for dietary information and she might have launched into an impromptu teaching session. Another sidetrack to avoid is jumping to premature solutions. There will be time for problem solving and health teaching later. The nurse should concentrate now on getting the data. It should be emphasized that getting complete data includes facilitating the patient in describing both content and feelings. For example, the nurse not only explored what

Mr. Brown needed to know before discharge but also how he felt about going home. If the nurse is taking notes and a patient begins to discuss pronounced personal feelings, it is helpful for the nurse to discontinue her note taking so that she can attend fully to the patient.[26]

During this phase, the nurse usually uses beginning nondirective statements and then becomes more directive as she defines an area. For example, the nurse in the next interaction is performing an initial assessment during a home visit to a newly referred maternity patient. She might ask the following questions, in discussing the mother's plans for feeding her baby, which illustrate moving from nondirective to directive levels.

> Nurse: What have you been thinking about in regard to feeding the baby?
> Jackie: I think I will bottle feed. I want Bill to be able to feed the baby whenever he wants to and enjoy the interaction that occurs.
> Nurse: Any other reasons?
> Jackie: I want to return to my work as soon as possible. Breast feeding a baby would be very difficult and potentially frustrating for both the baby and me with my schedule.
> Nurse: Have you purchased any formula or bottles yet?
> Jackie: No. I have some questions about the different types of bottles and nipples . . .

## Problem Solving Phase

At this time, the nurse's goal is one of guiding the patient's efforts at problem solving by helping the patient to identify and clarify the major problems, evaluate alternatives, and plan action. The nurse may have helpful information or know about resources of which the patient might not be aware, which she can appropriately introduce at this time.

## Closing Phase

The nursing goal during this phase is to evaluate the achievement of the goal of the interaction and to carry out any necessary followup if the goal was not met.

# The Communication Continuum

Nondirective and directive therapeutic communication techniques have been considered separately, but it is important to represent them as they really exist—as two ends of a therapeutic communication continuum. At the one extreme, the nondirective technique is initiated and directed by the patient with the nurse providing feedback and encouragement. At the other extreme, the directive technique is initiated and directed by the nurse with the patient primarily providing information. The nurse rarely employs exclusively directive or nondirective approaches. She probably interacts with others on different points along the continuum from nondirective to directive communication. The following points can now be elaborated:

1. The nurse may differ in regard to how directive she is with individual patients, based on how effectively the patient provides the nurse with verbal content. The nurse may also plan nondirective and directive contacts with one patient at different times.

2. During any one interaction with a patient, the nurse and patient may move back and forth on the continuum. For example, a nurse has initiated an interaction with the mother of a newly admitted child to obtain information needed during the child's hospitalization. At some point during the collection of data, the mother alludes to a matter of importance to her about which she apparently has many feelings. The nurse may become nondirective to facilitate the mother's initiative in discussing the area. Afterwards, she may return to more directive responses and questions.

3. The nurse will develop a unique style in communicating with patients which will include her personal philosophy on when to be directive and when to be nondirective.

4. It is frequently very helpful for the nurse to work from nondirective communication to progressively more directive communication. For example, during a nondirective interaction, a patient begins to express his fears about an approaching event. After allowing the patient to fully describe his fears, the nurse may want to become more directive because she may be able to identify what specific elements of the coming situation the patient is fearful about and, therefore, some specific nursing action might help alleviate the fear. This might not have been identified if the nurse had remained nondirective.

5. A common thread throughout the continuum is the problem solving phase. It is important to remember that the patient does not always get to problem solving. Ventilation or data collection may characterize the achievements of the entire interaction, depending on the needs of the patient and the skills of the nurse.

## POSSIBLE COMMUNICATION TECHNIQUES

The following information describes specific actions the nurse can take to facilitate therapeutic communication.

### Planning the Environment

Although the nurse may not always have control over environmental factors, if it is possible some modifications in the environment might be useful. An ideal place for therapeutic communication to occur would be private, comfortable, and free from numerous distractions. The nurse can survey the setting in which she practices to see if there are areas conducive to helping interactions. Even if the interaction will take place in the confusion and clutter of a busy hospital ward, there may be things which can help such as pulling curtains, reducing the volume of radios or televisions, attending to the patient's comfort, and planning a time to talk to the patient when interruption might be least likely. If the interaction is to occur in the patient's home, the nurse can plan a time when the patient or family might possibly be alone and initially attend to their comfort.

### Communicating Through the Visual Channel

Because of the tremendous amount of information communicated nonverbally, the nurse may wish to give some thought to what her nonverbal behavior and personal appearance communicate to the patient. The nurse may find the opinions of friends helpful. Watching several videotapes of herself may increase her consciousness of her appearance, facial expression, and body movements. Her facial expression is of utmost importance.

Ideally, if she wants to encourage communication, the nurse would desire to appear unhurried and attentive. She can do this by sitting down or putting herself at eye level with the patient somewhere near the boundary between the personal and social distance which most people find comfortable—around 4 feet.[1] Patients reportedly perceive that individuals who sit down have stayed with them longer than individuals who stand for the same length of time.

The nurse should strive for a relaxed body posture and avoid annoying mannerisms. She hopes to nonverbally communicate that nothing is more important to her at that moment than the patient. Some authorities suggest that one should lean slightly forward at the waist, maintain direct eye contact, and face the person squarely.[1] Another source suggests, however, that the face-to-face position is usually assumed by combatants while individuals intending to cooperate usually assume a side-by-side position.[9] The nurse might try both of these positions or an intermediate position and see which she prefers.

Without the appropriate nonverbal behavior, the nurse's verbal comments of willingness to help are for naught. Of course, nurses cannot always take time to "pose" for each interaction they have with another individual, but an awareness of the tremendous communicative value of their nonverbal behavior is important. Also, the nurse can use the above information to move into more attentive positions should a patient begin to discuss a topic which the nurse wishes to encourage. Because the nonverbal behavior of the nurse sends the largest portion of her message to the patient on the visual channel, it deserves considerable emphasis and attention. With some patients it is her only available channel.

## Communicating Through the Tactile Channel

Nurses use two types of tactile communication which can be considered separately. Nurses use tactile communication as a secondary component of many routine activities such as taking a blood pressure or applying a bandage. Nurses also use tactile communication as an independent method of communication such as taking a patient's hand or patting someone on the shoulder.

The nurse should be aware of what her use of touch in performing nursing activities may be communicating to the patient. Is her handling of another while giving care firm, rough, brisk, inconsiderate, uncertain, awkward, or gentle? Does she prepare the patient before pulling off tape, inserting a needle, or applying a cold solution? Does she treat a painful area with consideration while bathing the patient? Does she plan tactile communication to appropriately supplement other care measures such as giving the patient a backrub after administering a calming medication or repositioning a patient with pain to relieve incisional tension after administering an analgesic? Does she consider the measures just mentioned as substitutes for medications? The patient will be more influenced by the secondary tactile messages he receives or does not receive than by his visual assessment of her technical excellence in giving care.

The use of the tactile channel to communicate with patients as an independent component of care is assumed by the patient to be one of the fundamental tasks of the nurse who has long been associated with the "laying on of hands." It is very difficult to know exactly when and how to use touch as an independent action in nursing situations—especially with adults. The use of touch with children seems more spontaneous.

The nurse needs first of all to examine her own feelings about touch. It is worth stating again that our society is one wherein touch is carefully regulated. The nurse who wishes to use touch might be encouraged by the following points:

1. The nurse, as well as other health professionals, is allowed and probably expected to use touch with her patients; for example, she may apply a cool cloth to the feverish brow and steady the shoulders of the aged.
2. Patient studies have reported that patients frequently describe touch as significant, therapeutic, and desirable.

Therefore, the nurse should deliberately consider touch as a nonverbal nursing measure and as part of the communication process on the tactile channel and probably use it more frequently. The nurse must consider:

1. The age of the patient.
2. The sex of the patient.
3. The situation.
4. The tactile contact to be used.
5. The background of the patient.
6. The channels of communication available.
7. Her own feelings.

Each nurse must construct her own guides but the use of touch may be most uncomfortable when the patient is of the opposite sex and when the age of the patient is near the age of the nurse. Hands and arms seem to be the most acceptable agents of tactile communication as in giving pats, a hand squeeze, or putting an arm around someone's shoulders. Each of these may communicate different messages. The acceptable parts of the patient to be touched in independent action seem to be the hands, arms, or shoulders, and possibly the face, as in wiping away tears. Touch seems to be most appreciated in situations where the nurse is not a complete stranger. The nurse cannot fully know the background of the patient in regard to his cultural expectations about touch so she must be alert to determine if her touch was helpful or unhelpful. The need for contact comfort appears to be an inherent need of every individual beginning at birth and the nurse is in a good position to communicate her interest, support, and concern by touch. With many patients, communication through the tactile channel may be the most appropriate channel. There may be reasons to presume that touch is physically as well as psychologically therapeutic.[20]

## Communicating Through the Aural-Auditory Channel

Verbal and paraverbal messages can be used by the nurse to facilitate therapeutic communication. The philosophy inherent in the suggestions to be presented is consistent with that proposed by Carl Rogers and widely and abundantly adopted in nursing literature. The use of the techniques to be presented will give the nurse a place from which to start. There are other schools of thought on therapeutic communication which are becoming more influential and which will eventually become noticed in nursing literature. One must realize that adherence to Rogerian techniques is not the only road to helpful interactions. Each nurse should eventually become eclectic as she refines her own style based on her unique personality, the characteristics of the patients and families she works with, and her experience. Any pattern which is consistent with the goals of helpful interactions can be used. It would be very sad if all nurses talked and acted just alike. However, one must start somewhere and the following suggestions may be useful and effective in general nursing situations.

## ACTIVE LISTENING

Oddly enough, the most valuable aural-auditory communication technique one can possess is one which implies the absence of verbal or paraverbal activity. It should be clarified that listening is not something one does to use up the time while waiting to talk, nor is it synonymous with hearing. Active listening is a strenuous activity which includes:

1. Conscious or unconscious reception of auditory stimuli.
2. Comprehension of the message.
3. Interpretation and analysis of the meaning of the message.
4. Integration of the meaning of the message with other data.

The possibilities for errors in this system are numerous. The listener may not have heard the message. Or he may have heard the message but may not have been consciously aware of hearing it and thus did not comprehend it. The listener may inaccurately interpret the message due to the fact that the message was ambiguous, unfamiliar, unexpected, or incongruent with what he wanted to hear or expected. The listener may integrate the message incorrectly due to the influence of other data. For example, a speaker might say to the listener, "I feel much stronger today," but the listener may not correctly integrate the message because he has other conflicting data.

The listener usually makes a response after listening to a message. This might be immediate or greatly delayed. The message initiator is dependent upon the response given by the listener to know if his message was received and if it was understood accurately. Thus, the message initiator who receives no response or a greatly delayed response is likely to wonder if he was heard. The message initiator who receives an incongruent response is likely to wonder if he was understood. The message initiator who receives a nonspecific response such as a grunt is left puzzled over how he was received. The message initiator who receives from the listener a response which indicates that he was heard and understood is the freest to concentrate on sending more messages without concern over whether or how to send the message again. This response given by the listener to the message initiator is called feedback.

There are many ways to send feedback to the one who initiates a message on any of the channels. The nurse must learn to use feedback to indicate to the patient that the message was heard and understood, if it was, so that the patient can continue to initiate messages unobstructed.[36] One will notice that the verbal responses suggested for use by the nurse to facilitate communication all provide a degree of feedback. The nurse is most likely to be able to give accurate feedback only to the extent to which she learns to actively listen.

It is estimated that we listen with only 25 percent efficiency.[34] No one can correctly perceive everything but there are some ways to improve one's ability to actively listen. First, one can learn to eliminate or reduce obstructions to listening. Some possible blocks to listening and how to reduce them are given below.

1. Environmental distractions such as radios, traffic, and so forth. The nurse can reduce them if possible, move to another setting, or concentrate more fully on the message initiator.

2. Psychological noise such as anxiety and preoccupations. Concentrate on the patient more fully. The nurse should try to mentally repeat each sentence the patient is saying to reduce other thoughts.
3. Words or phrases used by the patient which are emotionally charged for the nurse so that she tunes out the patient or the rest of the message. For example, the patient describes someone as a communist or women's libber, uses unusual or obscene language, or expresses a strong opinion contrary to hers about politics or religion. The nurse can quickly tell herself that what she was struck by can be thought about later and return to following the rest of the communication as quickly as possible.
4. The patient who talks on and on profusely. One can try to avoid wandering away by mentally pretending to take notes as the individual talks.
5. Automatic sentence completing such as occurs when one listens only to the beginning of a sentence said by an individual and then finishes the sentence mentally without listening. This is a common occurrence and one can concentrate on the end of the sentence and listen particularly for the last word.

It has been estimated that an individual can seldom talk at more than 125 words per minute but that one can think at 600 words per minute, thus the nurse has time for performing the mental gymnastics mentioned and should still be able to listen accurately.[28] If the nurse forgets to listen, it is best to admit it to the patient and ask him to repeat what he just said. This will usually work out better than pretending that one was listening.

In addition to listening to what the patient is saying, the nurse listens to other things. One important thing to listen for is what the patient avoids saying. For example:

A community health nurse was working with a mother and her child who had a recently discovered convulsive disorder. The nurse had decided that the child was successfully medicated and that the family was capable of handling the situation and was ready to close the case when she realized that the mother had never used the words "seizure" or "convulsion." On her next visit she pursued the area with the mother and determined that the mother was very definitely denying the illness. The nurse did not close the case but developed new objectives instead.

The nurse also checks the agreement among verbal, paraverbal, and nonverbal messages based on her comparison between what she hears and what she sees. The patient who denies pain but appears strained as he lies unmovingly and tightly gripping the side rails may be attempting to avoid medication.

The nurse's skill at listening is probably the crucial element which determines whether the patient sees her as interested and concerned. The patient can tell in the first few minutes of the conversation if the nurse is listening actively to what he is saying.[34] If he feels she is listening, he is more likely to reveal important information than if he feels she is not listening. To be really listened to is a satisfying experience. It implies to the message initiator that he is important enough to be heard and understood. Being really listened to is probably a rare experience.[18] The nurse who makes a habit of active listening will be amazed at what she begins to hear. Before one can listen one must of course stop talking. Sometimes all the patient needs is to be listened to and understood. He desires nothing more.

An old story is told about a wife who complained to her husband because she had to do the laundry with an old-fashioned washing machine. The husband bought her a new machine, but soon she complained because she had to hang the clothes outside. The husband bought his wife an automatic dryer, but again soon she complained because she had to carry the clothes up and down the basement steps. The husband moved the washer and dryer upstairs, but soon the wife complained because there was so much laundry to do. Finally the husband in exasperation said, "What do you want? I've bought you a new washer, a new dryer and moved them upstairs. What more can I do?" The wife replied, "All I've ever wanted you to do was to listen to me and acknowledge that you understood what I did and appreciated it. I never really needed the other things."

## General Measures to Improve Verbal Communication

Before specific verbal techniques are presented, there are some general ways the nurse can improve the verbal messages she sends.

First of all, the nurse should consider how she speaks, and in particular her speech habits, voice quality, pitch, rate, and volume.[6] Listening to a tape recording of one's speech can be most revealing. If the nurse does not like what she hears on the recording, she can practice speaking more slowly, more distinctly, on a different pitch, and so forth until what she hears is more pleasing. Most speech characteristics are learned habits and can be altered. Patients find particularly annoying people who whine, rush their words, or speak either too softly or too loudly. If the nurse has a particular ineffective speech pattern, a course especially focusing on improved speaking habits can be beneficial.

The nurse can also facilitate verbal effectiveness by conscious efforts to:

1. Reinforce verbal messages by corresponding nonverbal messages.
2. Avoid the use of excessive medical jargon and complicated verbalisms.
3. Avoid slang terminology which may have unclear meanings.
4. State ideas as concisely, clearly, and understandably as possible.
5. Listen for the answer to the questions she asks.

## Openings

The following are guidelines for specific verbal responses which the nurse can make to the patient, coupled with appropriate paraverbal and nonverbal behavior which should lead to the facilitation of the patient's communication of messages. Responses which tend to be less directive[3] will be presented first.

### OFFERING SELF

One of the most effective ways for the nurse to initiate an interaction may be to indicate to the patient that she is available. This is especially useful in the beginning phase.

"I could sit and talk with you for a while if you would like."
"I have nothing to do for the next few minutes if you would like me to stay and talk."

### UNIVERSAL OPENERS

Because the nurse wants the patient to pick the topic which is most relevant to him, she can refrain from indicating the topic with remarks such as, "How are you feeling?" or "How was the surgery?" and instead use broad unspecified openers. These openers are useful in the beginning phase.

"How are things going?"
"How are you?"

## *Responses*

The following methods are used to provide feedback and to facilitate the patient's communication.

### ENCOURAGING VERBALIZATIONS

This can be done by remarks which are very brief and imply "Continue, I'm listening." These are especially useful during the beginning and content phases.

"Go on."
"Yes."
"Oh."
"And then . . ."
"Uh huh."

Nonverbal behavior alone can be used such as nodding, tilting the head, or leaning forward.

### RESTATEMENT

The nurse repeats almost the same words the patient used. This emphasizes what the patient said and may encourage him to continue. Restatement can be easily overdone. This is especially useful in the content and mood phases.

Johnny:     I couldn't sleep last night because I was so worried about my surgery today.
Nurse:     You are concerned about going to surgery?

### EXPLORING

This encourages the patient to explore an area in more depth. It is useful during the content phase when elaboration is needed. The nurse indicates to the patient what he can more fully explain.

"Tell me about your work."
"Can you describe your last labor and delivery?"
"You mentioned that your family has a history of bleeding disorders. Would you go into that more?"

### EXPRESSING ACCEPTANCE

This can be done to provide feedback to the patient that one heard and understood the message. It also communicates to the patient that the nurse is not negatively judging what the patient is saying, but can accept what is discussed. This is appropriate during all phases.

"I can understand why you walked out."
"I think I can appreciate how you felt about the accident."

## FOCUSING ON FEELINGS

This is done to encourage the patient to express his emotional feelings. The nurse verbalizes what the patient might be feeling. This is especially useful during the mood phase.

Jane:  My mother-in-law can be a pain in the neck sometimes.
Nurse:  You get annoyed with her?

Jack:  This just can't be happening.
Nurse:  You are still overwhelmed by all of this.

## CLARIFYING

This may be done to check the nurse's perception of the situation. This is sometimes referred to as validation. It is useful during all phases.

"Are you saying that . . ."
"Do I understand you to be saying . . ."
"Have I got this right? You . . ."

## SUMMARIZING

Putting previously discussed topics into a brief statement for emphasis or conciseness may help the patient to move toward resolution. This is useful during integration.

"So you have signed the operative permit and called your wife."
"You would like to quit work but you can't do without the money right now."

## Openings

The following techniques are usually considered to be more directive.[3]

## OBSERVATIONAL OPENERS

These are useful when opening the conversation. They differ from the openers previously presented in that they suggest the topic to be discussed. The nurse shares an observation she has made relevant to the patient.

"I noticed that you were up walking this morning."
"You seem anxious."
"You appeared reluctant to talk with me on my visit last week while your sister was here."

## SITUATIONAL OPENERS

The nurse uses situational openers to introduce the topic she wishes to discuss with the patient. These are useful during the opening phase.

> "I would like to talk to you about your reaction to physical therapy."
> "Could we spend a few minutes talking about what you expect to happen in clinic?"

## *Questions*

Asking appropriate questions is not as easy as it might at first seem. The following suggestions reveal the optimal characteristics of appropriate questions. These are usually used during the data collection phase.

### QUESTIONS THAT REQUIRE ELABORATION

It is best to avoid questions which can be answered by yes or no. This can lead to a pattern similar to a military inquiry. Most yes and no questions can be asked as questions which require elaboration instead.

> Yes or no question:
>   "Do you work?"
> Question requiring elaboration:
>   "Tell me about yourself."

> Yes or no question:
>   "Has Billy recovered from his accident?"
> Question requiring elaboration:
>   "How is Billy now since the accident?"

### QUESTIONS THAT DO NOT SUGGEST THE ANSWER

Questions should be worded so that the patient is not told how to respond by the nurse. Most statements in which the nurse suggests an answer can be stated otherwise.

> Answer suggested:
>   "I'll bet you will be glad to get home."
>   "It must be nice to have such helpful neighbors."
> More effective:
>   "How do you feel about going home?"
>   "How do you feel about your neighbor's concern?"

### QUESTIONS THAT DO NOT EVOKE THE SOCIALLY ACCEPTABLE ANSWER

Some questions the nurse might ask may lead the patient to reply as he thinks he should rather than as he really feels. These can usually be asked in a more effective manner.

Socially acceptable answer probable:
"Do you and your husband have a good marriage?"
"Do you miss your children while they are at camp?"
More effective:
"How has your relationship with your husband been?"
"How do you feel about having both children gone at camp?"

## QUESTIONS THAT DO NOT PRY

The nurse should seek information which she needs but she should not probe into the patient's private life out of curiosity. The nurse who believes a patient desires to discuss a personal area should be receptive but she can offer the patient a chance to still say no. In general, the nurse should not require the patient to tell her any information which he might later regret telling her or for which she has no legitimate need.[31]

Probing:
"Do you sleep with your boyfriend?"
"Why did your wife leave you?"
More effective:
"Would you like for me to go over some of this birth control information as a general review?"
"Would it help to talk about your wife's departure?"

## QUESTIONS THAT CALL FOR DETAIL

When collecting data, the nurse can use the following areas to help thoroughly explore a situation.[26] This is especially useful in collecting data about a symptom the patient is experiencing.

Location:
"Where does it hurt?"
"Can you point to where the numbness is?"
Quality:
"How would you describe the sensation?"
"What is the buzzing like?"
Quantity:
"How often does this happen?"
"Do your ears ring all of the time?"
"How much does it hurt?"
Chronology:
"When did you first notice this bruise?"
"What happened after you felt the muscle spasm?"
"Did you notice anything unusual before you fainted?"
Setting:
"Do you ever faint at work?"
"Where were you when this happened?"
Conditions:
"What happens to the contractions if you walk around?"
"Did this happen after eating any particular food?"
"Were you standing or sitting when you became dizzy?"
Associated factors:
"Did you notice any tiredness or weakness in general when you began to see double?"
"Were you sick at your stomach when you had the headache?"
"Have you recently had a sore throat?"

## "LAUNDRY LIST" QUESTIONS

Sometimes the patient lacks words to describe what he knows and he can be encouraged to be more specific if he is given some choices to select from.[13] The nurse will be less likely to put words in the patient's mouth if she gives several choices.

John:    I was upset for a long time after he left.
Nurse:    Do you mean you were upset for hours, days, weeks . . .
John:    Several days.

Betty:    I don't know how many of my pills she took. Here is the bottle. It wasn't full fortunately.
Nurse:    Would you say it was more like 10, 20, 50, 100?
Betty:    It was probably more like 20 or 30.

## UNDERSTANDABLE QUESTIONS

The nurse who finds that she has to explain the question should consider how she asked the question. The excessive use of medical jargon is often the problem.

Misunderstandable:
    "Did the baby have physiologic jaundice?"
    "Was the pain intermittent?"
More effective:
    "Did the baby's skin turn yellow after he was born?"
    "Does the pain come and go?"

## QUESTIONS THAT ARE SEPARATE

Ideally, each question should be asked individually and not grouped into clusters such as, "Tell me about your family, how many children you have, and what they are doing." The patient hardly knows what to respond to first. This could have been, "Tell me about your children."

Multiple question:
    "Would you like to come in this week or next week?"
    "Do you like your job, what do you do, how long have you worked there?"
Separate questions:
    "When would you like to come in?"
    "Tell me about your job."

## QUESTIONS THAT DO NOT ASK "WHY"

Why questions put the patient in a quandary because he is often unaware of his motive. Asking him a why question may encourage rationalization. Using why questions also reminds many of their childhood and implies criticism as when mother asked, "Why in the world did you do that?"[8,24] Most why questions could be better stated using who, what, when, where, and how.

> Why questions:
>    "Why weren't you at the clinic last week?"
>    "Why don't you test your urine regularly?"
> More effective:
>    "I noticed that you weren't at the clinic. How have you been?"
>    "How do you feel about testing your urine three times a day?"

## INDIRECT QUESTIONS

Changing a direct question into an indirect one may encourage the patient to verbalize beyond what is required to answer the question. Indirect questions hardly seem like questions.

> Direct questions:
>    "How do you feel about birth control?"
>    "What do you think would happen if you quit right now?"
>    "Do you think you need to see a physician?"
> Indirect questions:
>    "I wonder how you feel about birth control."
>    "You must have many thoughts about changing jobs right now."
>    "You must have considered seeing a physician."

# *Responses*

## OFFERING INFORMATION

This can be done when it appears that the nurse has some knowledge which might be helpful to the patient. She offers to share it with the patient at the appropriate time. Giving information may be overdone unless one remains sensitive to the idea that the patient needs to learn to solve his own problems. It is usually helpful in the problem solving phase.

> "I have worked for several years with parents whose children are fatally ill. I could share with you some of my ideas on living with a fatal diagnosis if you would be interested sometime."

> "I have just returned from a diabetes workshop and I could tell you some of the discussions I heard about teenagers with diabetes if you wish."

## REFOCUSING

This is done when the communication has progressed from a desired area to an area where data are not needed or relevant. With tact and politeness, the nurse suggests where the conversation should return to.

"Getting back to your health for a minute, do you have any allergies to foods or drugs?"

"You mentioned a few minutes ago that you might send your daughter to nursery school. I wonder what your thinking has been regarding that decision."

It should be remembered that the techniques presented are only guidelines. The nurse should strive to avoid overuse of these techniques. If the nurse can concentrate on the goals of therapeutic communication, she will come naturally to use appropriate openings, responses, and questions.

## COMMUNICATING IN SPECIAL SITUATIONS

In the course of a therapeutic interaction, the nurse may encounter some individual situations about which she may be uncertain. The following information suggests some general approaches to special situations which may be helpful.

### When the Patient Cries

Most of us feel uncomfortable when someone begins to cry. The nurse may experience a heightened anxiety when a patient cries as she wonders what she did to cause the crying and how to get the patient to stop. The social system of communication with which one initially is familiar dictates that one should not cry except in a few specific situations and that the appropriate social response to crying is something like, "Now stop crying. It will be all right." The nurse must first learn that crying is a healthy and normal mechanism for release of emotional tension. The patient should not be told to stop crying. The nurse should do what she can to reduce the patient's embarrassment by telling him that it is all right for him to cry, providing him with as much privacy from others as possible and providing him with tissues if necessary. Staying with the patient reinforces her words that the patient's crying is acceptable behavior. She should communicate to the patient that she is willing to wait until he finishes crying. The nurse who notices that a patient is about to cry should avoid her tendency to keep the patient from crying and might offer acceptance instead by saying something like, "You still feel like crying when you talk about your mother's death," or "You seem on the verge of tears. It's all right to cry if you feel like it."

### When the Patient Asks Personal Questions

Nurses are sometimes caught by surprise when a patient asks a personal question. The task of the nurse when the patient asks a personal question is to determine whether or not she wishes to answer the question and why the patient is asking the question.

If the nurse wishes to answer the question, she can do so simply and return the focus of the conversation to the patient promptly. "Yes, I like to ski. Do you ski?" If the nurse does not want to answer the question, it would be best for her to say so simply rather than to reveal information she wishes to keep private or to attempt to give an evasive answer. She can say, "I'd rather not talk about my religious beliefs. You were discussing having a tubal ligation. I wonder what you have considered about it," or "I'd rather not discuss that. I don't think my ideas on that are important here. What is important is what you think about premarital sex." Again, the nurse refocuses the discussion to the patient.

Some of the reasons that the patient might ask a personal question include:

1. Being sociable and friendly. "Where did you go to school?" These can be responded to at the level at which they were asked. It is especially important to refocus on the patient or the conversation may indicate to the patient that the nurse would rather talk about herself than him. The nurse can decide whether or not to answer these questions based on how she feels about revealing the information involved.

2. Wanting to determine if the nurse has the background to understand his situation. "Have you ever had surgery?" "Do you have any children?" These questions may arise spontaneously or within the context of a discussion. For example, a mother in labor who asks, "Do you have any children?" probably is trying to determine the nurse's personal familiarity with labor. These questions should be dealt with on the basis of helping the patient to clarify what he really is asking. "No, I've never had surgery. Are you wondering if I can understand how you feel about yours if I've never been through one?" "Yes, I've had two children. Are you wondering if I've been through labor?"

3. Curiosity. Sometimes the patient may be interested in finding out information about the nurse or others which the nurse should not divulge because it would violate her own rights or another's. These questions are best answered in a way that protects the others involved and politely indicates to the patient that the question was inappropriate.

| | |
|---|---|
| Mrs. Black: | What is the matter with that baby over there? I heard someone say that he was beaten. Is that true? |
| Nurse: | I can't answer that. Nor would I tell other parents or visitors about your child's condition. |
| | |
| Jack: | I've heard Dr. Burton has had four wives. Is that true? |
| Nurse: | You will have to ask him about that. It isn't really proper for me to discuss someone else's personal life. |

When the nurse is unable to determine why the patient asks a question, she can reply, "Why do you ask?"

## When the Patient Asks for Confidentiality

Occasionally a patient may desire to tell the nurse some information but he may first ask the nurse to promise that the information he is about to reveal will be kept confidential. The nurse cannot agree to this because she must share information she has learned if it is important to the health of others or the patient. In this situation, the nurse should clearly indicate to the patient that she cannot promise secrecy, specifically who the information he might tell her might be shared with, and who the information would not be available to. The patient must then decide if he can accept these conditions.

| | |
|---|---|
| Jill: | I think you will understand the mess I'm in. I think I have VD. If I tell you how I got it, will you promise not to tell anyone else? |
| Nurse: | I can't promise you that, Jill, because that information might be very important. I would have to share it with the other staff members at the clinic and they would also contact anyone whom you name as a sexual contact. I can assure you that your parents can never obtain any information from this health service. |

## When the Patient is Silent

Silence has a particular unnerving quality for the learner who is trying to develop skill in therapeutic communication. It may be helpful to distinguish between types of silences. The nurse can use nonverbal clues and consideration of the previous interaction to differentiate.

### THE THOUGHTFUL SILENCE

This usually occurs during an interaction where the patient is engaging in considerable reflection and thought. A silence usually precedes the presentation of an important piece of information. If the silence is interrupted, the important information may be lost. As a general rule, the nurse should not interrupt a thoughtful silence.[27]

### THE RESISTIVE SILENCE

The resistive silence occurs during an interaction when the patient does not want to discuss a topic or answer a question. It may arise quite unexpectedly. In general, the nurse might allow the silence to last for a short period of time to see if the patient is going to respond, and then deal with the silence through an observational opener:

"You have become very quiet. Can you tell me what you are thinking about?"

### THE EMOTIONAL SILENCE

When a patient is discussing a highly emotional subject he may become silent in an attempt to control his emotions. The nurse should allow the patient a period of silence and if the patient does not eventually speak, she can offer the patient the choice of continuing or not.

"I notice that this seems difficult for you to talk about. Would you like to discuss this more or would you like to change to another topic?"

### THE NERVOUS SILENCE

Sometimes, when the nurse and the patient are not familiar with each other and both are a little uncomfortable talking, a silence may occur when neither can think of something to say. This type of silence can become more anxiety producing the longer it lasts, so the nurse should interrupt it when she feels it is increasing the anxiety level.

The nurse may find that she is initially very uncomfortable with silence and that she interrupts it after only a few seconds. As she gains experience, she will be able to tolerate longer periods and she should work toward this.

## When the Interaction is Interrupted

Absolute freedom from interruptions is unlikely in most situations. The nurse who must leave a patient during a therapeutic interaction either because she or the patient is called away should tell the patient when she will return and make a mental note about what was being discussed. If it is possible, the nurse might summarize the discussion briefly before she leaves. When she returns, she can refocus the interaction at the place where it was interrupted.[35]

## When the Patient Uses Lay Terminology

Patients will often use a variety of lay terms which the nurse may assume she understands. Some examples of these lay terms include nervous breakdown, enlarged heart, stomach flu, hot flashes, head cold, heartburn, nervous stomach, fits, and hives. Until the nurse clarifies what the patient means by these terms, it is best to use the patient's terms when talking to the patient rather than exchanging the proper medical term which she thinks the patient is referring to. She can clarify the terms he is using by asking for descriptions of the term.

"You mentioned that you felt very depressed. Can you describe this depression?"

## When the Patient Talks On and On

Nurses will occasionally encounter patients who can talk nonstop for hours and hours. Although the nurse may realize the importance of providing the patient with a chance to verbalize, she may find her boredom or annoyance growing and her listening decrease as she listens to volumes of irrelevant information. There are two things the nurse might wish to try in these situations. First, she could inform the patient from the beginning of how much time she can spend talking with him. For example, she might say, "I have 20 minutes left to spend talking with you this morning before I must leave. What would you like to talk about?" She can warn the patient just slightly before the time is up. "I have to go in a few minutes. Is there anything else you specifically want to discuss?" Setting limits may help her feel less abused by the patient. The patient just might become more serious about using the time available to better advantage. This is also helpful when the patient always waits just until the nurse is about to leave before bringing up what he wants to talk about.[31] Second, the nurse could use refocusing to help the patient stay on the topic.

Wilma:   I have a lot of trouble living by myself. You know my sister, Cara, comes to visit me each week to clean my house. Her husband just died and she's very lonely. Her children are all far away. One lives in Minneapolis and one moved to California. The one in California is one of those . . .
Nurse:   Could we get back for a minute to how you manage living alone? What do you do about meals?

Interestingly, elderly individuals sometimes engage in a "life review" which is different from the rambling conversation described. This should be encouraged as it is seen as a summary operation that the individual goes through in preparation for death.[5]

## When There Is Disagreement Between What the Patient Says and His Behavior

The nurse may encounter situations where the patient says one thing but does something quite different in actuality. In these situations, the nurse may wish to confront the patient with what she has observed. This must be done very carefully. It is suggested that the nurse must earn the right to confront a patient by having first developed a well established relationship with the patient.[1] The nurse should remember that all of us display some degree of inconsistency between what we say and what we do in areas of our lives. The nurse should confront a patient only when the inconsistency he is displaying is serious and is adversely affecting his wellness and the nurse believes he is ready to face the inconsistency.

Confrontation can be easily overdone. It may give the nurse a feeling of superiority to go around pointing out inconsistencies in others' behavior—while ignoring her own. But properly used, within an established relationship, confrontation may serve a useful purpose. A nurse who plans to confront a patient should consider timing carefully because she and the patient must be available after the confrontation to deal with the consequences. If the patient denies the inconsistency, the nurse should probably let the matter go until she feels he is more ready to explore the area. The nurse should try to state the confrontation objectively with specific data and without anger or vindictiveness in her voice.

> "Becky, I've been coming here every week for two months to teach you how to give your own insulin injection. You tell me you want to do it and yet you don't seem to pay attention to what I say and you admit that you don't practice any of the steps during the week. Is there something about learning to give your injection that we should talk about?"

## When the Patient is Avoiding Reality

There may be instances in which a patient is denying one aspect of a situation which is very important to his wellness. The nurse may wish to remind him of the reality of his situation in the hopes that more realistic problem solving will occur. Similar to confrontation, introducing reality must be done carefully, within an established relationship, when the patient is ready to face the situation, and with concern for timing. And, as in confrontation, if the desired result is not achieved, the nurse should let the matter drop for the present.

The following statements by the nurse represent attempts at introducing reality.

> "It seems to me that you would like to forget about the accident and lead your life as you always have, but some things are going to be different, aren't they?"

> "I get the feeling that you would like to ignore how your father feels about your marriage, but you will have to face him sometime, won't you?"

## SOME UNHELPFUL COMMUNICATION TECHNIQUES

Presented here will be some communications which the nurse might make which are usually very unhelpful in a therapeutic interaction. Ironically, many of these are in common usage in social intercourse so that "unlearning" them is often difficult because the nurse is so accustomed to using them.

## Nonspecific Reassurance

"Everything will be all right." "Things always work out for the better." These statements offer the patient nothing concrete on which to build hope. They also may communicate to him that his concerns are irrelevant and best ignored. He probably will not express them again and the nurse will not learn what he is particularly concerned about.

Specific reassurance, however, can be useful if given at the right time. For example, "I have heard other patients who have had amputations talk about this type of pain. They have told me that it gets less bothersome in a few days." "I think the medicine you were taking for your arthritis might be causing you to be dizzy. Now that you have stopped the medication you may notice less dizziness."

## Nonspecific Praise

"You're such a good mother." "You are always so kind and thoughtful." Unspecific praise usually leads the recipient to deny the praise because he can think of many reasons why he does not deserve the praise. Specific praise is more useful to the patient because he can accept it more readily. Specific praise should be used only when it can be sincerely given because the patient will easily spot phoney compliments. Some examples of specific praise are: "I think it really is a good idea to spend a half hour with each child when you get home from work the way you do," and "You have walked twice as far today as you did yesterday."

## Pep Talks

"We've got to get you up and going. There's no reason to let this get you down. You've been through worse things than this without batting an eye. Now let's get some sunshine in here . . ." Pep talks are not really inspiring and are probably of more benefit to the nurse than to the patient because she can deny how the patient feels and present a veneer of enthusiasm which she expects him to adopt. Leave the pep talks to the coaches.

## Personal Examples

The nurse is sometimes tempted to tell the patient about a similar experience she has had in the belief that it will be helpful. The patient may in reality feel closed out and that the nurse would rather talk about herself. He will probably not believe that her situation was just like his. If she indicates in her personal story her courage and persistence, he may feel even more demoralized. If the nurse feels she has a story that would be helpful because it was so related, she might allude to her experience briefly and let the patient decide if he is interested. She may be able to relate her personal experience to specific reassurance. For example she might say, "I remember being nauseated after I had my surgery. It went away by the next morning. I hope yours does also."

## Urging

"Why not go over there right now and get started on this?" Often urging is done in conjunction with excessive advice giving. The nurse probably senses that her patient is resistant to her advice and tries to counteract his resistance with her own persistence. If the nurse finds that she is continually engaging in efforts to strengthen a patient's determination to do something, she should reflect on the situation. Is she acting on a goal she has for the patient which the patient doesn't share? Has she taken over ownership of the patient's problem? Excessive urging is likely to ultimately result in discouragement because the nurse is usually setting herself up for failure.

## Moralizing

"This low salt diet is for your own good. Sneaking potato chips in the canteen is a miserable insult to all of us here who want to help you." Moralizing is a frequent temptation to nurses if they feel they have a divine calling to enlighten others when their health is at stake. Being a nurse does not give one the right to preach to others what they should do and then become their superego when they do otherwise. Nurses seem especially likely to moralize to children and teenagers. Moralizations can be identified by the fact that they remind the patient of moral "shoulds" and "oughts" which the nurse feels should guide his behavior. The nurse in the first situation would most likely have been more helpful if she had confronted the patient calmly without delivering a sermon as a bonus. "I notice that you were eating potato chips in the canteen even though you know you are on a restricted sodium diet."

## Claiming the Patient's Feelings

"I know just how you feel." "I know exactly what you are going through." Although the nurse may think she is expressing empathy and acceptance, the patient is likely to feel that his feelings have been dismissed. He believes that no one can feel exactly like he does and those who tell him that they do cannot really understand. The nurse could use a response which would more likely imply empathy and acceptance if she has been listening carefully while allowing the patient to own the feeling. "I think I understand why you feel that way," "I can appreciate why you feel as you do about what you have been through."

## Cliches

"It will all come out in the wash." "Every dog has his day." "Every cloud has a silver lining." Sometimes one can get in the habit of responding to others through a series of meaningless and trite phrases which add nothing to the conversation. They may imply to the patient that he is talking to a computer programmed to respond randomly with wise sayings. When the nurse is tempted to use cliches, she might remember one herself: "When in doubt, leave it out!"

## COMMUNICATING IN PROBLEMATIC SITUATIONS

Some situations will be described where the nurse and the patient or family member have a problem because of the nature of the interaction which has developed between them. The suggestions to be given are appropriately used when the other individual is consistently meeting his needs at the expense of the nurse's needs. They are rather drastic measures not to be taken lightly. These techniques are based on the assumption that improved communication can lead to an improved relationship.

### Helping Others to Cease Manipulative Behavior

The nurse may experience situations in which the patient has learned to be manipulative or, in other words, to get the nurse to do things she does not believe she should do. If the nurse finds that she feels abused or misused in an interaction and ends up agreeing to do things which she does not want to do, she might want to consider learning some skills to counteract manipulation. First consider what is occurring in this interaction.

> Ms. Wiggins has repeatedly treated Betty more like a servant than a nurse. Today is no exception.
>
> Ms. Wiggins: Say, Betty, I was wondering if you could do me a little favor. I am all out of these mints and I do so enjoy having them when my evening visitors come. Would you be so kind as to stop at a drugstore tonight and pick up another tin for me?
>
> Betty: Well, I don't know, Ms. Wiggins. I have a lot to do tonight.
>
> Ms. Wiggins: It would only take a minute of your time. I hate to have to ask you but you have always been so sweet to me. You are about the only nurse here who really seems to care if I live or die.
>
> Betty: Thank you, Ms. Wiggins, but I don't really go by any drugstores on my way home.
>
> Ms. Wiggins: There must be one not too far from you. I wouldn't ask you if I thought I couldn't depend on you. It is so difficult for me to be asking people to do all of these things for me, but what can I do—being so helpless here.
>
> Betty: I just don't know if I can find time tonight.
>
> Ms. Wiggins: You finish work at 3:30, don't you? Maybe you could ask the head nurse to let you leave early since you are going to do something for a special patient of yours.
>
> Betty: I don't think I could to that because I have to give report. Couldn't your husband bring them?
>
> Ms. Wiggins: Oh, he probably would forget or get the wrong ones. Anyway he is so busy I hate to bother him. Now let me get you some money. Be sure you bring back the receipt . . .

Ms. Wiggins is skillful at manipulation and she probably knew that the compliments and the plays for sympathy would be especially effective.

### Learning to Say No

What can the nurse do when a patient asks her to do something she does not believe she should do? First of all, she should say, "No," definitely and unequivocally. The nurse shouldn't be trapped by plays on her conscience or fairness. She is the only one who need

judge her own behavior. She doesn't need to ｊ
justify her decisions except to herself. The examp
learn to say no without guilt, excuses, or offerin

Connie has been visiting Ms. Elliot for several months. Th
Elliot has managed to convince Connie to do a number c
problem is that Connie feels sorry for Ms. Elliot because sh
four children are constantly out of one crisis and into anot
them to clinic appointments, picked up a child at school
dental school, and even babysat one night. Connie has the
relationship has not achieved a proper level. Worst of all, M
Connie has decided that she will say "no" to Ms. Elliott c
something against her philosophy of community health n

Nurse: I'm sorry. The tr
Roy:   I guess. Why
Nurse: It's a way o
Roy:   Now be
Nurse: I'll b
Roy:   O
Nurse:
Ro

48

| Connie: | Hi, how are you today? |
|---|---|
| Ms. Elliott: | Come in. Boy am I glad to see you. |
| Connie: | Oh? |
| Ms. Elliott: | Yes. I'm in a terrible mess. Joey is ill with another strep throat. The doctor phoned in a prescription for him at the drugstore on the corner. Can you run down and get it before we start our visit? |
| Connie: | No. |
| Ms. Elliott: | (Somewhat surprised) I already told them you would be coming. They said it could be added to my bill. It's all ready. All you need to do is run in and get it at the back. Couldn't you go? |
| Connie: | No. |
| Ms. Elliott: | Why not? I wouldn't ask you except I have no way to get there and I can't leave these two kids here alone. What am I going to do? |
| Connie: | I don't know. |
| Ms. Elliott: | You could be there and back in 5 minutes. I have a lot of other problems right now. This ovarian cyst I have is causing me terrible pain. I'm afraid I need an operation. You've always been such a help to me. I knew you were the one person I could count on. |
| Connie: | I just can't. |
| Ms. Elliott: | That doesn't make any sense. You have a car; you would be here an hour anyway. What is the matter with you? Are you sick today or something? |
| Connie: | No, I'm not sick. |
| Ms. Elliott: | Are you mad at me because I wasn't home last time you came? |
| Connie: | No. |
| Ms. Elliott: | Well, what is it? |
| Connie: | There is nothing wrong. I just don't want to get the medicine. |
| Ms. Elliott: | Well, can I take your car? |
| Connie: | No. |
| Ms. Elliott: | I didn't think so. (Sigh) Well anyway, did I tell you that Jacqueline needs glasses . . . |

So why make such a big deal over a small errand? The important thing is that Connie believes that she should not get the medicine and she has resisted being manipulated into doing so. It is probable that if Connie continues to resist Ms. Elliot's manipulation, the relationship may become quite different. Connie probably will not dread visiting Ms. Elliot in the future now that she feels she is able to uphold her own convictions.

## Learning to Defuse Criticism and Advice

Some individuals engage in manipulative behavior which uses criticism as the main technique so that the nurse is often forced into a child ego state. For example:

Roy:   You are certainly late enough this morning.

ffic was bad. Are you ready to have your dressing changed?
o you always put on that apron? It looks silly.
protecting you and me.
careful when you tear off that tape. I don't know why you always put so much on.
careful. I didn't want your dressing to fall off.
ch! Stop! Don't you know that hurts?
I'm sorry. Tell me when I can go ahead.
Don't put so much on this time. Why do you have to have such cold hands?

urse: I'm sorry. It's cold outside. (Struggling to control her irritation)
Roy: Be careful. That sticks. Can't you figure out how to put that on so it won't stick?
Nurse: I'm doing my best. (Said through clenched teeth)
Roy: The nurse who came last Saturday didn't hurt me a bit . . .

When this situation exists, meaningful communication is unlikely unless the nurse uses techniques to move the interaction to a more adult-to-adult level. One way to defuse persistent and unjust criticism and advice when it is interfering with an interaction is to acknowledge and agree with the comments. This also helps the nurse to resist becoming defensive. The criticism should decrease and the conversation refocus.

In the next situation, Hilda is continually complaining and criticizing. No one has been able to experience even one satisfactory exchange on other than a parent-to-child level. Staff anger and resentment are running high and prayers for a speedy discharge are offered daily. Melissa has decided to try to defuse Hilda's criticisms today in the hopes that she might be able to move to another type of interaction with Hilda.

Hilda: Oh! You are my nurse today. I was wondering when someone would appear to get this tray out of here.
Melissa: You have barely touched your food.
Hilda: No one could eat this stuff. The coffee tastes like it was warmed up from last night.
Melissa: It could have been.
Hilda: And those scrambled eggs. Just look at how pale they are.
Melissa: They do look pretty tasteless, don't they?
Hilda: They're powdered! And who could eat bacon like that swimming in grease?
Melissa: You're right. It does look greasy.
Hilda: I don't know what has happened to this hospital. It used to be that a stay here was marvelous. Things have gone downhill around here.
Melissa: You could be right.
Hilda: You just don't get the care. When I was here before, I got a backrub every night. Nurses don't know how to give backrubs anymore.
Melissa: You are probably right.
Hilda: You've never even offered me a backrub.
Melissa: No, I haven't, have I?
Hilda: You dash out of my room at your first chance.
Melissa: I do that, don't I?
Hilda: (Beginning to study the nurse's face) And most of the nurses look like tramps now with that long hair and pantsuit uniforms.
Melissa: We probably do.
Hilda: You're acting sort of peculiar this morning.
Melissa: Am I? That could be.
Hilda: No one seems to pay much attention to me.
Melissa: We probably do act that way.
Hilda: Sometimes a person really needs someone she can talk to.
Melissa: I'm sure you're right. Is there something you would like to talk about?
Hilda: I've been wondering if you can tell me about this next test I'm scheduled to have . . .

Excessive advice can also force the nurse into responding from a child state. In the next example, Terry uses agreement to deal with advice from her clinical supervisor who has been helpful but tends to expect Terry to live her life the way she thinks it should be lived. Most of their previous discussions have ended in an argument. This interaction is included to show that defusing criticism and advice can be useful in other than nurse-patient situations.

Mildred: Have you decided if you are applying to graduate school for this fall yet?
Terry: Just about.
Mildred: Well, I hope you don't. You should stay here and get more experience. You baccalaureate grads are so far behind when you come.
Terry: You could be right.
Mildred: I don't want you to make another mistake like going off to take that other course.
Terry: That could have been a big mistake.
Mildred: You can always go to grad school later when you get too old to work very hard. I don't know what they teach there anyway. It would be a waste of your time.
Terry: That might be.
Mildred: You can learn so much here. Think of the experience you would gain if you took the opening on permanent nights.
Terry: You could be right.
Mildred: (Beginning to look confused) I've been around long enough to know. Graduate school is for those nurses who haven't got what it takes.
Terry: That could be.
Mildred: Well, I hope you make the right decision. (Beginning to study Terry's face)
Terry: So do I. We'll just have to wait and see.
Mildred: (Pause) I would hate to lose you. We need some new blood around here.
Terry: I'm sure you do.
Mildred: I can't sell you on permanent nights, can I?
Terry: No.
Mildred: Well, I tried. I really hope you don't leave. I don't know what will happen to my ideas about primary nursing if you aren't here to help me . . .

Notice that Mildred eventually stopped telling Terry what to do based on what was supposedly best for Terry but finally started to level with Terry about her real reasons for not wanting Terry to leave. One might speculate that a new relationship may develop between Terry and Mildred based on more adult-to-adult communication and fewer attempts by Mildred to manipulate Terry into what Mildred wants under the guise of advice.

## Helping Others to Send Clear Communication

Occasionally a situation may develop where the patient controls the behavior of the nurse by carefully worded insinuations. For example:

Peter: You look sleepy this morning. I'll bet you were out running around with some guy all night.
Nurse: I wasn't out very late.
Peter: Well, I hope you are awake enough to know what you are doing. Maybe you had better get someone else to help you hook me up for dialysis.
Nurse: I can do it.
Peter: Wednesday that male nurse hooked me up. He really knew what he was doing. They should have more male nurses down here.
Nurse: Bill is off today. (Through clenched teeth)
Peter: Now are you sure that goes there?

The interaction might have gone differently if the nurse had known how to deal with insinuations. One technique is to ask the patient if what he is insinuating is what he means.

This should eventually lead the patient to realize how ridiculous his insinuations sound and to abandon his insinuation technique in favor of more direct statements. This is how it might have worked with Peter.

Peter: You look sleepy this morning. I'll bet you were out running around with some guy all night.
Nurse: Are you saying that I shouldn't date?
Peter: No, of course not. I hope you are awake enough to know what you are doing. Maybe you had better get someone else to help you hook me up for dialysis.
Nurse: Are you saying that you are afraid I won't do it right?
Peter: No. No. Last week that male nurse hooked me up. He really knew what he was doing. They should have more male nurses down here.
Nurse: Are you saying that you think male nurses are better than female nurses?
Peter: Oh, of course not. Boy, you are really jumping to conclusions today. It's just that I get so nervous when I go on this contraption.
Nurse: It's scary?
Peter: It sure is . . .


## Nurse-Physician Interaction

It is indeed sad that nurse-physician interactions could be placed under problematic interactions, but this is often the case. It is predictable that much of the communication between the physician and the nurse will be parent-child due to many factors such as sex roles, historical influences, and cultural expectations. However, the most productive mode would be adult-to-adult because this is the type of interaction which allows both individuals to process data clearly and problem solve accurately.[21,34] The nurse who wants to communicate on this level with physicians may find the techniques just presented helpful in promoting adult-to-adult interactions if a situation exists where parent-to-child interactions predominate. The following examines a problematic situation.

Dr. Rogers is a pediatrician who admits patients to the pediatric unit where Maggie is the head nurse. Maggie anticipates Dr. Roger's daily arrival with foreboding. Dr. Rogers never is pleased with anything. His criticism, mostly about petty things, are hurled loudly and indiscriminantly. Maggie is usually near tears by the time he leaves. She rarely has the courage to ask questions or offer her comments about situations where she feels she has something important to contribute. She usually vents her frustrations on her staff the rest of the shift and a burning pain in her epigastric region is becoming more persistent. Dr. Rogers is adept at using insinuations, criticism, and other manipulative techniques. After talking with her clinical supervisor, Maggie decides to apply some relationship improvement techniques in the next interaction with Dr. Rogers. The clinical supervisor has conducted role play sessions to allow Maggie to prepare for her encounter. This is how the next visit from Dr. Rogers goes.

Maggie is talking with a mother when she hears:
Dr. Rogers: I need a nurse down here!
Maggie:     Coming, Dr. Rogers. Good morning.
Dr. Rogers: How come I can never find a nurse at this desk?
Maggie:     We never seem to be here, do we?
Dr. Rogers: No. I have to go looking around in patients' rooms almost every time I come up here.
Maggie:     Are you saying that we shouldn't be in patients' rooms?
Dr. Rogers: Of course not. But I don't have time to waste. Where are my charts?
Maggie:     I'll get them for you. Here you are.
Dr. Rogers: There is one missing here. That Kenton kid.
Maggie:     You're right. It isn't here.

Dr. Rogers: Is it too much to ask—to have my charts here when I come in? I haven't got time to stand here while you run around and look for them.

Maggie: We always mess that up, don't we?

Dr. Rogers: You sure do. Well, let's go.

Maggie: I'm not going on rounds this morning.

Dr. Rogers: Why not?

Maggie: I don't want to go, that's all.

Dr. Rogers: Do you expect me to carry these charts around by myself?

Maggie: I don't know.

Dr. Rogers: Who is going to write down all the orders?

Maggie: I don't know. I would like to talk to you when you get finished. (Dr. Rogers disappears down the hall, muttering to himself. When he returns . . .)

Maggie: I would like to talk to you.

Dr. Rogers: Can't you leave me a note? I'll look at it tomorrow.

Maggie: I'm sure you would, but I would like to talk to you today.

Dr. Rogers: I'm very late. You nurses have no appreciation for my schedule.

Maggie: You're probably right. But I would still like to talk to you.

Dr. Rogers: (Sighs) What is it then?

Maggie: Please step in here. (Closes door) It's about one of your patients, Beth Comstock. I think she might be pregnant.

Dr. Rogers: What! When did you take up medicine? You must be mistaken!

Maggie: That could be.

Dr. Rogers: She's only 15. I've known her all her life and her family goes to my church.

Maggie: Are you saying that she couldn't be pregnant?

Dr. Rogers: No. Of course she could be. You must be wrong.

Maggie: That could be.

Dr. Rogers: What ever gave you the idea that she is pregnant anyway?

Maggie: She has many of the presumptive signs of pregnancy such as . . .

Dr. Rogers: I know what they are! Don't you realize I went to medical school. You don't need to list them.

Maggie: You're right. I should realize you are a doctor.

Dr. Rogers: Why didn't you tell me this sooner? Good Lord, I've sent her to X-ray! You had better get a pregnancy test on her right away.

Maggie: You're right. I sent one yesterday as soon as I thought of the possible pregnancy.

Dr. Rogers: You did! Without an order!

Maggie: Yes. I felt certain you would want one right away.

Dr. Rogers: Yes, of course. I wonder how far along she is—if she is pregnant.

Maggie: I figure about 4 months.

Dr. Rogers: Oh you do, do you? Is it a boy or a girl?

Maggie: (Laughing) I'm not sure yet.

Dr. Rogers: What a mess. Thank you for pointing this out. I never even thought about it, but it does make sense. You just can't think of everything.

Maggie: I'm sure you can't.

Dr. Rogers: Well, call me at the office as soon as anything comes back.

Maggie: Yes, I will.

Dr. Rogers: I have to be going.

Maggie: Just one more quick question. Can we send Judy Kempster to physical therapy? She's . . .

Maggie had survived the morning without her usual agony, nor had she resorted to coy suggestions as she had been taught in her educational program. She even began to enjoy her interactions with Dr. Rogers, which she and her supervisor referred to as "the taming of Dr. Rogers" because of the opportunity to practice her interactions skills. It was not long before Dr. Rogers commented one day, "You're running this place a lot better lately. It used to be a mess up here" to which Maggie replied, of course, "You're probably right."

Those who wish specific information on skills such as those just described should consult the reference by Manuel Smith on assertiveness training. It is possible to teach these skills to patients who need them for personal relationship improvement. For example, one nurse was working with a 20-year-old male who was having an extremely difficult time emancipating himself from his parents. His father used continual criticism and constant advice and his mother used plays for sympathy to manipulate him to plan his life around theirs. The nurse taught the patient some assertiveness techniques and helped him prepare to use them by role playing his parents for him. The son was eventually able to vastly improve his relationship with his parents and respected them and himself much more as a result.

## COMMUNICATING WITH CHILDREN

It is common for learners of communication skills to express special concern when they are first faced with the task of talking with children. Before suggestions are given for communicating with children of various ages, some suggestions are in order about how not to talk to children. For some reason, adults sometimes use some very strange verbal techniques with children, which will be discussed briefly.[14]

### BABY TALK

"Let's go get on our jammie wammies. It's time to go to beddie bye." Baby talk encourages the child to learn improper speech and misarticulations. It also does not provide appropriate vocabulary stimulation. The child who learns baby talk may be laughed at by other children later when his speech is inappropriately immature.

### UNIVERSAL "WE" AND "OUR"

"Let's go take *our* bath now." "*We're* getting sleepy, aren't *we*?" The use of "we" and "our" when "you" and "your" is meant is untruthful. The child may wonder why the nurse does not get in the tub!

### DISMISSING FEELINGS

"That doesn't hurt." "You'll get over it." Even adults who take the feelings of other adults seriously may feel that a child's feelings are not nearly as important. It would be more helpful to say, "I know it hurts."

### TALKING ABOUT THE CHILD AS IF HE WERE NOT PRESENT

"Does Johnny like school this year?" said to Johnny's mother while Johnny stands there. Ask Johnny.

## FUTURISMS

"If you don't take your medicine, you'll never get better." "If you don't eat your carrots, you won't grow up to be big and strong." The nurse cannot predict the future and the child knows it. The child may never eat a carrot and yet become big and strong or he may eat millions of carrots and not become big and strong. The child is not motivated by futurisms.

## COMPARISONS

"See, Barbie isn't crying while her stitches are being taken out. She has many more than you do. Why can't you be big and brave like her?" The child could not care less about Barbie. His attention is focused on himself. The comparison does not allow him to understand what is happening to him. It is unlikely to lead to his being "big and brave."

## IMPLYING CHOICE WHERE NONE IS INTENDED

"Do you want to take your medicine?" The child is later confused when he discovers he really has no choice. Say instead, "It's time to take your medicine now."

## SQUELCHING NEGATIVE FEELINGS

"You really don't hate your sister. Now go give her a big kiss." "You didn't really mean that. Now tell him you're sorry." The child is being told to lie about how he feels. Help the child to deal with the feeling instead. "Sometimes your sister makes you very angry." "You're very annoyed with him right now."

## LABELING THE CHILD

"You are a brat." "Bad boy." "Isn't she a devil?" It is more useful to the child if you comment on his behavior and not label him in general. The child should know specifically what he has done. "I won't let you play in this playroom if you hit other children." "Crayons are not for writing on the wall." The child needs to learn that he is a respected person who sometimes does objectionable things, but that does not mean that he is "bad." It is probably best to avoid using the terms "bad" and "good" altogether.

## PROMISES

"I promise I'll come back in an hour and we can go to the canteen." First of all, it is difficult to make a promise which one guarantees not to break. In the example above there are many possible reasons why the nurse might not be able to do as promised. Secondly, making a promise implies to the child that the nurse's word is only trustworthy when she does promise. Does that mean that she is usually untrustworthy?

## BRIBES

"If you do your exercises, I'll bring you a surprise on my next visit." "If you are good while your mommy sees the doctor, we'll find some candy for you." Children need to learn that certain behaviors are expected and necessary without the promise of a reward. In addition, offering a bribe tells the child that the nurse does not really expect the desired behavior or else she would not be adding an incentive to counteract the expected failure by the child. It is not helpful to encourage children in an attitude of "what's in it for me."

## *General Suggestions for Communicating with Children*

Some suggestions for communicating with children in general can be elucidated.

1. Children of all ages benefit from verbal stimulation and should be talked with as much as possible and encouraged to verbalize. Cognitive development is related to vocabulary and verbal ability although no one is sure exactly how.

2. A child's receptive ability is in general more advanced than his expressive ability so that the nurse can talk about and explain to a child more than she might think based on his communications to her.

3. Children have "emotional contagion" due to their sensitivity to nonverbal behavior. It is felt that they may be able to absorb the emotion of a highly charged situation without understanding the emotion. This can lead to confusion and fear. For this reason, the child may need to be shielded from some situations which might occur in a health care setting because of this. And the nurse should realize that they may feel afraid and not know why.

4. Children are very astute observers of nonverbal messages. It is futile for the nurse to try to fool them with words which disagree with her nonverbal behavior.

5. Children often send complex coded messages and the nurse may need to devote considerable effort to guessing the hidden meaning. A child who tattles on another child may be trying to find out what would happen if he accidentally did the same thing. A child who shows the nurse an "ugly" picture another child drew may be asking if it is all right for him to make ugly, mean pictures.

6. Children do not think with adult-like reasoning and logic. For example, some children around the age of 6 are worried about injections primarily because they are afraid all of their blood will come out—a proposition which seems ridiculous to an adult. The child has his reasons for feeling as he does. He sees the drop of blood forming over the needle hole. If he wipes it away, another one appears. He has no idea how much blood he has to spare. Trying to explain to him with adult logic why he will not bleed to death is an exercise in futility. The nurse will be more successful if she simply covers the needle hole with a bandaid which the child is sure will help. The nurse who works with children can collect many examples of children's logic and develop interventions which are effective at the age level of the child.

7. Children are by psychological design more egocentric than adults. For this reason,

the nurse will not get very far by trying to play on the young child's sense of pity. "If you don't drink this juice I'm going to be hurt." Nor will the child benefit much from observing things which do not directly relate to him. Watching a doll or another child get a cast will not prepare 5-year-old Tom very well unless *he* plays with the plaster, feels the temperature and weight, and so forth.

8. Children can be prepared for painful or stressful events and will cope better than if they are unprepared. Preparation must be appropriate to the age level of the child and is best done by someone they trust. It should be given just shortly before the event is to occur so the child does not have time to fantasize the event out of proportion. The preparation should be honest, simple, and concrete. The nurse should not dwell on the unpleasant aspects nor should she minimize them. The child should be told how he can participate. "I am going to draw a sample of your blood which we need to see how your medicine is working. You can help me by holding very still. You can say anything you want to but you must hold very still. Now watch what I am going to do. This cotton ball has alcohol on it. Does that feel hot or cold? . . ."

9. Children usually are familiar with communication through the tactile channel and the nurse should plan tactile contact as part of her care.

## Communication Guidelines for Specific Ages

In addition to what has already been said, the nurse who wishes to develop expertise in communicating with children must be aware of the psychological makeup of children of various ages. Only the most brief of suggestions can be given here as an example of how one might go about applying this knowledge.

### INFANTS AND TODDLERS

Because the infant or toddler often needs much tactile contact and visual and auditory stimulation, the nurse should talk to him, carry him around, and place him where he has things to handle and look at. The infant or toddler will talk back if he is encouraged.

### PRESCHOOLERS

The preschooler communicates through play. He may indicate his thoughts by what he does with and to his toys.[30] The nurse can communicate to him best through play. For example, the nurse who wants to prepare a preschooler for a trip to the dentist could pretend that Teddy Bear is going to the dentist and create a little scenario to illustrate all that happens with the child actively involved.

### SCHOOL-AGE CHILDREN

The school-age child has an increasing ability to express himself verbally and a decreasing egocentricism. The school-age child is also more sophisticated at using play materials and can play expressively. An indirect approach to help the school-age child express his feelings is often useful, such as having the child draw a picture and then telling the nurse about it. School-age children often respond well to talking with the nurse through a hand puppet. The child may say things indirectly through the puppet that he would not express otherwise.[23] Play is therapeutic for the child and the nurse should learn how to facilitate nondirective play.[30]

## TEENAGERS

Teenagers are usually adept at verbal communication and can talk for hours. They will frequently directly express their feelings to others their age. They are often exquisitely introspective. Some silent and nonexpressive teenagers will become quite animated and vocal when working with a teenage group on an art activity. The nurse might plan to use groups when communicating with teenagers because they seem to find considerable safety in numbers. The nurse must work at avoiding parent-child interactions. Some teenagers who do not possess high degrees of verbal skill may express themselves well through an art medium.[19] The telephone is also very important to teenagers—maybe because it provides intimacy with peers and privacy from parents without too much physicial closeness.[15]

## THE COUNSELING ROLE OF THE NURSE

If nurses can learn and use the techniques of therapeutic communication, can they be considered as counselors? The answer is probably yes but with some qualifications. Because of the lack of specific background in counseling which most nurses have, the nurse should probably restrict her counseling efforts to situations where the patient is experiencing a stressful but potentially self-limiting problem in one area but does not have severe or long-standing emotional problems or social problems such as alcohol or drug abuse.[30,31] For example, the nurse might appropriately work with patients or families who have sought her help and are mentally healthy, but are experiencing well defined situational problems such as the death of a meaningful friend or relative, a divorce, unemployment, an unexpected pregnancy, a major life decision, adjustment to a serious illness, or adjustment to marriage or parenthood. The nurse's intervention may help them face the current problem without developing a more overwhelming problem. In these situations, the nurse may want to see the patient for a limited number of regular sessions over a period of a few weeks and help him to focus specifically on the problem. The nurse who finds a problem which is beyond her competency should not hesitate to refer the patient to a competent counseling service. The nurse who finds herself frequently in counseling situations should plan to improve her counseling abilities by workshops, courses, and independent study.

## WHERE TO START

The nurse who desires to increase her communication effectiveness will not be able to do so overnight. Some suggestions as to how to begin with a step-by-step approach might be in order.

A good place to start is to decide that she really wants to hear and understand what her patients are saying even though it may mean abandoning some of her earlier ideas about communication. She can then concentrate first on active listening. The nurse who tries to hear what the patient is saying will probably begin to use patient focused social communication and to hear cues. She will begin to adopt unconsciously appropriate nonverbal behavior which will facilitate the patient's responses. If she finds that she can repeat to a patient in different words what he has said and he agrees, she is probably listening appropriately. As she tries to understand, she will begin to use techniques which facilitate the patient's responses.

Next, the nurse can begin to identify situations where her listening is blocked and plan ways to overcome the blocks. She can tape her interactions or record them in writing to see where points occur where her listening or responses were adequate or inadequate. Unfortunately, many learners become overly concerned about memorizing specific communication techniques such as reflection or clarification and their use of them often sounds staged. If the nurse can concentrate instead on what she is trying to achieve in each phase, the appropriate responses will probably fall into place naturally. For example, when a patient is in the content stage of a nondirective interaction, the nurse can remind herself that she wants to understand fully his story and structure her responses accordingly. Then when she feels she understands his story, she plans her responses to determine his feelings about what he has just discussed, and so forth. She can also remind herself that she should not be worrying about answers to his problems right now. That will come later.

The nurse will eventually be ready to concentrate specifically on responses. Sometimes learners overuse one response such as restatement. Initially, clarification tends to be underused. In other words, one tends to assume they know what the patient is saying when they may not. Clarification is rarely overworked.

Later the nurse may want to give particular attention to how she uses the visual and tactile channels of communication. It is difficult to analyze one's own nonverbal behavior and the opinions of a friend or videotape may help.

Learning to cope with special situations such as crying and silence will come later. The learner should not feel too discouraged if she initially is not completely competent in all circumstances. For example, she may find that she is particularly uncomfortable with crying or silence. She can try to slowly increase the period of time she can tolerate crying or silence and look for improvement towards expertise.

Dealing with problematic interactions should probably not be done until one feels competent in therapeutic communication because the techniques presented for problematic interactions should be used when one has not been able to achieve satisfactory communication through the usual techniques, and they are designed to lead to the more optimal communication patterns.

Attempting therapeutic communications with a small group is a still more advanced skill and will require additional practice and reference to resource material.

## SOME SUGGESTIONS FOR SELF-EVALUATION

The following areas should be considered by the nurse in evaluating her communication techniques.

## General Communication

1. Is there agreement between verbal, paraverbal, and nonverbal behavior?
2. Is active listening used?
3. Is the speech pleasant and distinct?
4. Is the voice quality pleasant and nonirritating?
5. Can the nurse move from directive to nondirective communication appropriately?
6. Is the environment planned to enhance communication.
7. Are the patient's verbal, paraverbal, and nonverbal communications considered?
8. Is communication kept on an adult-to-adult level?

## Therapeutic Communication—Nondirective Focus

1. Is social communication patient focused?
2. Are cues listened for and responded to?
3. Are the patient's attempts to communicate facilitated?
4. Is the patient allowed to arrive at his own solutions or resolutions?
5. Is the patient provided with feedback which acknowledges that he was understood?
6. Is the overuse of specific techniques avoided?

## Therapeutic Communication—Directive Focus

1. Is the purpose of the interaction explained?
2. Does the interaction progress from broad openers to more specific questions?
3. Is the discussion refocused when necessary?
4. Are questions phrased to the best advantage?

## Therapeutic Communication—Other Situations

1. Can the nurse remain with patients who cry and communicate acceptance?
2. Are personal questions handled appropriately?
3. Are patients who ask for confidentiality answered honestly?
4. Are types of silences distinguished and responded to appropriately?
5. Are interruptions handled properly?
6. Is the conversation refocused when the patient rambles excessively?
7. Are patients confronted or encouraged to face reality only within an established relationship and with respect for timing?
8. Are unhelpful techniques avoided?
9. Can the nurse recognize when the patient or others are meeting their needs at her expense and employ techniques to alter the interaction?
10. Is communication altered appropriately for the age of a child?
11. Are unhelpful responses avoided with children?

## *Tactile Communication*

1. Is the use of touch planned while performing nursing activities which involve personal contact?
2. Is touch used to communicate with patients as an independent action appropriately?

# AN EXAMPLE OF THE USE OF THE COMMUNICATION PROCESS

The following is a short nondirective interaction which a nurse had with a patient. This interaction is included to demonstrate how one nurse approached therapeutic communication. Not everyone would have used exactly the same approach. This interaction is not included because it was perfect.

The patient, Becky Martin, was on a maternity unit after a miscarriage in the fifth month of pregnancy. The nurse-clinician involved visited the patient two days after the miscarriage in the afternoon. She had had no previous contact with the patient.

Nurse: Hello, may I come in? My name is Ms. White.

Becky: Sure, have a seat. (Patient appears tired. Eyes are swollen and red.)

Nurse: I noticed that you have just had some visitors. Would you like me to come back later?

Becky: No, that's okay. I'm not tired.

Nurse: I will only stay a few minutes. How are things going? (Sitting down in the chair nearest patient.)

Becky: Okay, I guess. The doctor said I could go home Sunday morning if everything goes all right. (Patient moves hands rapidly, talks rapidly. Hint of nervous laughter in her voice.)

Nurse: (Nods)

Becky: I guess I'm doing okay so far. It's just one of those things.

Nurse: Just one of those things?

Becky: Losing the baby. You hear about these things but you never expect them to happen to you. We were so surprised when I got pregnant. Then we got used to the idea. Everything seemed to be just fine until I started bleeding.

Nurse: When was that?

Becky: Last week. My husband, Bob, called the doctor and he told me to go to bed. I bled a lot and finally started to get crampy pains. I never realized at first what it might mean and then I began to get worried.

Nurse: About . . .

Becky: About losing the baby. Bob called the doctor again Thursday and he said to bring me to his office. Then everything happened so fast. I never expected the pains to hurt so much.

Nurse: The labor contractions?

Becky: Yes. And they wouldn't let Bob stay with me after they brought me here because there was another woman in the room. I didn't know what was going on half of the time. The nurses wouldn't tell me anything. And those medications they give you! Dr. Jones kept telling me not to worry and that everything would be all right.

Nurse: (Nodding) And then . . .

Becky: Then they took me to the delivery room and told me they were going to put me to sleep so I figured the baby wasn't going to make it because Dr. Jones had told me earlier that I could be awake when I delivered. When I woke up they let Bob come see me and he told me that the baby had been too little to live and that it was a boy. (Eyes filling with tears)

Nurse: You feel sad about losing the baby.

Becky: Yes. Everyone is trying so hard to be cheerful and I know I shouldn't cry but I just can't seem to get over this. (Beginning to cry)

Nurse: (Closes patient's door) I can understand why you feel sad. You've had a real disappointment. (Returns to chair)

Becky: This is the first time I've cried in front of anyone else. Bob tells me that the important thing now is for me to get better and put all of this behind us.

Nurse: Forget about the pregnancy and the baby?

Becky: Yes. He wanted to have the baby buried before I got home but I told him I wanted to see the burial.

Nurse: You'd feel better if you did?

Becky: Yes. I guess I want to tell the baby goodbye.

Nurse: Did the doctor let you see the baby?

Becky: No. I asked if I could but he said that babies that small don't look very pretty. What would the baby have looked like?

Nurse: Have you ever seen a premature baby before?

Becky: Yes, I saw a picture of one in a booklet once. They look like little peanuts with wrinkles and big eyes. I guess that's what our little boy would have looked like. (Smiling a little)

Nurse: (Nodding)

Becky: I wish he could have lived. It's difficult after going through the hard part and not having a baby to take home to show for it.

Nurse: (Nodding)

Becky: It seems so hard to believe it all happened. I awaken at night and for a minute I think the baby is kicking, and then I remember. I think the burial will make it seem more definite. I guess that's why I want to go. Bob said they have real nice little caskets for babies. The minister of our church is going to do a little graveside service. He came to see me this morning so we have that all taken care of. I've never seen a baby buried before. I never thought it would be my own.

Nurse: It is hard to believe.

Becky: Yes. I don't think we will try to have another baby for a while. Dr. Jones said that we could any time after a few months but I think I want to wait until I've had plenty of time to get this off my mind.

Nurse: (Nodding)

Becky: If it just hadn't been a boy. We were going to name him Robert Thomas so I guess that is the name we will give him for the burial.

Nurse: It seems harder because you wanted a boy so badly.

Becky: It really does. I guess we can always have another boy some day. Maybe having a child later will work out better anyway. We weren't sure how we were going to manage financially right now.

Nurse: So you think this might be better in the end?

Becky: Yes. It seems hard to believe right now but losing the baby may have been a blessing in disguise. The doctor said there was nothing wrong with the baby. He was perfectly formed.

Nurse: You seem pleased about that.

Becky: Yes. I'm glad he wasn't deformed or something like that. I guess things could have been worse. At least we're still young and we have plenty of time to start a family. And we know we don't have any problems getting pregnant—even with an IUD!

Nurse: You feel even though it hurts a lot now it will work out.

Becky: Yes. I think it will. I'll be glad when I can get home and get our lives back to normal. We have a lot of remodeling on our house we wanted to do and now I guess we can think about doing it again.

Nurse: That should keep you busy.

Becky: That's what Bob says. He tells me he is going to teach me how to do it all so he can supervise!

Nurse: That should be interesting.

Becky: Yes, it will.

Nurse: Well, I should be going. I'm glad I got to come see you.

Becky: Thank you for coming. I hope you'll come back again before I go home.

Nurse: I could do that. I'll see you later then.

Becky: All right, goodbye.

Nurse: Bye.

## SUMMARY

The nurse will have many opportunities to use the communication process in her practice regardless of the setting she works in. She needs to understand the goals of therapeutic communication and how it differs from social communication. She needs an understanding of message components, levels of communication, and message channels and how to use this knowledge to increase communication effectiveness.

Communication which is therapeutic can range from nondirective to directive depending on the characteristics of the situation. There are specific techniques which can be used to facilitate effective communication such as planning the environment and using visual, tactile, and aural-auditory channels. Different techniques may be necessary in special situations, in problematic situations, and when communicating with children. Skill in the use of the communication process does not occur automatically but requires practice and study.

# REFERENCES

1. Anthony, W. A., and Carkhuff, R. R.: *The Art of Health Care.* Human Resource Development Press, Amherst, Mass., 1976.
2. Argyle, M., and Dean, L.: "Eye contact, distance, and affiliation." Sociometry 28:289, 1965.
3. Benjamin, A.: *The Helping Interview.* Houghton Mifflin, Boston, 1974.
4. Berne, E.: *Games People Play: The Psychology of Human Relations.* Grove Press, New York, 1964.
5. Butler, R.: "The life review: An interpretation of reminiscing in the aged." Psychiat. 26:65, 1963.
6. Cohen, M. S.: "Easy to listen to." Am. J. Nurs. 66:1999, 1966.
7. Condon, W. S., and Sander, L. W.: "Neonate movement is synchronized with adult speech: Interaction participation and language acquisition." Science 183:99, 1974.
8. Edinburg, G. M., Zinberg, N. E., and Kelman, W.: *Clinical Interviewing and Counseling: Principles and Techniques.* Appleton-Century-Crofts, New York, 1975.
9. Egolf, D. B., and Chester, S. L.: "Speechless messages." Hearing and Speech Action 43:12, 1975.
10. Ekman, P., and Friesen, W. V.: "Nonverbal leakage and clues to deception." Psychiat. 32:88, 1969.
11. Ekman, P., and Friesen, W. V.: *Unmasking the Face.* Prentice-Hall, Englewood Cliffs, N.J., 1975.
12. Fiedler, F. E.: "Factor analyses of psychoanalytic, non-directive and Adlerian therapeutic relationships." J. Consult. Psychol. 15:32, 1951.
13. Fowkes, W. C., and Hunn, V. K.: *Clinical Assessment for the Nurse Practitioner.* C. V. Mosby, St. Louis, 1973.
14. Ginott, H. G.: *Between Parent and Child.* Macmillan, New York, 1965.
15. Group for the Advancement of Psychiatry: *Normal Adolescence.* Scribner, New York, 1968.
16. Hall, E.: *The Silent Language.* Doubleday, Garden City, New York, 1967.
17. Harris, T. A.: *I'm OK—You're OK: A Practical Guide to Transactional Analysis.* Harper & Row, New York, 1967.
18. Jourard, S. M.: *The Transparent Self.* Van Nostrand, Princeton, N.J., 1964.
19. Konopka, G.: *Adolescent Girl in Conflict.* Prentice-Hall, Englewood Cliffs, N.J., 1966.
20. Krieger, D.: "Therapeutic touch: The imprimatur of nursing." Am. J. Nurs. 75:784, 1975.
21. Lange, S. P.: "Transactional analysis and nursing," in Carlson, C. E., and Blackwell, B. (eds.): *Behavioral Concepts and Nursing Intervention.* J. B. Lippincott, Philadelphia, 1978.
22. Lewis, M.: *Infant Speech.* Routledge and Kegan Paul, London, 1951.
23. Linn, S.: "Puppets and hospitalized children: talking about feelings." J. Assoc. Care Child. Hosp. 5:5, 1977.
24. MacKinnon, R. A., and Michels, R.: *The Psychiatric Interview in Clinical Practice.* W. B. Saunders, Philadelphia, 1971.
25. Mehrabian, A.: "Communication without words," in *Readings in Psychology Today.* CRM Books, Del Mar, Cal., 1969.
26. Morgan, W. L., and Engel, G. L.: *The Clinical Approach to the Patient.* W. B. Saunders, Philadelphia, 1969.
27. Murray, R.: "Therapeutic communication: Prerequisite for effective nursing," in Murray, R., et al.: *Nursing Concepts for Health Promotion.* Prentice-Hall, Englewood Cliffs, N.J., 1975.
28. Nichols, R.: "Listening is a 10-part skill." Nation's Business, July, 1957.
29. Pluckhan, M. L.: "Space, the silent lanauge." Nurs. Forum 7:386, 1968.
30. Pothier, P. C.: *Mental Health Counseling With Children.* Little, Brown and Company, Boston, 1976.
31. Singer, E.: "The counselor role of the nurse." Presented at the Continuing Education Program, University of Cincinnati, College of Nursing, 1976.
32. Smith, E. C.: "Are you really communicating?" Am. J. Nurs. 77:1966, 1977.

33. Travelbee, J.: *Intervention in Psychiatric Nursing: Process in the One-To-One Relationship.* F. A. Davis, Philadelphia, 1969.
34. Veninga, R.: "Defensive behavior: Causes, effects, and cures." J. Environ. Health. 37:5, 1974.
35. Wicks, R. J.: *Counseling Strategies and Intervention Techniques for the Human Sciences.* J. B. Lippincott, Philadelphia, 1977.
36. Wilson, L. M.: "Listening," in Carlson, C. E. (ed.): *Behavioral Concepts and Nursing Intervention.* J. B. Lippincott, Philadelphia, 1970.

## BIBLIOGRAPHY

Bakdash, D. P.: "Becoming an assertive nurse." Am. J. Nurs. 78:1710, 1978.
Blondis, M. N., and Jackson, B. E.: *Nonverbal Communication With Patients.* John Wiley, New York, 1977.
Fiedler, F. E.: "The concept of an ideal therapeutic relationship." J. Consult. Psychol. 14:239, 1950.
Fox, M. J.: "Talking with patients who can't answer." Am. J. Nurs. 71:1146, 1971.
Freund, H.: "Listening with any ear at all." Am. J. Nurs. 69:1650, 1969.
Goldin, P., and Russell, B.: "Therapeutic communication." Am. J. Nurs. 69:1928, 1969.
Loesch, L. C., and Loesch, N. A.: "What do you say after you say mm-hmm?" Am. J. Nurs. 75:807, 1975.
Moniz, D.: "Putting assertiveness techniques into practice." Am. J. Nurs. 78:1713, 1978.
Peplau, H. E.: *Interpersonal Relations in Nursing.* G. P. Putnam's Sons, New York, 1952.
Rodger, B. P.: "Therapeutic conversation and posthypnotic suggestion." Am. J. Nurs. 72:714, 1972.
Rogers, C. R.: *On Becoming a Person.* Houghton Mifflin, Boston, 1961.
Ruesch, J.: *Disturbed Communication.* W.W. Norton, New York, 1967.
Smith, M. J.: *When I Say No, I Feel Guilty.* Bantam Books, New York, 1975.
Ujhely, G. B.: "What is realistic emotional support?" Am. J. Nurs. 68:758, 1968.
Underwood, P. R.: "Communication through role playing." Am. J. Nurs. 71:1184, 1971.
Veninga, R.: "Communications: A patients' eye view." Am. J. Nurs. 73:320, 1973.
Walke, M. A.: "When a patient needs to unburden his feelings." Am. J. Nurs. 77:1164, 1977.
Watzlawich, P., Beavin, J., and Jackson, D.: *Pragmatics of Human Communication.* W.W. Norton, New York, 1967.

# CHAPTER 2

# THE HELPING PROCESS

Almost all individuals who enter nursing do so in part out of a desire to "help" others as a primary or important motivational factor. Through the life experiences they have had, beginning nurses usually already possess some helping skills. This chapter will examine the process by which one helps others with the goal of helping the nurse begin to develop, refine, or expand her helping attitudes and skills. The chapter on the communication process was discussed first because the skillful use of the communication process is important in helping.

Helping is often erroneously thought of as something instinctual or elementary in complexity.[39] However, as will be seen, using the helping process is a complex, challenging, and sophisticated use of self in the best interests of another.

The helping process can be most simply defined as an interaction between two individuals in which one individual focuses on facilitating the other to enhance his personal growth and functioning. This interaction has been referred to by many names such as the interpersonal process, the therapeutic relationship, and the nurse-patient interaction. Forming a helping relationship is often implied in statements frequently encountered in nursing literature such as "developing rapport" and "providing emotional support." The use of the helping process by the nurse with a patient is often conceived of as the core of nursing practice because the ability of the nurse to form a helping relationship may influence all other activities the nurse attempts with the patient and family.

The helping process is not something a nurse does to a patient, but rather something she does with the patient. It is initiated by her on the patient's behalf. It focuses on helping the other person to accomplish a goal by facilitating his own efforts in that direction. Thus, the nurse can be thought of not as one who pushes, solves the patient's problems, or establishes goals for the patient, but rather as one who serves the patient as his helper or advocate.

The advocacy role implies a far different focus than many individuals may associate with nursing. Some may more readily visualize nurses (and health care workers in general) as authority figures who know what is best for patients and subtly, or not so subtly, pressure them into wanting it also. In fact, the physician is often thought of as a father figure, the nurse as a mother figure, and the patient as childlike.[7,46] The advocacy role implies that the patient is on an equal adult–adult level with the nurse.

The nurse who functions as an advocate or helper relates to the patient in a way that allows her to use her skills and knowledge to work with him in defining his goals and achieving them as they relate to his health.[16] A large part of her input will be related to increasing his knowledge about himself: his concerns, resources, capacities, and options. She will avoid telling the patient what he should do and doing for the patient what he can do for himself. She lets him fully choose his actions and she accepts his choices. She realizes that the patient and not the nurse is responsible ultimately for the patient's health.[11]

The helping process is used, therefore, when for some reason a patient needs an advocate because he is temporarily unable to cope with his health needs without one. This might occur when a patient is in a state of conflict or crisis, unfamiliar with his surroundings, facing a stressful situation, or diminished in coping abilities due to a threat such as illness or change in his situation. The nurse helps the patient to accomplish what he would not be able to do alone.

As mentioned previously, a large part of what the helping nurse does is related to increasing the patient's knowledge of himself. She serves as a source the patient uses to fully explore himself, reveal himself maybe as never before, become comfortable with himself, and plan change in his behavior. This is not as easy as it sounds as will be seen as helping is further explored.

The nurse gains personally from use of the helping process in several ways. She learns about herself as she learns about another. She identifies how she is similar and how she is different. She learns about new and different experiences which she may never have herself.[49] She clarifies her knowledge of herself. She experiences satisfaction in helping another to succeed. She grows in her abilities to relate to others meaningfully.

The helping process is not easy to learn. It is not subject to cold statistical analysis nor based on hard and fast rules. It lies in that "iffy" area of nursing which is elusive and often easy to dismiss as unquantifiable. There is a lot that has been learned about helping, however, and the nurse can now use helping as a legitimate process and need not think of the helping process as just a vague, rhetorical platitude to "provide support."

While using the helping process lies within the area of nursing which concerns emotional comfort and care, one should not overlook the significance of the patient's emotional state on the physical processes of the body. Although Western thought separates the mind from the body in many respects, it is known that one's psychological state can greatly influence physical illness and healing.[25] The nurse, probably more than other health care practitioners, has unique opportunities and the knowledge to combine physical care measures aimed at promoting the physical integrity of the body with helping measures aimed at promoting emotional integrity.

The nurse who learns to use the helping process will be providing for the patient and family a service which is greatly in demand. Some consumers of health care are becoming vocal in asking for care by providers who are not only technically competent but who also care about them as individuals. Much of the current dissatisfaction of consumers of health care is due to a lack of this feeling that the health care provider cares. Use of the helping process by health care personnel should promote this feeling.

The nurse is only one of many individuals who uses the helping process. Ministers, counselors, physicians, teachers, and social workers, among other professionals, often attempt to help others with a specific formal process. Less formally, parents, spouses, and friends function as helpers at times, although they may be unaware of using a specific process.[5]

## Helping Interaction and Social Interaction

Most beginning practitioners of nursing are naturally more skilled at social interaction than they are at helping interaction. There are important differences between social interaction and helping interaction. These differences are highlighted in Table 2-1. Details of these differences will become more explicit later.

The fact that these two modes of interaction have been separated does not mean that they are always mutually exclusive. A social interaction may become a helping interaction if one participant expresses a need for help and the other participant initiates a helping interaction. Similarly, a helping interaction may become a social interaction after one person has been helped. The point is that the two are intended for different purposes.

Because most beginning nurses are usually more adept at and familiar with social inter-

**TABLE 2-1.** A comparison of characteristics of social interactions with characteristics of helping interactions

| Social interaction | Helping interaction |
|---|---|
| Mutual sharing of ideas, experiences, and feelings by both participants. | Focus by helper on ideas, experiences, and feelings of individual seeking help. |
| Purpose of friendship, socialization, enjoyment, using up time, etc. | Purpose of helping one participant enhance personal growth and functioning. |
| Both participants may meet needs within interaction. | Focus is on the needs of the one seeking help and not on needs of the helper. |
| Either participant may choose to initiate or discontinue interaction. | Helper assumes professional responsibility to promote interaction. |
| Use of social communication skills predominates. | Therapeutic communication skills and helping skills predominate. |
| Participants may shift or exchange roles during interaction. | Helper maintains consistent approach and role. |
| Content for discussion determined by either participant. | Individual seeking help provides content. |
| Little emphasis on evaluation of interaction. | Helper and the one seeking help both evaluate interaction. |
| Subjective feelings expected. | Helper strives to be objective about the interaction. |
| Content discussed superficially usually with avoidance of issues of personal significance. | Focus on significant personal issues. |
| Advice and suggestions freely given by either participant. | Helper refrains from advice and suggestions but facilitates problem solving by individual seeking help. |
| Participants react naturally to each other. | Helper committed to managing her behavior to promote the optimal benefit for the one seeking help.[10,16,17,23,37,39] |

action, they may find it difficult initially to engage in helping interactions. The nurse may detect resistance within herself to changing the way she relates to others. She may feel most comfortable relating to patients and families as she does to her friends. While this practice may not actually harm the patient, it is not likely to accomplish as much for the patient as might be possible. For a few nurses, helping interactions will seem natural and easy, but for many it will be a struggle to alter comfortable and familiar ways of focusing on others.

## PHASES IN THE HELPING PROCESS

Four phases have been identified which individuals usually pass through in the course of a helping process. The nurse needs an understanding of these phases so that she can assess what stage she and the patient are in, and there are special challenges in each phase which the nurse must plan for. These phases are the beginning phase, the transition phase, the working phase, and the termination phase.

### The Beginning Phase

The beginning phase occurs after the nurse has initiated an interaction or offered to interact with a patient. This may be formal with a written or verbal contract, but is usually as informal as "May I sit and talk with you for a while?" One characteristic of the first phase is possible anxiety for both patient and nurse.[42] The patient may be anxious over what is expected of him and what the nurse may think of him among other things. The nurse may be anxious over performing in a helping role and worried about rejection by the patient. The anxiety of one may be communicated to and intensified by the other.

The nurse can help abate her own anxiety somewhat by preparing for her contact with the patient. She can reflect on how she will introduce herself, explain her purpose, talk to the patient, and so forth. The nurse can do several things to decrease the patient's anxiety if it is excessive. She can plan her behavior to not increase the patient's anxiety and she can help the patient to recognize and cope with his anxiety. Specific information on reducing anxiety can be found in the chapter on anxiety.

Another characteristic of the initial phase is orientation.[37] The nurse gives the patient information he needs to understand who she is and what her purpose is for interacting with him. This information will vary considerably depending on the situation in which the nurse is working with the patient. The nurse at this time is attempting to become oriented to the patient. In particular she assesses the patient's health, goals, and needs, and his expectations of her.[10]

A third characteristic of the beginning phase is the building of a personal relationship with feelings of security and trust for both individuals. The patient must decide if the nurse is trustworthy, truthful, reliable, understanding, and helpful.[26] The communication skills and other attitudes and skills the nurse has used with the patient will be crucial in determining how the patient perceives the nurse at this point.

The hazards of this stage include developing predominantly a pattern of social interaction rather than helping interaction, failing to establish a bond of mutual trust, and a lack of common understanding about the patient's goals. The length of this phase varies according to the situation.

## The Transition Phase

This phase is present in some helping processes but not in all. If it occurs, it is characterized by testing and ambivalence by the patient. The patient in this phase is vacillating between true involvement with the nurse and rejection of help. He may behave one way on one contact and quite another way on another occasion. Often his ambivalence is seen within one contact in that he initially reacts indifferently to the nurse but warms to her as the contact progresses. However, at the next contact, he may again react indifferently.

This phase can be difficult for the nurse. She may experience frustration at her inability to win the patient's trust. At other times she may feel that she is finally getting somewhere only to have the next contact with the patient go badly. No one enjoys being rejected or treated inconsistently. The nurse is likely to respond with hostility and anger to the patient. If she can remember that the patient's behavior is a reflection of his uncertainty, the interaction may be able to survive this stage and progress to the next phase.

This phase can have three outcomes. The patient and nurse may move to the next phase, the relationship will become permanently fixed at this level, or the relationship may be terminated by mutual agreement, often under the convenience of a good excuse. If the relationship becomes permanently fixed in the transition phase, there is usually mutual withdrawal of both patient and nurse from each other. This can occur even though the contact continues for years.

Patients who are likely to move through a transition phase include those who have had negative experiences with nurses or other health care workers in the past, those who have trouble trusting others, and sometimes young children.

The hazard of this stage is that the nurse may not be able to tolerate the patient's ambivalent and testing behavior and, therefore, abort the relationship. The nurse needs to seek support and encouragement outside of the patient situation.

## The Working Phase

In this period, the nurse helps the patient to learn about himself, determine if changes are needed, and practice change.

She helps him to learn about himself by listening and using her communication and helping skills to facilitate his exploration of himself. She helps him talk about how he perceives himself and others, how he copes with problems, what he values, what supports are available to him, how he handles feelings, and how he relates to others.[8,48] She uses her skills to perceive how the world looks to the patient—his frame of reference.[13]

The nurse during this stage becomes symbolically a mirror in which the patient can safely look at himself and what led to his present situation. She tries to understand the patient's frame of reference, and in so doing the patient learns about himself. She is nonjudgmental so he need not be defensive. She accepts what he reveals so he can also. She remains positive about what he can become. She attends to him fully and consistently so that he experiences her involvement and interest. He develops a feeling that another individual cares deeply about him, what he has been, and what he is becoming. He develops a feeling of safety within the interaction.[43] This experience may be totally new to him. For many individuals in this busy world, it is rare to have anyone really listen, let alone listen, understand, and seek to know one better.

Several therapeutic benefits may occur within the working phase for the patient.[33] The patient may find that mere verbalization of his feelings is beneficial because once they are in words, they can be examined. He may feel support and optimism because he is doing something about difficulties which had seemed overwhelming at times. He may experience insight into situations that he never understood before and join together aspects of his experience which he did not realize were related. He may gain awareness of half-buried situations and feelings which he had denied before. He may begin to use these new knowledges to change aspects of his behavior—cautiously at first. As he becomes aware of himself and more comfortable with his identity, energy which has been used to deceive himself and others is free to be used in other ways. He may begin to see others in a different perspective also. He may recognize ways in which some of his behavior causes him problems and desire to change some aspects of his behavior. He may begin to do this first with the nurse before he attempts it in the real world. He may learn how he makes decisions or when he fails to make them.[23]

From his new base of self-knowledge, he may reevaluate his strengths and weaknesses and develop a personal inventory of assets which increase his ability to cope with adversity.

As a result, his life can become more fulfilling and meaningful. He may begin to focus on helping others. His priorities and life goals may change slowly or be reoriented. His confidence in himself may increase.

The nurse may provide the patient with specific resources during this phase if she has information which the patient appears to need or want. Resources must be offered in a way that allows the patient to accept or reject them according to his needs.[45] For example, a patient who is particularly troubled by obesity and wishes to lose weight can be given information on resources related to losing weight but he must feel free to not use the information and the nurse must accept his choice. This is not easy, needless to say.

Unfortunately, not every helping interaction will have such profoundly positive outcomes. What has been described is the ideal working phase. But even if the ideal is not reached, a helping interaction has great potential for facilitating the personal growth and functioning of another.

The working phase is very difficult for both the patient and the nurse. The patient may be disappointed initially when he learns that the nurse has no magic solutions and that he is expected to find his own answers.[23] He may experience, in addition to the positive reactions described, uncertainty and anxiety as he looks at himself. At times he may be so overwhelmed that he withdraws for a period of time and avoids working on his self-discovery. At other times he may experience grave feelings of failure as he gains new insights into his behavior. He may cling more strongly to denial of significant facts as his awareness threatens to increase.

The nurse lives through these ups and downs with great expenditures of her own emotional energy. She in addition must struggle to remain in the role of participant-observer so that she can guide the interaction with the patient in the way she feels will be most helpful. In addition, the nurse is often challenged during this stage with significant revelations of her own. As she experiences the patient's frame of reference, she begins to feel that he is a lot like her regardless of their more superficial differences. In other words, she recognizes the vast commonalities they share. They are both human, have joys, sorrows, pain, love, achievements, and failures. She experiences this as closeness to the patient. As the patient discovers himself, the nurse learns more about herself too. She sees ways that she is the same as him and ways that she is different. Each helping interaction can be a significant experience in learning to know herself. This, along with the feeling of closeness and involvement, is emotionally draining. She needs support from individuals outside of the situation to recharge her emotional batteries.

The hazards of this stage are numerous. The nurse may forsake her reflective role and instead resort to giving advice as an authoritarian "parent." This diminishes the patient's learning opportunities. She may lean too much into the participant role and become lost in subjectivity to the extent that she is unable to guide the interaction and it goes nowhere. She may lean too heavily into the observer role so that she does not interact appropriately and warmly. The patient may expect too much from the nurse and refuse to work on solving his own dilemmas. He may be looking for magical solutions or seeking help with an impossible situation.[23]

Some difficulties in the interaction between the patient and the nurse may occur at this time due to a process called *transference*. This refers to a process in which the patient unconsciously relates to the nurse based on an earlier pattern of interaction which he had with someone else.[48] The nurse comes to symbolize someone else and the patient reacts to her as if she were that other person. How he reacts depends on the relationship he had with the other person she symbolizes. He is unaware that this is occurring. The nurse can only identify transference with difficulty. There is currently disagreement over what to do if it should occur. Children frequently develop transference towards an adult helper who symbolizes a parent.[42]

The working phase is usually the longest phase of a helping interaction.[42] The length depends on the depth to which the interaction progresses.

## The Termination Phase

The termination phase can be summarized as usually one of conflicting emotions for both patient and nurse, not unlike sweet sorrow. In an interaction of great depth, the patient is usually anxious to get on with his life yet sad to leave the source of such significant learning. The nurse is pleased with the patient's progress and excited to see him ready to try the world on his own, yet she will miss seeing someone she was involved with and cared about. Both experience anticipation mixed with grief at parting. The secret to successful resolution to this phase lies in recognizing and providing for this ambivalence.

Ideally, the patient and nurse have known when termination was coming, have had a successful working phase, and have time to discuss parting. This optimal gradual lessening of ties and transfer of interests to others is referred to as termination with resolution. In essence, the normal termination should be considered a form of the grief process.[34] Usually termination is a mild, temporary, grief-like reaction. Some characteristics of the grief reaction may occur such as mild amounts of preoccupation with the lost object, some anger, withdrawal, and eventually, restitution. One's reaction to termination may be somewhat colored by feelings associated with past separations and losses. Therefore, termination may evoke sadness and anxiety for some or pleasure, relief, and a sense of pride for others.[23]

Termination does not always occur in an ideal manner, however. Termination may occur abruptly if a patient moves, leaves the hospital, dies, or if the nurse must leave abruptly due to illness, moving, and so forth. This often leads to frustration and sadness.[42] Similarly, the patient and the nurse may use various mental mechanisms to cushion themselves for the parting:

1. Either the patient or nurse may deny that the relationship was very significant in the first place.
2. One may begin to react negatively to the other as evidenced by subtle critical comments and attacks.
3. Either may propose a good excuse to prolong the interaction such as new problems to be dealt with.
4. They may psychologically withdraw from each other.
5. They may plunge into another interaction which seems to replace the present one.[34,42]

These reactions and abrupt termination are not as desirable as the normal resolution described previously and are forms of termination without resolution and the main hazard of this phase of the interaction.

To plan for a successful termination, several things may be helpful.[23,34,40,42] In some situations it is possible to be clear from the beginning about how long the helping interaction will last. The nurse might say, "I will be visiting weekly until December" or "I will be the nurse taking care of you most evenings as long as you are on this unit" or "You can come to see me until we both decide that you no longer need my help." Similarly, occasional references can be made to the fact of eventual termination. If the nurse's role with the patient has been identified clearly, the time for termination will be recognized more easily. As the working phase comes to conclusion, it is helpful often to plan for a specific time to accomplish termination. During this time, no new material should be worked on but rather the nurse and patient should review what has happened, what the patient's plans are for the future, and discuss how they both feel about the end of the interaction. It may be prudent to inform the patient of other sources of help should they be needed now or later.

Although termination is painful, the advantages of the interaction for the patient and nurse should hopefully outweigh the disadvantages which arise from the necessity of having an ending to the interaction. And both the nurse and patient will always carry a little part of each other in their memories.

## ATTITUDES CONDUCIVE TO HELPING

Certain attitudes exhibited by the one who tries to help another have been identified in the literature as useful for the nurse to strive to develop. These will be described. Most of these concepts are based on the philosophy of Carl Rogers.[43–45]

### Nonjudgmental Attitude

A nonjudgmental attitude implies that the nurse refrains from evaluating the patient's appearance, behavior, attitudes, beliefs, and motivations. Being totally nonjudgmental is rarely if ever achieved. Allport comments that a helper looks at a client through a unique set of eyeglasses. The lenses have been ground by his textbooks and teachers.[3] And probably by his previous life experiences.

In the process of growing up one has been taught to evaluate others and, in some situations, not to do so would potentially be harmful. The problem is that one has usually developed a very narrow set of criteria by which others are judged. Thus, individuals who are not a lot like the nurse herself are likely to be seen as deviant. Because most nurses are from middle class backgrounds, middle class values and attitudes are seen as normal and expected. This then leads to three responsibilities for the nurse who wishes to become less judgmental.

First the nurse should become aware of what judgments she makes and she should learn what criteria she uses to judge others, i.e., what her values are.[27] For example, is she especially concerned with appearance, style of dress, and body intactness? Is she suspicious of individuals whose religion differs from hers? Does she place value on saving money, accumulating material possessions, cooperating, working hard, planning, achieving, competing, trusting experts, delaying gratification, and pursuing educational goals?[1,38] Does she believe in marriage only when individuals can assume total financial responsibility and sexual relations only within marriage? The task of exploring one's values is a lifelong pursuit. Most nurses will find it a struggle to just recognize that they have middle class values which are very different from many of the values of their patients. Recently considerable attention is being given to a process called values clarification.[20,52,53] The nurse may be able to benefit by attending workshops or classes and by reading about values clarification.

Secondly, the nurse can reflect on where her values came from.[27] Why are they as they are? Where did she learn them? Sometimes she may realize that a few of her values are irrational.

Thirdly, after the nurse has clarified and explored her values, she can reflect on whether she can allow others the freedom to have different values.[27] This does not mean that she changes her values, but that she accepts that others have the right to values different from her own. If she can accept this, then she may be able to work with others with values different from hers without evaluating whether their values are better or worse than hers. When she has accomplished this, she is on the road to becoming less judgmental. This approach recognizes that she may never reach total objectivity about the patient she works with, but she can reach for respect for differentness and a less evaluative approach to looking at others. She can learn to be more tolerant and learn to enjoy learning about others who behave and think differently.

Being nonjudgmental would be shown in behaviors which communicate to the patient or family:

1. I won't look down on you because you choose to lead your life differently than I do.
2. I don't assume that my values and my way of doing things are better than your way—only different.
3. I will not attempt to impose my values on you or force you to act like me because I respect your right to your own value system.

A nurse struggling to achieve a nonjudgmental attitude is illustrated in the following incident.

Marcy was a teenager whom the school nurse had always admired. Marcy was interested in becoming a nurse and had consulted with the nurse on several occasions related to her career plans. The school nurse was very surprised when Marcy, who was now a senior, sought her out for information on pregnancy testing. She related to the nurse that she believed she might be pregnant and wanted to know for sure. The nurse found herself thinking about Marcy differently than before. She had lost some of her respect for her because she had been sexually active. On reflecting on her feelings, she realized that Marcy had a right to feel different about teenage sexuality than she did. Nor should she attempt to pressure Marcy into doing what she would have done in the same situation. The nurse had to work at accepting Marcy's behavior but she was eventually able to relate to her again with positive feelings and respect although she might never value what Marcy did.

Becoming less judgmental is not a one time activity. The issue is revived each time a nurse experiences a situation in which her values are in conflict with those of another.

## Accepting Attitude

Another attitude worth cultivating is one of acceptance of the one seeking help. Acceptance of another implies that the other individual need not behave in a certain way or refrain from certain behaviors to be accepted. Instead, the nurse accepts him in his entirety on his own terms and not hers.[5,54] This does not mean that the nurse intellectualizes about the behavior which the patient exhibits.[51] Rather, she allows him the freedom to choose his own behaviors.[54]

As was true for being nonjudgmental, being absolutely accepting of all other individuals is not possible. And, as with the task of becoming more nonjudgmental, the nurse has to work at being accepting of some patients by becoming aware of the behavior she initially reacts to as unacceptable, deciding why she feels it is, and then granting the patient freedom to behave as he chooses.[54] She learns to go beyond her initial reaction.[16] It is also crucial that she learns to accept herself. This implies knowing herself: her strengths, weaknesses, and potentials. When she knows who and what she is, she is less likely to see reasons not to accept others.

Acceptance is shown in nursing behaviors which communicate:

1. I will not require you to behave in a certain way to please me. You can be yourself.
2. I will not ask that you earn my approval by changing to meet my standards. I will approve of you as you are.
3. I accept your behavior as the most appropriate for you.
4. I will not attempt to make you regret what you may have done.

Unconditional acceptance is hinted at in the old adage, "Parents love you only when you're good but grandparents love you even when you're bad."

## Positive Regard

To regard another positively means that one respects the individual as a person of dignity, potential, and inherent worth.[2] Positive regard is present when the nurse considers each patient as responsible and capable.[8] Regardless of the patient's status in life or his situation, he is thought of as one with full personhood. This means that the nurse does not relegate a patient to subhuman status because he might be unconscious, a criminal, intoxicated, elderly, or retarded.

Achieving positive regard is not always easy in the dehumanized mechanistic settings often found in health care organizations.[16] Our society does not always place equal value on all individuals. Often those who are dying, psychologically ill, retarded, unhealthy, or nonproductive are seen as inferior. Because nurses are so involved with health, those who disregard their health according to her standards or are apathetic may be regarded negatively. This would include those who excessively eat, drink, and smoke and those who contract social diseases.

The nurse must struggle to analyze her rank-order classifications of people, and work to dissolve them. After she recognizes what her beliefs are about others, she must recognize the consequences of these beliefs as revealed in her actions.[16] Positive regard for another is demonstrated through behaviors which say to the patient:

1. I will be sensitive to your privacy, requests, questions, and feelings.
2. I will treat you with my highest respect regardless of your status in the eyes of society.
3. I will relate to you with a positive viewpoint toward what you may become.
4. I will not judge your worth or compare your value to others.
5. I will not impose on you my solutions to your problems as if you were unaware of what is best for you but respect your right to choose what is best for you.

The opposite of positive regard is shown by a lack of concern for the patient's feelings, experiences and potentials, and by avoidance and rudeness.[2,16]

## SKILLS CONDUCIVE TO HELPING

In addition to cultivating a nonjudgmental attitude and attitudes of acceptance and positive regard, the nurse who wishes to develop expertise in use of the helping process can learn skills which have been related to helping. These too are mostly based on the work of Carl Rogers[43–45] and that of Robert Carkhuff.[4,13]

### Empathy

Understanding another requires the use of empathy which may be thought of as a process which allows one to explore the inner core of another's experience while remaining one-self.[8] Empathy is a skill which requires a special kind of comprehension of the situation, feelings, and reactions of another. Almost all individuals are capable of a certain amount of empathy in some situations and at some times. For example, one may easily understand how a close friend feels when she is sad or happy. Learning to feel empathic with individuals one does not know well requires refining this complex skill.

There are several steps to empathic understanding. First, empathy requires that one temporarily put aside his own mental preoccupations so that he can concentrate as fully as possible on another.[6] Achieving understanding requires mental effort.

Secondly, the nurse explores with the patient his situation so that she can experience his situation as if she were actually involved in it. She remains always separate from the patient's situation, however, and intellectually objective. This may be thought of as a specific type of detachment from the patient.[39] As she enters the patient's world, he becomes no longer an "it" but a "thou."[17] She tries to imagine what the patient may have experienced and felt. She uses reflective comments to assure her understanding.[4,30] She does this by guessing at what the patient is feeling and responding with a statement which verbalizes the patient's possible feeling and the area of concern. She might say, "You felt disappointed that the medicine didn't solve the problem?" or "You were happy your child was included in the study?" She uses tentative statements so that she avoids putting words in the patient's mouth. This requires using all of her cognitive abilities to grasp the significance of the situation to the patient and responding with her best interpretation. She is saying, "I hear you."[8] She must remain sensitive to corrections in her perceptions by the patient.[5] She realizes that one can rarely perfectly understand another.

Thirdly, she avoids anything which would block further verbal comments from the patient.[2] This might occur if she did not listen, gave reassurance such as, "I'm sure your husband will forgive you," or made insensitive comments such as, "I know just how you feel."

Lastly, she avoids becoming immersed in the patient's emotion to the extent that she loses her objectivity. This is referred to as sympathy. If she were to do this, she would hamper her effectiveness in some ways.[32] She would no longer be able to validate how well she is perceiving what the patient is experiencing because she would be lost in her own feelings and would probably project them to the patient. She would lose her ability to focus on the patient because she would become focused on herself and her feelings. As a result, she would learn much less about the patient.

The crucial difference between sympathy and empathy lies in the fact that with empathy the nurse tries to understand how she would feel if she had the patient's experience or situation. In sympathy, the nurse passes beyond this as if she did have the experience.[8] Often students in nursing more easily develop empathy with patients than some more experienced nurses who have become less understanding.[2]

Empathy is communicated to the patient in behaviors which say:

1. I will try diligently to understand how you perceive your situation.
2. I will tell you what I think you are experiencing and ask for your validation.
3. I will not let myself be overwhelmed by your situation so that I become useless to you.

The following represents part of a conversation between a nurse and a patient in which the nurse works to develop empathic understanding. Notice how the nurse searches for the patient's feelings.

Suzy:  My mom never listens to me—just talks, talks, talks.
Nurse: You feel sad that you never get to say what you want?
Suzy:  Yes. Especially when I have something real important I need to discuss with someone. Some of the other kids talk with their parents all the time.
Nurse: You feel jealous because you can't?
Suzy:  Yes. Barb tells her mother everything. Even about her dates. She says her mother never hassles her.
Nurse: You feel jealous of Barb in a way because she's got someone to talk to.
Suzy:  She's got a father too. (Sigh) . . .

## Being Congruent

Another helping skill involves striving for congruency or agreement between one's verbal and nonverbal behavior. To be noncongruent would be to say one thing verbally while saying the opposite nonverbally. Being congruent requires that the nurse develop the ability to monitor how she is reacting to the patient. No problem exists when she feels predominantly positive towards the patient because she will probably naturally evidence these feelings in her verbal and nonverbal behavior. A problem exists when she is reacting with negative feelings towards the patient. She will most likely communicate her reaction to the patient nonverbally, but at the same time use verbalizations that deny her underlying feelings. This causes a confusing situation for the patient.[5] He perceives the nurse as saying all the right things but her nonverbal behavior readily communicates that she is not being genuine with him. The nurse who is not in touch with her "gut level" reactions to patients is not usually aware of her duplicity. The nurse who keeps in touch with her feelings will be more likely to notice when her verbal and nonverbal behaviors are becoming noncongruent and this is the first step in becoming congruent.

Next, when one does notice the beginning of negative feelings, there are several things which can be done. One might try to examine these negative feelings to determine what has aroused them, if they are rational, and if they can be dissipated. For example:

> One nurse had a particular dislike for individuals who cursed habitually in normal conversation. She often became annoyed with patients who did so without consciously realizing what was breeding her annoyance. When working with one man, this nurse noticed her angry feelings building after each contact. Outside of the situation she reflected on what was causing her anger at the patient. She eventually related her anger primarily to his continual cursing. She was then able to regain a more positive feeling towards the patient because she had now more definitively identified the source of her annoyance. She could then work on acceptance of her patient's language style even though she wasn't pleased with it.

This approach may not lead to the alleviation of negative feelings but it may help to lessen them.

Another approach upon discovering negative feelings towards a patient is to avoid a pretense of positivity towards the patient and instead discuss what one is feeling with the patient involved.[5] This must be done in a way that is not aimed at attacking or harming the patient. The following example illustrates how one nurse attempted to deal with annoyance towards a patient rather than attempt unsuccessfully to hide it from herself and the patient.

> A nurse had been caring for Mr. Ryan for several days. She dreaded her contacts with him because in her opinion he was flirtatious and made seductive comments. She ignored the situation and attempted to remain polite. Finally she realized that she was operating with a facade of interest and friendliness towards Mr. Ryan when in actuality she felt neither. She waited for an appropriate situation and then initiated a discussion of the situation with a verbalization which was congruent with what she was undoubtedly expressing nonverbally: "I feel very uncomfortable when you joke about my 'sex appeal,' Mr. Ryan, because I wonder if I have led you to believe that my interest in you is more than a professional interest?"

This approach must be taken carefully and the nurse must allow time to fully explore the situation with the patient.

Another approach to deal with negative feelings is to avoid situations where one must continuously work with patients to whom one is likely to react negatively. For example, if a nurse is not particularly fond of teenagers, she should avoid a career as a nurse in a high school. This sounds almost too obvious but sometimes nurses who do not know themselves have done similar things. The nurse who is in tune with her reactions will know those she is likely be effective with and those she is likely to have trouble with.

Being congruent then requires first a sensitivity to one's inner reactions because if these are at variance with what one is attempting to portray verbally, the patient senses a confusing message. Secondly, being genuine means cultivating consistency between what one feels internally and what one expresses verbally. If a patient senses noncongruence, he is likely to question the nurse's trustworthiness.

Congruence is demonstrated in behaviors which communicate to the patient:

1. I will level with you and not say things to you which I don't feel.
2. I will not hide behind a professional mask or role but I will be a genuine human being.
3. I will accept my responsibility to work on recognizing and accepting the behavior to which I react negatively.

The opposite of being congruent is evidenced by behaving in ways unrelated to one's actual internal feelings.[2] For example, if a nurse pretends concern for a patient when she feels none, she is playing a role and developing a facade.[16]

## Attending

Attending implies focusing on the patient with mind and body. The person who wishes to attend to another would first prepare by assuring the other's comfort.[4] This might involve taking his coat, offering a chair, adjusting pillows and lights, decreasing distractions, and other polite behaviors. She might show polite interest in the patient before the interaction. "How was your trip here?" "That coat certainly looks warm; is it?" "What book are you reading?" Humor is often appreciated too. One new mother repeated over and over to friends with glee this statement by a nurse as she was being discharged with her new baby: "We try to teach all the babies in the newborn nursery to stay awake all night and sleep all day so that when they go home their new parents won't forget they are there!"

Similarly when the nurse wishes to closely attend to a patient she needs to prepare herself mentally by putting aside her preoccupations as much as possible. Sitting down closely to the patient, leaning forward, facing the patient, and maintaining eye contact all show attention.[4] She communicates that the most important thing she has to do at the moment is to exclusively listen to the patient.

Attending then is shown by behaviors which communicate to the patient:

1. I will arrange for this interaction beforehand.
2. I will devote my entire attention to you and listen carefully.

Behaviors opposite of attending would include looking away from the patient, withdrawing, maintaining distance, actively creating or responding to distractions, and ignoring the patient.

## Being a Participant-Observer

Another skill which is useful in helping interactions is to be a participant-observer. This is one who interacts in the situation freely yet is continuously monitoring the conditions of the situation and guiding the interaction.[22] The nurse observes and participates simultaneously.[39]

There is a continuum of interaction with the total participant at one end, participant-observer in the middle, and total observer at the other end.[12] The difficult middle ground as participant-observer consists in responding naturally and obtaining adequate information from the patient without becoming so involved that one loses sight of the direction of the interaction. The nurse usually must learn to both participate and observe while interacting with a patient. She probably will tend at first to become involved as a participant to the extent that she forgets to also observe.

Behaviors which indicate that the nurse is a participant-observer communicate to the patient:

1. I will not become so involved in what we are discussing that I am unable to control underlying facets of our interaction.
2. I will not withdraw from our interaction to concentrate on observing.

## Concreteness

Concreteness means that the nurse helps the patient to discuss fully and specifically his concerns.[2] The nurse must use careful communication skills to ensure concreteness. The opposite of concreteness is encouraging the patient to talk in vague generalities and abstractions. The patient is often not totally aware of the exact basis of his discomfort or worries or is unable to verbalize them. When he is helped to be concrete, he often can explore and come to an understanding of his specific concerns.[2] A specific concern is often easier to cope with than a vague sense of concern. The following illustrates how a nurse helped a patient be more concrete.

> Patient: I'll be glad when this is over. I know it's best to be awake but I wish I could be put to sleep.
> Nurse:   You're concerned about being awake while the surgeon does the biopsy?
> Patient: Yes. If I could just go to sleep, it would all be over when I woke up.
> Nurse:   This way you'll have to live through the whole thing?
> Patient: Exactly. I will know what is happening.
> Nurse:   You would rather not know what he is doing?
> Patient: Well, it's not really that, I guess I'm afraid I will be able to feel what he is doing.
> Nurse:   You're worried that you will feel things even though he deadens the area?
> Patient: Yes. Especially when he cuts my skin. What if my skin is not deadened enough and I feel the knife?
> Nurse:   That would be the worst part? Feeling the knife?
> Patient: Yes. I guess that is what scares me. And really, I know it is not going to be that bad. I've had a local anesthetic before and it was great. But I still have this fear that it might not work this time. Do you think I could tell the doctor about this?
> Nurse:   Would you feel better about the biopsy if you did?
> Patient: Yes, I really think it would help. Just talking about it makes me feel better somehow.

Behaviors which lead to concreteness communicate:

1. I will help you fully explore what you are feeling.
2. I will realize that you need help in being concrete because you may not fully know what your concern or feeling is.
3. I will avoid jumping to conclusions about what you are saying.

## Trustworthiness

The nurse hopes that the patient will learn to trust her. However, the approach she must take is first to be trustworthy herself.[42] She is trustworthy when she is initially trusting of herself.[50] This implies that she is aware of herself and comfortable with what she sees within. Secondly, she engages in behaviors which may lead the patient to trust her. These include being courteous, reliable, predictable, consistent, dependable, discrete, and congruent.

Of course, despite her best efforts, not all patients or families may be able to trust the nurse. In these situations the nurse has to continually demonstrate her trustworthiness while seeking to become aware of how the other individual is perceiving her. This situation may well occur when the nurse does not fully trust the patient. He will react in kind and not trust the nurse. Behaviors which are likely to lead patients to feel not trusted are ones associated with "checking up" such as probing to see if the patient is keeping appointments, taking his medicine, following his diet, and so forth.[26] An alternative approach is shown when the nurse allows the patient to determine how he will manage his health care needs and defines her role as one who educates him to his needs but respects his final judgments.

Trustworthiness is then fundamentally based on being trustworthy which depends on trusting both oneself and the other person. The opposite of being trustworthy includes being suspicious and doubting.

Behaviors indicative of trustworthiness communicate:

1. I will learn to trust myself.
2. I will trust you to manage your life without being suspicious.
3. I will behave in ways that will allow you to count one me.

The attitudes and skills previously described have as their purpose eliciting a certain response from the patient. Hopefully, people respond to each other according to the law of reciprocity.[26] This implies that if the nurse approaches the patient with respect and acceptance, the patient will tend to respond to the nurse in kind. Hopefully her behaviors will communicate to the patient that she accepts him and considers him a valuable and worthwhile individual. She communicates that she wishes to understand him and avoids judging him. The patient experiences her as a caring, respectful, interested, genuine, accepting, nonevaluative person. This should lead the patient to respond with openness and trust. If this occurs the nurse will be able to learn much more about the patient and her attempts to help should be effective as a result. The opposite result would be that the patient withholds from the nurse all or most relevant information so that nothing of significance can be accomplished in the interaction.

## VARIATIONS IN HELPING INTERACTIONS

As not all helping interactions are alike, some possible differences will be described.

### Helping Relationships and Helping Encounters

The previous material has focused primarily on a type of interaction which probably would take a period of several months to accomplish. This is sometimes referred to as a helping relationship and represents the fullest application of the helping process. Does this mean that a nurse cannot help patients whom she has contact with only once or for only a few times? While a nurse cannot help each patient she cares for with a prolonged full fledged helping relationship, she can still accomplish positive goals in brief contacts. Short applications of the helping process are sometimes referred to as helping encounters. They are essentially the same as the lengthy relationship described except that they are shorter and of less depth. For example, in one contact a patient and nurse may become oriented briefly and superficially to each other, work on an issue which the patient presents in some detail, and terminate their encounter. Such brief interactions can actually accomplish a lot if the nurse is skillful.

Raul, a foreign student, came to the health service on a large campus and asked to have his blood pressure checked. The nurse-practitioner noticed what appeared to be symptoms of high anxiety. As she talked with him she discovered that he was under considerable stress. His native country was engaged in a civil war and he found himself taking the side of the present government while the other students on campus from the same country were on the side of the revolutionaries. This led him to feel very isolated. He was having trouble getting information from his family and worried about their safety. He was afraid that his studies were being affected by his inability to concentrate. The nurse listened attentively and empathetically. Raul talked for about 25 minutes and gradually became more relaxed. As he left, he thanked the nurse for her understanding. The nurse invited him to return whenever he wanted his blood pressure checked again or wished to talk.

She did not see Raul again until two months later. He again returned to have his blood pressure taken. This time he talked with her again for about 15 minutes. The government in his native country had been overthrown. He believed that his family was safe, however. Again, as he left, he expressed his gratitude to the nurse for taking the time to listen to him.

Nurses often remark that they do not want to get involved in meeting patients' emotional needs because it takes too much time. Actually much can be accomplished in a short period of time. If the nurse is involved in direct physical care, often she can use that time with the patient to great advantage as a helping encounter. The pressures nurses often feel to manage machinery and complex treatments can interfere if the nurse permits them.[16] To avoid this requires that the nurse become comfortable with the physical aspects of her care so that she can concentrate on the patient and respond appropriately.

## The Helping Process with Groups

The helping process is traditionally assumed to be a one-to-one interaction. However, a nurse can use the attitudes and skills of helping and communication skills with small groups to achieve the goal of furthering personal growth.[5] Groups might be composed of patients, coworkers, small classes, or family members.

Mr. and Ms. Marsh were faced with a grave prognosis for their youngest daughter. The nurse arranged to make a home visit so he could talk with the family. The family responded to the approach well and asked him to come back again. He planned his visits to use the helping process with the family members as a group.

Obviously, working with a group rather than just one person is more of a challenge to the nurse. She must strive to tune in to the varied needs and reactions of several people and divide her time among all individuals.

Groups have some special helping potentials.[24] The nurse should strive to maximize these. Group members can often give to each other a sense of "universality" that is often most comforting. The patient feels, "I am not the only one." Group members can give each other specialized information which the nurse might not know. As the nurse models helping attitudes and skills, often other members of the group begin to use them in their relationships with each other unconsciously. In other words, they begin to try to understand each other more fully, react genuinely to each other, express acceptance, and so forth. Group interaction can lead to a sense of altruism for some members who experience gratification in being helpful to another. A sense of group cohesiveness can develop which increases the member's sense of supportive help. An individual may believe that there are several caring individuals with whom he can safely be himself.

Many groups have the potential for becoming helping groups. For example, some "self-help" groups such as Alcoholics Anonymous and parents' groups are cited as being extremely helpful to many participants. The nurse can influence this potential for helping groups if she demonstrates helping behavior in the group and the group members copy her behaviors. Nurses are beginning to use the helping potentials of groups more and learn the necessary skills of group leadership. Recently groups have been reported as useful with obese teenagers, smokers who desire to quit, new widows, and unwed pregnant mothers.

## The Helping Process with Children

Developing a helping interaction with a child presents some special challenges. Adults often have difficulty restraining their tendencies to judge and evaluate children. They also are likely to have difficulty understanding the child's frame of reference which may seem absurd. Not uncommonly, adults predominantly give much advice and make decisions for children. The nurse will have absorbed many of these attitudes and will need to attempt to free herself from them so that she can interact with children in a different way.

### THE BEGINNING PHASE

Because children are often very perceptive of nonverbal communication, the nurse must realize that much of what the child learns about her will be based on how she uses touch and physical contact. Is her contact gentle and safe or rough and threatening? Are contacts always associated with pain and discomfort? Can she be trusted to keep her word?

### THE TRANSITION PHASE

Children are likely to test the nurse just before they decide that they can completely trust her. They may unconsciously engage in a forbidden activity to see her reaction. She must remember that if she can withstand this stage, she may be able to be more helpful to the child eventually.

### THE WORKING PHASE

Learning the child's frame of reference is difficult but important. In order to be helpful, the nurse needs to develop empathetic understanding of how the child sees his world. Depending on his age, he may view the world in a self-centered fashion. He may develop unjustified interpretations of what is happening around him and engage in fantasy.[35] He often interprets illness or hospitalization as punishment.[36] He likely cannot comprehend the necessity for painful treatments or diet and physical limitations. Often he is unable to clearly communicate how he is reacting. This places on the nurse the responsibility of developing sensitivity to the child and seeking to understand how he is perceiving his situation. It may be useful to provide play materials through which he can reveal his perceptions and fantasies.[9] Having the child tell a story may also provide quantities of information.[41]

 If the child is in the hospital, feelings the nurse is likely to uncover include homesickness, separation anxiety, fear or anger, and the loss of self-identity.[9] If the child is out of his natural environment, his anxieties may be reduced by following his usual routines, helping him maintain close contact with his parents, preparing him for coming events appropriately, encouraging the use of comfort items, and relieving physical discomforts.[9,15,35,36]

The child will usually use play activities to work through his problems and gain self-awareness. The nurse observes his play and maybe interprets to him what he seems to be saying. This must be done when the child seems ready to face each issue. Safe opportunities can be provided for the appropriate expression of negative feelings which he may be punished for expressing with parents. The nurse accepts the child's feelings, allows the child to work through his problems, and encourages him to make his own decisions. She counteracts the experiences he may have had of being judged and always told what to think and do. She may wish to subtly demonstrate to the parent helpful ways of interacting with the child which communicate acceptance, positive regard, empathy, and so forth. The study by Pothier contains additional information about helping children through play activities.[42]

## THE TERMINATION PHASE

Termination with children can occur with or without resolution. The child may likely be angry or despair when the relationship must end. Hopefully the child's parents can replace the nurse and learn to help their child as she did.

## DANGERS TO AVOID IN HELPING

Some dangers await the nurse who attempts helping relationships. Each nurse has unresolved conflicts and concerns which she has brought to adulthood from her childhood. These can lead her to behave in certain situations in a biased way based on distorted perceptions. She may react to a patient on the basis of a previous experience which has been revived in the present situation but which has nothing to do with the present situation. This is referred to as countertransference.[48] This is especially likely when working with a child who may evoke long forgotten conflicts by his behavior, or when a patient reminds her of a sibling or a parent or herself. The nurse does not recognize that her response to the patient has been exaggerated by her own unresolved feelings.

To reduce countertransference, the nurse must be on the lookout for exaggerated reactions to patient situations. She can ask herself what past situations she is reminded of as she works with the patient. The best way to detect countertransference is probably through consulting with another person about her interaction.

Another danger involves the possibility that the helpful nurse may develop unconscious rescue fantasies. She may see herself as saving another from some horrible fate by her benevolent actions and she may feel antagonism towards others whom she feels have contributed to the patient's unfortunate state. Her antagonistic feelings may then be evidenced in her behavior towards the source of her feelings. She may even unknowingly encourage the patient to adopt her attitude. For example, a nurse working with young children may develop rescue fantasies especially if she believes that the child has been harmed or neglected by the parents. If she treats the parents with subtle hostility and turns the child against the parents, she seals off the child's greatest source of future help. It would be more useful for her to accept the parents' behavior and work on reorienting them to help their child.[47] Other patients who may evoke rescue fantasies include those she believes have been rejected by others such as a wife whose husband has left her or an elderly individual whose children assume little responsibility for him. Rescue fantasies can hamper the patient's development of independence.

The nurse can look for rescue fantasies by checking to see if she is developing hostility towards another individual significant to the patient or reacting to the patient as a victim of others. Discussing her interaction with another objective listener is likely to uncover rescue fantasies as well.

Another danger is in developing a pseudo-helping focus. This can lead the nurse to unduly probe into the patient's life to learn "the dirt." The nurse who does this may brag to others about what she knows about the patient and about how others come to her for help. She may not consider an interaction a success unless the patient becomes emotionally distraught or cries. She may find comfort unconsciously in knowing that others have important problems so that her problems may seem more insignificant as a result.

The nurse can check for a pseudo-helping attitude by asking herself for whose benefit she engages in helping interactions and what she is trying to accomplish. If she feels a compulsion to tell others what she has found out about a patient, she should entertain the notion that she may be engaging in a pseudo-helping interaction to meet her needs and not the patient's.

Another hazard awaits the nurse who does not meet her needs for acceptance and esteem from interactions with friends and peers in social situations. She may turn to patients to meet these needs. She may structure the patient interaction so that she will receive gratification of her needs from the patient.[39] It is unlikely that she can form a successful helping interaction because she is focused on herself. She may be likely to keep the patient in a dependent state.[21] This allows her to feel needed.

The nurse can discover if she is meeting her own needs in a helping interaction by reflection and by discussing the interaction with another person who understands the goals of the helping process.

## THE NURSE AND THE HELPING PROCESS

The therapeutic use of oneself in the helping process requires much from the nurse. Helping patients may not be a highly rewarded activity since it is difficult to measure any tangible benefits in some situations. The nurse needs encouragement from others to engage in helping interactions. In addition, once a nurse learns to help others, she may begin to readily use the skills involved in everyday contacts with other professionals, health team members, and with individuals outside of her professional life. The nurse will find that her expertise in using the helping process can influence her life positively. Her relationships with others may become more meaningful as she learns to become involved and to care. Others may become more humanistic because of her example. On the other hand, she may need to learn when she can be helpful and when she must protect her energy and self-system by referring others to someone else. No one person can be continually other-focused.

The nurse who becomes a helping person needs to develop her own support system.

She cannot continue to give to others when she has unmet needs of her own. She should look for sources of support at work and at home. One way to develop supportive relationships is by providing support to others so that they will be sensitive and responsive when one needs them. Professional counselors and supervisory nursing personnel may also be good resources.

The responsibilities of the nurse to increase her self-knowledge have been mentioned but cannot be overemphasized. One who knows herself perceives others more objectively and accurately.[29] Therefore, the nurse strives to be in touch with who she is and what she values. She must learn to accept herself. She must learn her limitations. There will be individuals whom she cannot help and situations in which she cannot be helpful.[16] She may have learned to agonize over her weaknesses and deny her strengths. She may need instead to make a personal inventory of her strengths and forgive herself for her weaknesses.[54] Thus her philosophy becomes doing the best she can with what she is rather than becoming immobilized with concern over what she is not. One who accepts herself is more likely to accept others.[54] Growth groups, if available, may be helpful.[14]

The nurse who wishes to become a helping person should seek out an environment where she will be facilitated in this respect. Nurses who are accepted, trusted, and encouraged to grow in self-understanding are more likely to relate to patients in the same way. An environment where there is competition, criticism, and an emphasis on task completion above all else is not conducive to the nurse's development of helping interactions with patients. If the nurse is a student, she needs a situation in which she experiences positive relationships with her teachers if she is to learn to form helping relationships with patients.[28]

It may sound as if every helping interaction would look identical. Actually each helper develops her own unique style and, since each patient is unique, no two interactions will be alike. This makes the helping process difficult to learn because one cannot exactly model what another helper does.[16] It also adds variety and interest because no one can ever predict how a helping interaction will end before it begins.[16]

Studies of helpers seem to suggest that there are no common personality traits of successful helpers. There do appear to be certain attitudes they hold. For example, successful helpers seem to have accurate perceptions of others, of themselves, and about how people learn.[18,19]

## WHERE TO START

The nurse must realize that developing skill in helping others requires experiential learning. Study can give guidance but skill requires practice. Fortunately, opportunities to practice helping attitudes and skills abound in the nurse's private and professional life. She may find it easiest at first to try out her helping skills with those she knows because she may be less anxious than when with patients. In addition, role playing situations and videotaped situations may be helpful tools.[2] Some nurses find it easiest at first to work with patients when they are free from direct care responsibilities while other nurses find it easier to have something to do for the patient as they interact. Helping encounters are probably easier to conduct at first but the nurse should also find situations in which she can carry out a long term helping relationship. Working with groups and with children may be most difficult and require more study and practice.

## SOME SUGGESTIONS FOR SELF-EVALUATION

The following questions are suggested to help the nurse evaluate her use of the helping process.

### Developmental Phases

1. Can I help the patient cope with excessive anxiety in the beginning of a helping interaction?
2. Do I properly orient the patient to my role?
3. Do I obtain the patient's goals?
4. Can I accept ambivalent behavior as a necessary reaction for some patients?
5. Do I facilitate the patient in disclosing himself?
6. Do I allow the patient to control his life?
7. Do I plan for termination to promote resolution?
8. Do I avoid mentalisms which promote nonresolution?

### Personal Attitudes

1. Do I work towards becoming nonjudgmental by learning my values and allowing others to have theirs?
2. Do I work to accept others who differ from me?
3. Can I respect and think positively towards others regardless of their present situation?

### Professional Skills

1. Can I use empathy with my patients?
2. Am I congruent in my interactions with patients?
3. Do I recognize and deal with negative feelings towards patients?
4. Do I attend carefully to patients?
5. Am I able to be a participant-observer with patients?
6. Is my communication directed towards achieving concreteness?

### General Concerns

1. Do I recognize the importance of the helping process by planning helping encounters and relationships with patients?
2. Do I strive to maintain predominantly helping interactions rather than social interactions with patients?

3. Do I use even limited time with patients to conduct a helping encounter?
4. Can I function as a helper with small groups of individuals?
5. Do I recognize how my attitudes may interfere with helping interactions with children?
6. Do I use attitudes and skills conducive to helping with children appropriately for their age?
7. Do I work to discover if I am developing countertransference, rescue fantasies, or a pseudo-helping interaction while working with patients or using patient interactions to meet my own needs?
8. Do I use the helping process in my personal life without overextending myself?
9. Have I developed a personal support system?

## AN EXAMPLE OF THE USE OF THE HELPING PROCESS

The following example illustrates a helping relationship which a nurse had with a patient. Only parts of the interaction which related to a particular theme have been portrayed.

Mr. W. was a 73-year-old widower who lived alone in a residential area of a small city near a college campus. His house had been converted into a duplex with the top floor rented to three college students. He lived on the ground floor and stored belongings in the basement. Mr. W. had been admitted to a hospital after a tenant found him in the basement following an apparent fall down the stairs. He was physically debilitated on admission but recovered progressively and returned home in one month. The hospital nurse initiated a community health nursing referral because she believed that there might be problems with safety in the home, so someone could assess Mr. W.'s diet and other health practices, and in order to assure assessment of the healing areas on his legs.

The community health nurse planned her first visit to explain her purposes to Mr. W. and to learn about him as a person. She introduced herself, explained where she was from, and explained that she had been asked to see Mr. W. to see how his legs were healing and to see if he needed any help now that he had returned home. She explained that she would visit regularly unless they agreed that her visits were not needed.

Mr. W. seemed puzzled by the concept of a nurse outside of the hospital but was receptive to the nurse and showed her his healing abrasions on the anterior surfaces of both legs. The nurse had the perception that Mr. W. was lonely, and although he was glad to be back home, he missed the human contact he had had in the hospital.

The nurse found out that Mr. W. had been a widower for 10 years. He ate irregularly and what appeared to be mainly prepared foods from cans such as ravioli, spaghetti with sauce, soup, and beef stew. The home itself was incredibly cluttered with possessions. Even a brief glance around the living room revealed electrical hazards and hazards likely to lead to falls such as loose scatter rugs. The nurse noticed a kerosene lamp perched precariously on a stack of books on a rickety table.

Mr. W.'s socialization consisted primarily of listening to the radio in the mornings and watching TV in the evenings. He visited with a few old neighbors on occasion but the neighborhood was becoming predominantly rental property as his old friends died or moved away. Mr. W. had social security income, rental income, and a retirement income from the nearby college where he had taught. He owned his home and his expenses were few. He seemed financially secure.

Mr. W. got some exercise by walking to a grocery store several times a week and to the bank when necessary. He had no car. When he needed to make trips downtown he paid his renters to drive him there or took a city bus. Mr. W. seemed somewhat forgetful but oriented and alert.

The nurse used reflective comments to encourage Mr. W.'s verbalizations about his health and his present life situation. She summarized later that he seemed somewhat unhappy with his present living environment but did not seriously entertain any ideas of a change because his house and his mass of possessions were very important to him.

On the next visit, the nurse planned to focus on assessing Mr. W.'s health and on learning more about him as a person. She decided to wait on working with him on the hazards in the home and his diet until she and Mr. W. knew each other better. To begin working on improving his living environment right away might indicate to him a lack of acceptance.

When she arrived for the second visit, Mr. W. greeted her warmly but had forgotten that she was coming. Mr. W. was convalescing well from his fall as indicated by the healing abrasions on his legs. The nurse noted that his diet must be somewhat adequate because he was healing well. He had been out walking twice that week. As the visit progressed, Mr. W. discussed his problems with his renters, the decline of the neighborhood, and his concerns over the future prospect of not being able to care for himself in his home. In view of the fact that Mr. W. had alluded on the first visit to similar topics, the nurse proposed that this area of concern was quite meaningful to Mr. W. She encouraged him to continue further. He explained that the fall had really scared him. He mentioned that if he had fallen one week earlier, no one would have found him because the students who were his renters would have been gone on Christmas vacation. The nurse listened carefully and facilitated Mr. W.'s discussion of his worries. Mr. W. also talked of his loneliness since his wife's death. As he talked he became quite sad and near tears. The nurse tried hard to develop empathy for Mr. W.'s situation. She encouraged him to be concrete, and he responded readily. Before she left, she noticed that the kerosene lamp had been moved to the kitchen table where it looked more stable.

The nurse continued to visit Mr. W. regularly. His legs healed well. Mr. W. talked more at each visit about his life and present situation. The nurse felt that they were now in the working phase of the helping process. It seemed that Mr. W. trusted the nurse and was ready to share his concerns and fears. Mr. W. was never bitter about his situation, but rather sad. The nurse noticed that in a way he seemed to be anticipatorily grieving for what he knew he would someday have to lose. Mr. W. never actually mentioned moving from his neighborhood or home nor did he refer to dying—only being unable to care for himself. On the seventh visit the following conversation occurred.

Mr. W.: I guess I'm too set in my ways to adjust to a nursing home.

Nurse: (Surprised to hear Mr. W. mention a nursing home) You would be unhappy in one?

Mr. W.: Yes. I've been to see a friend in one. They had everybody lined up in beds like little stuffed dolls. That's no place for me.

Nurse: You're worried that you would be stuck in bed all day?

Mr. W.: Yes. And the food looked like the stuff they feed to babies—all mashed up. I don't want to live that way.

Nurse: It makes you sad just to talk about it.

Mr. W.: I would rather they take me out and shoot me than put me in a place like that! Still, I don't know what I would do if I got sick and couldn't cook or take care of my affairs.

Nurse: You're afraid there is no other choice besides a nursing home like you visited?

Mr. W.: Yes. No other choice.

Nurse: Have you ever been to see a retirement community?

Mr. W.: Aren't they just glorified nursing homes?

Nurse: There are some differences. Maybe you would like to visit one here in town sometime to see what it looks like?
Mr. W.: Maybe so. (Changing subject)

For the next several visits Mr. W. never brought up the subject of leaving his home again. The weather was improving, the sidewalks were clear of snow and ice, and Mr. W. seemed rejuvenated by the lengthening days. The nurse used this period of time to talk to him about his diet. After collecting a week's sample of menus, she recommended to him that he increase his intake of vegetables and also have citrus fruits and juices more regularly. She talked with Mr. W. about how he could carry out her suggestions and how he felt about them. She did not specifically check to see if he had followed through because she believed that the final decision on changing his diet was his.

As spring approached, Mr. W. abruptly asked the nurse for the name of a local retirement center. He stated that he might call and reserve a time to see the facility some day. The nurse discussed with Mr. W. what he wanted to know and what he expected to find out.

The nurse made several other visits before the subject was mentioned again. Mr. W. asked the nurse if she had ever been in the retirement center. The nurse wanted very much to relate all of the positive factors about the center she could think of to Mr. W. However, she wanted to be sure that Mr. W. took his time in reaching his own decisions so she made her remarks brief. She had secured a pamphlet from the retirement center and she gave it to him to look at. Mr. W. glanced at it only momentarily and laid it aside on a table.

Mr. W. then mentioned that he was having problems with the city fire department. It appeared that a few years before a tenant had reported his house to the fire chief as a fire nuisance. The fire chief had visited and required him to clean up the basement. Since then, he believed that the fire department had him "on their list." A neighbor had told him that the fire chief had been at his door one day when he had walked to the store. The nurse helped him talk about his reactions to this new problem. His approach to the situation was one of avoidance. He had told his renters to not let anyone in and he planned to never answer the door if the chief came back again. The nurse had a great deal of difficulty accepting his response to this problem because she was worried about the fire hazards in the home too. She decided that she could not be congruent without voicing her reaction.

Nurse: I understand why you want to avoid the fire chief but do you think you can?
Mr. W.: No. (Sigh) I'll have to clean up the basement sooner or later.
Nurse: That must be discouraging.
Mr. W.: Yes. Why does he care how I live anyway? I wish he would just leave me alone.
Nurse: You feel the fire chief is interfering in your life?
Mr. W.: Yes, he sure is. I'm not as strong as I once was. I don't know how I can get all those newspapers and cans moved. I'm tired of taking care of all those things. I've got to think of something. Maybe I could get . . .

The nurse and Mr. W. then went on to consider ways that Mr. W. could get his basement cleaned out. The nurse was anxious to discuss some of the electrical hazards on the ground floor but decided that this was not the time.

On the next visit the nurse found that Mr. W. had been visited by the fire chief but had managed to get his basement cleared out before he came. He was very gleeful over having "beat him to the punch." With this problem behind him Mr. W. was prepared to enjoy the summer to the hilt. He frequently walked to campus and spent his afternoons dozing on a park bench. The nurse continued to pay him occasional visits. She brought him a booklet on "common electrical hazards in the home." She asked Mr. W. if he ever worried about the mass of extension cords running around in the rooms. He seemed unimpressed with the problem.

As fall changed into winter, Mr. W. began to spend more time inside. On one visit when the weather was chilly, damp, and windy the nurse found that Mr. W. was having problems with his new renters. He looked tired and discouraged. He was upset about a new electric rate increase. He confessed that he had slipped on a scatter rug and had fallen down but had not hurt himself badly. The nurse and Mr. W. talked for some time. Mr. W. was depressed and angry. As the nurse was leaving, he asked her if she would take him to see the retirement community if he paid for her gasoline. He was very discouraged about the prospect of another winter, hassles with noisy renters, and the possibility of another fall. The nurse felt that Mr. W. needed her presence and support to face seeing the retirement community. She also suspected that he wanted her to come because otherwise he was afraid that he would keep putting it off and never go. The nurse agreed to go but left it up to Mr. W. to make all the arrangements and to call her office to inform her of the time.

Two weeks later, the nurse accompanied Mr. W. to the center. Mr. W. gave the impression of one who was trying to act uninterested but was absorbing a lot. The nurse took him home and stayed to talk with him. Mr. W. did not want to discuss the visit to the center but talked about other things.

The nurse did not visit until two weeks later. She was somewhat surprised and yet had half expected the fact that there was a "For Sale" sign in the front yard. Mr. W. was very busy sorting through his possessions and deciding what to take to the retirement center and what to sell. It appeared that he had not yet found anything which he did not plan to take. The nurse found out that he had contacted the center a few days previously and arranged to become a resident. His son was coming to help him move. He was sad about leaving his home and neighborhood and yet seemed determined to make the best of his situation. He was to move in as soon as he had his house sold and his affairs wrapped up. He was worried over selling his property in the middle of the winter and almost seemed hopeful that maybe it would not sell. The nurse allowed Mr. W. to talk about his move and reminisce about his home. She explained to him that she would not be able to visit him officially once he moved to the center. He expressed his unhappiness at this information and they discussed the eventual parting.

Mr. W.'s property did sell quickly and within a month he was at the center. The nurse called him and asked to make a visit at the center. She found him looking somewhat ill at ease with his ancient possessions among the modernistic surroundings of the center. He had made two new friends and seemed to enjoy visiting with them. He was still hesitant to enter into many of the center activities but he did take the shuttle bus to a shopping center twice a week. Mr. W. took the nurse on a tour of the facility although she had seen everything with him previously. He seemed pleased with the meals in the dining room although the nurse noticed that he had a hoard of canned food from the grocery store in his room. Mr. W. talked about missing his old home and the neighborhood. He did state that he liked having people around to visit with. He said he was going to the store to get some new shirts to wear because everyone dressed up for dinner and he wanted to be in style. The nurse believed that this possibly indicated a sense of belonging and identification with the center.

The nurse eventually told Mr. W. that she had to leave. Mr. W. rose to shake hands with her—the only time he had ever done so. The nurse had grown fond of Mr. W. during their months of contact and she told him how much she had enjoyed getting to know him and how much she would miss seeing him regularly. Mr. W.'s eyes filled with tears and he could not speak. The nurse too was next to tears. She squeezed his hand, wished him well, and asked to drop in again sometime when she was near the center. She felt a sense of loss which followed her all day.

The nurse often thought of Mr. W. as she drove near the college area where he had lived. She did stop to see him again in the center after he had been there six weeks. He was obviously glad to see her and full of stories about the center. He seemed very popular with several ladies, one of whom would not leave his side. Mr. W. again shook hands with the nurse as she left. Mr. W. expressed his gratitude to her for all her visits and told her how much he had enjoyed having her talk with him. He told her that she had helped him more than she would ever know. Although it was hard to say goodbye again, she was encouraged by having seen Mr. W. settled and content.

## SUMMARY

The skillful use of the helping process can help assure that contacts nurses have with patients and families in any setting are used to optimum advantage. Helping requires the sophisticated and controlled use of oneself through the acquisition and demonstration of helping attitudes and the application of helping skills. A helping interaction may progress through the phases of beginning, transition, working, and termination and may range from a prolonged relationship to a brief encounter.

Each helping interaction will be unique in focus, progress, and outcome because of the interplay of characteristics of both the helper and the one seeking help. Learning to use the helping process requires continual practice and reflection.

The nurse who develops competence in use of the helping process will find that other activities she attempts with patients and families will be enhanced because of the rapport she had gained with them. For this reason, the ability of the nurse to use the helping process is crucial to all areas of her practice. The nurse will find her ability to be helpful to others through application of a specific process useful in her personal life as well.

## REFERENCES

1. Aguilera, D. C., and Messick, J. M.: *Crisis Intervention: Theory and Methodology.* C. V. Mosby, St. Louis, 1978.
2. Aiken, L., and Aiken, J.: "A Systematic approach to the evaluation of interpersonal relationships." Am. J. Nurs. 73:863, 1973.
3. Allport, G. W.: "Psychological models for guidance," in Torrance, E. P., and Strom, R. D.: *Mental Health and Achievement.* John Wiley and Sons, New York, 1965.
4. Anthony, W. A., and Carkhuff, R. R.: *The Art of Health Care.* Human Resource Development Press, Amherst, Mass., 1976.
5. Barrett-Lennard, B. T.: "Significant aspects of a helping relationship." Mental Health (Canada), Special Suppl. 47:1, 1965.
6. Baumgartner, M.: "Empathy," in Carlson, C. E. (ed): *Behavioral Concepts and Nursing Intervention.* J. B. Lippincott, Philadelphia, 1970.
7. Bayer, M., and Brandner, P.: "Nurse/patient peer practice." Am. J. Nurs. 77:86, 1977.
8. Benjamin, A.: *The Helping Interview.* Houghton Mifflin, Boston, 1974.
9. Blake, F. G., et al.: *Essentials of Pediatric Nursing.* J. B. Lippincott, Philadelphia, 1970.

10. Boland, M. et al.: "The nurse-patient relationship in the nursing process," in Murray, R. et al.: *Nursing Concepts for Health Promotion.* Prentice-Hall, Englewood Cliffs, N.J., 1975.
11. Braden, C. J., and Price, J. L.: "Encouraging client self-discovery." Am. J. Nurs. 76:444, 1976.
12. Byerly, E. L.: "The nurse researcher as participant-observer in a nursing setting." Nurs. Res. 18:230, 1969.
13. Carkhuff, R. R.: *Helping and Human Relations.* Holt, Rinehart and Winston, New York, 1969.
14. Ceriale, L.: "Facilitated unfolding of human relations skills in the baccalaureate nursing student." Nurs. Educat. 1:11, 1976.
15. Chadwick, B. J., Pflederer, D., and Ray, M. A.: "Maintaining the hospitalized child's home ties." Am. J. Nurs. 78:1360, 1978.
16. Chapman, J. E., and Chapman, H. H.: *Behavior and Health Care: A Humanistic Helping Process.* C. V. Mosby, St. Louis, 1975.
17. Clemence, Sr. M. V.: "Existentialism: A philosophy of commitment." Am. J. Nurs. 66:500, 1966.
18. Combs, A. W.: *The Professional Education of Teachers.* Allyn and Bacon, Boston, 1965.
19. Combs, A. W., and Soper, D. W.: "Perceptual organization of effective counselors." J. Consulting Psychol. 10:222, 1963.
20. Corcoran, S.: "The value of values in nursing education." Image 7:5, 1975.
21. Dyer, W. G.: "The nurse-patient system relationship," in Reinhardt, A. M., and Quinn, M. D. (eds.): *Family-Centered Community Nursing: A Sociocultural Framework.* C. V. Mosby, St. Louis, 1973.
22. Dyer, W. G.: "Working with groups," in Reinhardt, A. M., and Quinn, M. D. (eds.): *Family-Centered Community Nursing: A Sociocultural Framework.* C. V. Mosby, St. Louis, 1973.
23. Edinburg, G. M., Zinberg, N. E., and Kelman, W.: *Clinical Interviewing and Counseling: Principles and Techniques.* Appleton-Century-Crofts, New York, 1975.
24. Fochtman, G. A.: "Therapeutic factors of the informal group." Am. J. Nurs. 76:238, 1976.
25. Frank, J. D.: "The medical power of faith." Human Nature 1:40, 1978.
26. Gibb, J. R.: "Climate for trust formation," in Bradford, L. P., et al.: *T-Group Theory and Laboratory Method.* John Wiley and Sons, New York, 1964.
27. Goldsborough, J. D.: "On becoming nonjudgmental." Am. J. Nurs. 70:2340, 1970.
28. Gunter, L. M.: "The developing nursing student: Part III. A study of self-appraisals and concerns reported during the sophomore year." Nurs. Res. 18:237, 1969.
29. Jourard, S. M.: *The Transparent Self.* Van Nostrand, Princeton, N.J., 1964.
30. Kalisch, B. J.: "What is empathy?" Am. J. Nurs. 73:1548, 1978.
31. Kalkman, M. E., and Davis, A. J. (eds.): *New Dimensions in Mental Health-Psychiatric Nursing.* McGraw-Hill, New York, 1974.
32. Katz, R.: *Empathy: its Nature and Uses.* Collier-Macmillan, London, 1963.
33. Kelley, R. L.: "Brief psychotherapy," in Soloman, P., and Patch, V. D. (eds.): *Handbook of Psychiatry.* Lange Medical Publications, Los Altos, Calif., 1971.
34. Kelly, H. S.: "The sense of an ending." Am. J. Nurs. 69:2378, 1969.
35. Kunzman, L.: "Some factors influencing a young child's mastery of hospitalization." Nurs. Clin. North Am. 7:13, 1972.
36. Langford, W. S.: "Children's reactions to illness and hospitalization." Feelings and Their Medical Significance (Ross Laboratories) 8:1, 1966.
37. Manaser, J. C., and Werner, A. M.: *Intruments for Study of Nurse-Patient Interactions.* Macmillan, New York, 1964.
38. Milio, N.: "Values, social class, and community health services," in Reinhardt, A. M., and Quinn, M. D. (eds.): *Family-Centered Community Nursing: A Sociocultural Framework.* C. V. Mosby, St. Louis, 1973.
39. Peplau, H. E.: "Professional closeness." Nurs. Forum 8:343, 1969.
40. Phillips, B. D.: "Terminating a nurse-patient relationship." Am. J. Nurs. 68:1941, 1968.
41. Piche, J. C.: "Tell me a story." Am. J. Nurs. 78:1188, 1978.
42. Pothier, P. C.: *Mental Health Counseling With Children.* Little, Brown and Company, Boston, 1976.
43. Rogers, C. R.: *Client Centered Therapy.* Houghton Mifflin, Boston, 1965.
44. Rogers, C. R.: "The interpersonal relationship: The core of guidance," in Rogers, C. R., et al.: *Person To Person: The Problem of Being Human.* Real People Press, Lafayette, Calif., 1967.
45. Rogers, C. R.: *On Becoming a Person.* Houghton Mifflin, Boston, 1961.
46. Sarosi, G. M.: "A critical theory. The nurse as a fully human person." Nurs. Forum 7:349, 1968.
47. Scharer, K. M.: "Rescue fantasies: Professional impediments in working with abused families." Am. J. Nurs. 78:1483, 1978.
48. Snyder, J. C., and Wilson, M. F.: "Elements of a psychological assessment." Am. J. Nurs. 77:235, 1977.
49. Stephanics, C.: "My involvement with a young family," in Hall, J. E., and Weaver, B. R. (eds.): *Nursing of Families in Crisis.* J. B. Lippincott, Philadelphia, 1974.

50. Thomas, M. D.: "Trust," in Carlson, C. E., and Blackwell, B. (eds.): *Behavioral Concepts and Nursing Intervention.* J. B. Lippincott, Philadelphia, 1978.
51. Travelbee, J.: *Intervention in Psychiatric Nursing.* F. A. Davis, Philadelphia, 1969.
52. Uustal, D. B.: "Searching for values." Image 9:15, 1977.
53. Uustal, D. B.: "Values clarification in nursing: Application to practice." Am. J. Nurs. 78:2058, 1978.
54. Wolff, I. S.: "Acceptance." Am. J. Nurs. 72:1412, 1972.

## BIBLIOGRAPHY

Brown, M., and Fowler, G.: *Psychodynamic Nursing.* W. B. Saunders, Philadelphia, 1971.

Emerson, L.: "There's always time." Am. J. Nurs. 67:1857, 1967.

Goldsborough, J. D.: "Involvement." Am. J. Nurs. 69:66, 1969.

Hall, J. E.: "Growth: A transcending experience, in Hall, J. E., and Weaver, B. R. (eds.): *Nursing of Families in Crisis.* J. B. Lippincott, Philadelphia, 1974.

Hoyman, H. S.: "Models of human nature and their impact on health education." J. School Health 44:374, 1974.

Kemp, R.: "Ambivalence," in Carlson, C. E. (ed.): *Behavioral Concepts and Nursing Intervention.* J. B. Lippincott, Philadelphia, 1970.

Peplau, H. E.: *Interpersonal Relations in Nursing.* G. P. Putnam's Sons, New York, 1952.

Pope, M.: "Thoughts from an artificial nurse." Am. J. Nurs. 75:248, 1975.

Powell, J.: *Why Am I Afraid To Tell You Who I Am?* Argus Communications, Chicago, 1969.

Price, J. L., and Braden, C.: "The reality in home visits." Am. J. Nurs. 78:1536, 1978.

Redman, B. K.: *The Process of Patient Teaching in Nursing.* C. V. Mosby, St. Louis, 1976.

Schmidt, J.: "Availability: A concept of nursing practice." Am. J. Nurs. 72:1086, 1972.

Shetland, M. L.: "The responsibilities of the professional school for preparing nurses for ethical, moral and humanistic practice." Nurs. Forum 8:17, 1969.

Sobel, D. E.: "Love and pain." Am. J. Nurs. 72:910, 1972.

Varela, J. A.: "Solving human problems with human science." Human Nature 1:84, 1978.

Von Bergen, R.: "Intensive family health work." Nurs. Outlook 11:202, 1963.

Yura, H., and Walsh, M. B.: *The Nursing Process: Assessing, Planning, Implementing, Evaluating.* Appleton-Century-Crofts, New York, 1973.

# CHAPTER 3

## THE PROBLEM SOLVING PROCESS

The skilled use of the problem solving process is a crucial element in professional nursing practice. It is an instrument which enables the nurse to fully use and apply the knowledges and skills she has to appropriate situations; it is an instrument which exposes areas where new knowledge is needed. This chapter will focus on describing the problem solving process, suggesting how the nurse can develop competence in use of the process, and exploring the relevance of problem solving to the future of nursing.

Although nurses have been solving problems since the beginning of nursing history, widespread recognition of a problem solving process specific to nursing did not emerge until the mid 1960s.[30] One will find other terms in the literature which basically refer to the same process such as the "deliberative process"[29] and the "nursing process." For the sake of simplicity, this process will be referred to as the problem solving process since it focuses on solving problems. The term "nursing process," currently very popular with nursing educators, will not be used. The nurse uses many processes such as the communication process, the problem solving process, the leadership process, and the helping process to name only a few. It seems inappropriate to refer to any one process used in nursing as *the* nursing process.

The nurse who wishes to learn to problem solve is not starting without considerable experience. Individuals are faced continuously, beginning shortly after birth, with decisions, to some of which they apply the problem solving process. For example, most individuals must decide daily what clothing to wear. One usually quickly considers such things as the weather, the season, the expected activities of the day, and the options available. Later, one frequently evaluates the appropriateness or inappropriateness of his choices through thoughts such as, "I should have worn a heavier coat," or "I'm glad I wore my jeans." One is rarely aware that he has been problem solving because it is often an automatic and repetitive mental activity.

Nurses use problem solving strategies continuously, usually without much awareness. But the fact that nurses all know how to problem solve does not mean that they cannot learn to do so more effectively. Of course, all of the actions nurses take are not based on the problem solving process. Some actions one takes may be based on the use of habitual action. For example, one may repeatedly have a specific breakfast due to habit although there are other options available. This use of routine solutions can occur in nursing when the nurse reacts automatically to a situation with an habitual action. For example:

> An aide told the nurse that Ms. Rogers was complaining of pain. The nurse prepared Ms. Rogers' pain medication and administered it to her without any further assessment or additional reflection on the alternatives. The action was routine—any patient complaining of pain received a pain medication if available.

The additional dimensions in this situation which the nurse could have explored are numerous and well known to most nurses.

Another course of action may be to dismiss or ignore opportunities for problem solving. In this mode one does not use a routine solution but rather fails to notice the necessity to decide. For example, one may ignore the weather outside in the morning and end up wearing inappropriate clothing. Ignoring problems can happen in nursing situations.

> Jody, who had a newly applied cast, complained of a peculiar numb sensation in her fingers. The nurse ignored her comments. Later, it was discovered that Jody's cast was too tight and some nerve damage had occurred.

Obviously, applying routine solutions or ignoring problems can limit the effectiveness of nursing action. The quality of nursing practice might be elevated and the level of wellness of the patients and families the nurse serves be improved if nurses learned to consciously and consistently apply the problem solving process to the situations they encounter. The nurse can learn to do this by learning more effective problem solving techniques, becoming more consciously aware of opportunities to problem solve, and by learning how to substitute problem solving behavior for automatic behavior.

## AN OVERVIEW OF THE PROBLEM SOLVING PROCESS

The problem solving process as used in nursing is adapted from the scientific method but it has some distinctive characteristics of its own and it continues to be refined and embellished. Although the phases of the process are in reality practically inseparable, they can be considered separately for the purposes of analysis. Briefly they are:

1. Assessment: Problems are identified and defined.
2. Planning: Actions to alter the problems are determined.
3. Intervention: Actions are carried out.
4. Evaluation: The effectiveness of the process is determined and further action delineated.

Each of these phases will be examined in more detail later.

The use of a systematic process to guide action is not unique to nursing. For example, the physician uses the scientific method in a slightly different way with a different focus and with different terminology. Consider the following steps used by the physician as an example of how other disciplines utilize the problem solving process.

1. A history, physical examination, and possibly diagnostic tests are obtained and a diagnosis established.
2. A medical plan of care is determined which may include dietary prescriptions, medications, surgical intervention, changes in activity, and so forth.
3. The medical plan of care is implemented.
4. Progress is assessed through the use of followup examinations and possibly repeated tests; a revision of the plan is done if necessary.

Systems analysis is recently receiving considerable attention by many disciplines. Notice these components of a system and their relatedness to the steps of assessment, planning, intervention, and evaluation.

1. Input: receiving phase concerned with storing and absorbing information, energy, or material.
2. Thruput: a processing phase concerned with changing input into output.
3. Output: an outcome phase concerned with producing a result or product.
4. Feedback: a monitoring phase concerned with evaluation and regulation to guarantee appropriate results. Feedback then can become part of input to begin the system again.[23]

## THE PHASES OF THE PROBLEM SOLVING PROCESS

The steps in each phase of the problem solving process will be examined individually although one must remember that in practice this amount of specificity may not be desirable or feasible.

## Assessment

The specific steps which can occur in the assessment phase are as follows:

1. Data are collected about the patient or family.
2. The data are analyzed for the presence of suspected problems.
3. Specific data are collected to reject or validate the presence of each possible problem.
4. Problems are organized into nursing diagnoses.
5. Resources of the patient or family are identified from the data.

### Data Are Collected About the Patient or Family

The data collection step begins the moment the nurse has the initial contact with an individual or family and continues as long as the relationship continues. Much of the data the nurse collects will come directly from the patient or family. This requires that the nurse have expertise in observation, communication, interview skills, and in relationship skills. The amount of data she receives can be very much proportional to the trust the patient feels in her.[6] Initially it is helpful if the nurse performs a focused assessment in which she enters the situation specifically to look for certain pieces of data. It is rarely profitable to enter a situation just to "see what you can see." This focused assessment may involve looking at data from a large area or from a very limited area. For example, a nurse may enter a home to assess how well a newly diagnosed elderly male diabetic is adapting to his situation in general or to assess only how he is doing with insulin injections.

Considerable attention is being given to the area of focused comprehensive assessment in nursing. Many nursing assessment guides have appeared in the literature which delineate comprehensive nursing data to be collected on patients.[16,17,24] Most of these guides are designed to be used on the first contact with a patient. While these guides vary they focus on collecting broad information from which the nurse can delineate physical, emotional, and social needs as related to nursing. Some of the areas usually covered include appearance, personal identification data, and personal preferences related to activities of daily living such as diet, hygiene, rest, elimination, and mobility. Data are usually included on the meaning of illness and treatment, social and cultural factors, and possibly an assessment of functional abilities. Other areas covered may be significant religious preferences, teaching needs, orientation, medications taken, and physical needs of significance. If the patient is a child, information is often included in addition on what activities the child can perform for himself, his nickname, common words in his vocabulary, and so forth.[4,13,18,23,24] The nursing assessment is not a selected rehash of the physician's history but rather a tool with a different focus—that of uncovering nursing information and not necessarily medical information.

The use of a prepared assessment guide may be possible in some situations. Often nurses who are concerned with a common patient population can prepare an assessment guide specifically to focus on gathering the data they need. For example, the community health nurses in one agency prepared an assessment guide to use on visits to prenatal patients which facilitated comprehensive collection of data about the progression of the pregnancy and also allowed space for specific assessment topics to be added for each patient as needed.

The use of focused comprehensive assessment guides has many advantages. First, they help to insure that the assessment will be comprehensive and that areas will not be forgotten. If the nurse collecting the data is skilled at interviewing, the collection of data may help to make the patient believe that the nurse is interested in him. The use of a prepared guide which can be placed with the patient's permanent record so that it can be shared with others helps to communicate information and avoid repetitious collection of identical data by others. Lastly, an assessment guide can provide a data base to which later observations can be compared.

Unfortunately, there is unlikely to ever be one specific nursing assessment guide which will be useful for all nurses in all situations. Consider the different types of data needed by a school nurse in a high school, a nurse in a newborn intensive care nursery, and a nurse working with elderly nursing home patients. A nurse may need to develop her own assessment guide or adapt an existing one to her needs. It should:

1. Be relevant to the population she works with.
2. Include material which will identify not only problems but also resources.
3. Allow for rapid assessment of many areas in general and then more detailed assessment of a specific area in particular when warranted.
4. Provide for the collection of data about all relevant aspects such as physical, social, and emotional needs and resources.
5. Allow for the identification of possible problems as well as those already in existence or resolved.
6. Guard against observer's bias as much as possible because one tends to see what he expects to see based on cultural background, education, and experience.[12]

For any one contact with a patient or family the nurse will improve her collection of data if she plans ahead the particular topics she wishes to assess. For example:

A school nurse was preparing to see a child's mother. The child was repeatedly inattentive in class, listless, and not achieving at her potential level. The nurse jotted down the following topics she hoped to obtain information on:
   Rest and exercise child receives at home.
   Diet eaten by child at home.
   Behavior of child at home.
   History of present behavior.
   Past medical history.
   Recent medical care.
   Relationship of child to family members.

Other sources of data exist in addition to the patient and family. The nurse may obtain data from other nurses, other health team members, records, and other individuals such as friends, relatives, or neighbors.

Developing skill at data collection requires practice. The nurse will need to use several senses—hearing, sight, smell, and touch—appropriately. For example, with a patient with a possible wound infection she may hear what the patient says, see how the wound appears, smell any relevant odors, and feel the skin around the wound with regard to temperature and consistency.

It is especially important for the nurse to distinguish between subjective and objective observations. Objective observations are measurable and can be readily confirmed by another observer.[14] They are concerned with reality.[12] For example, a blood pressure reading is measurable and another nurse can duplicate the observation with little chance of much difference in data. Subjective observations are not measurable usually and are specific to only the person experiencing the data.[14] They concern the thoughts and feelings of another.[12] Pain, for example, is subjective. The nurse observing a patient who says he is experiencing pain cannot exactly interpret the patient's behavior as that consistent with pain, measure the pain, or even know if it is reality. Therefore, observations reported by the patient which cannot be objectively confirmed are considered subjective. Examples of things which patients may report which are subjective include pain, itching, nausea, shame, discouragement, fear, and bitterness to list only a few. Similarly, the nurse is making a subjective observation when she draws a conclusion about a patient's behavior which is not measurable or readily observable by another. Examples include stating that a patient is anxious, depressed, uncomfortable, restless, or shy. Obviously, objective observations provide a much stronger foundation for problem solving than subjective ones. Unfortunately, however, as much of nursing practice focuses on subjective states of patients and families, nurses do make and need to make subjective observations. The nurse may use three safeguards when dealing with subjective data:

1. She can attempt to correlate the subjective information provided by a patient with objective data. For example, if a patient comments that he has pain, does his behavior evidence those objective behaviors commonly associated with pain?
2. She can validate the subjective interpretations she makes with patients and families if appropriate. For example, if a patient seems depressed to her, she can ask him if he is.
3. She can attempt to record her observations in objective terms if possible and avoid subjective ones as much as possible. A different meaning may later emerge if she allows herself this freedom. For example, a nurse thought that a patient was anxious. She avoided recording this and instead described in her notes the behavior she was seeing—tense facial expression, quick reactions, increased muscle tone, etc. Later on reviewing her data she realized that the patient might instead be experiencing pain which he later validated.

It should be stated that the knowledge base of the nurse is very important because often it affects her observations.[13,30] For example, a nurse who is a knowledgeable about cystic fibrosis and its medical treatment is likely to make more specific and relevant observations when admitting a child with cystic fibrosis to a pediatric unit and about the family dynamics than a nurse who has little knowledge about the condition. Similarly, a community health nurse who understands toxemia of pregnancy may make more careful observations than one who remembers little about it. It behooves the nurse to strive continuously to increase her knowledge in all areas of nursing because assessment is such a vitally important part of practice.

## Data Are Analyzed for the Presence of Suspected Problems

The next step in the assessment phase of the problem solving process involves analyzing the data the nurse has collected for possible patient or family problems. Problems are events, conditions, or situations which obstruct or interfere with an individual's or family's functioning and possibly with their wellness. For example, the loss of a job by the principal wage earner in a family may lead to considerable changes in a family and possibly a change in health status. Thus unemployment in this situation is a problem with many manifestations. A smashed finger can also be a problem in that it interferes with functioning. Problem identification is a very challenging aspect of the process. Data can be analyzed in several fashions to determine possible problems.

The nurse might begin by listing the possible problems which were presented by the patient or family members. These possible problems may be in various states of refinement varying from well defined to vague. These possible problems should receive careful attention from the nurse because they represent the concerns and perceptions of the persons she serves.

Next the nurse can look for inconsistencies in the data between what was observed in the situation and what is normal which will illustrate problem areas. A 2-year-old child who was observed to neither walk nor feed himself is inconsistent with the normal growth and development of a 2-year-old child. A reddened, hot, painful, swollen incision with thick gray drainage is not consistent with the normal appearance of an incision five days postoperatively. A mother who lays her newborn baby in precarious positions, calls the baby "it," and holds the baby as little as possible is evidencing behavior which is not consistent with the normal behavior of new mothers. The nurse should list any inconsistencies she discovers as possible problems. For example, in the instances mentioned, a nurse might have listed as possible problems "questionable normal growth and development," "possible infected incision," or "potential failure of maternal-infant bonding."

Another way to uncover problems involves grouping relevant pieces of data together. While each piece of data is important, there are often some pieces of information which seem especially significant to the nurse but the meaning may not become clear until some of them are checked for association. One nurse pulled out from her assessment the following pieces of information about a young mother she was working with:

1. Mother states she is continuously fatigued.
2. Husband works two jobs and sleeps most of the time he is home.
3. Mother is raising four young children—two of her own and two of her sister's.
4. Mother states she has no outside activities away from home except shopping and church occasionally.

From the grouping of these observations, the nurse listed as a possible problem "possible social isolation from other adults." The nurse's ability to synthesize relevant cues into possible problems is, of course, highly influenced by her knowledge base, her interests, and her cognitive abilities. The skills needed are developed by study and practice. Assigning meaning to pieces of information is referred to as inferring.[13]

Possible problems may also be discovered by looking for data which do not exist. In this mode, one can search for the lack of expected pieces of information.[27] For example:

Mr. Welch had been found accidentally to have suffered a mild unnoticed myocardial infarct and was hospitalized for a few days for further evaluation. The nurse caring for Mr. Welch realized as she was analyzing her assessment data that several behaviors typical of young men who were in Mr. Welch's situation were absent in Mr. Welch's behavior such as anxiety, depression, and self-restriction of activity. Thus, the nurse considered "denial of illness" as a possible problem.

Another area of concern involves determining possible potential problems. The nurse looks for indications which she associates with the possibility of future problems. The association of some pieces of data with a potential problem is very automatic in some cases. For example, most nurses working with a young mother expecting her second child would automatically identify sibling rivalry of the first child as a potential problem to be listed. Other indications are less obvious and require more thought.

Another source of possible problems for the nurse to consider involves identifying expected problems. Rarely do individuals have any particular problem without its causing other problems. For example, rarely does one have a physical problem without an accompanying emotional component, or an emotional problem without a physical component.[30] For this reason, the nurse looks for problems which will logically relate to other problems. For example, a female patient having a mastectomy would be expected to possibly have a problem related to change in self-concept. A young unmarried teenage girl who is in the early months of an unplanned pregnancy would be expected to possibly have a problem with her parents' acceptance of the pregnancy. One does not know if these problems do in fact exist until further action is taken but they are good bets as possible problems.

Still another way to discover possible problems is for the nurse to look at her own actions and feelings in the patient situation. She may consider what she is doing in relation to the patient or family.[26] She reflects on what the patient asks for most often and what takes up most of her time with the patient or family. In addition she considers how she reacts to the patient. For example, if she feels anxious or depressed after being with the patient, the patient may be experiencing these emotions covertly and may be communicating them to her. This exploration of her own feelings and reactions may alert her to covert problems of significance.

During this stage, the nurse looks for facts and objective truths in order to identify possible problems but there is also a place for the use of her intuitive perceptions. This intuitive ability is often described by nurses in statements such as, "I don't know why but I have this feeling that there is something wrong in the relationship between this mother and her child." Often one's intuition is based on actual cues he has perceived but which were of such insignificance as to not be consciously noticed. These are referred to as subliminal cues.[13] One's intuition can be used to advantage as a starting point for more data collection. The nurse does this by asking herself, "What have I seen which has led to this feeling?" Intuitively perceived possible problems, therefore, deserve further consideration. However, one should be hesitant to rely on the use of intuition alone in problem solving.

In summary, possible problems are identified by the patient and family, by analyzing the data for inconsistencies, by grouping relevant pieces of information, by looking for the absence of expected information, by checking for information which indicates the possibility of potential future problems, by listing expected predictable problems, by reflecting on one's reactions to the patient, and by searching for intuitive perceptions.

## Specific Data Are Collected to Reject or Validate the Presence of Each Possible Problem

After the nurse has listed all suspected problems, she can begin to prove or disprove each problem. The physician also engages in this stage of problem solving. It is referred to in medicine as ruling out or ruling in medical impressions before forming a diagnosis. While the nurse engaged in a comprehensive assessment before, the data collected now will be more problem specific.[27] This phase is best carried out after some initial planning is done by the nurse in which she identifies the data she now needs. Some problems can be validated quickly. Others require more involved efforts.

Several methods can be used to validate or negate possible problems. One method is further observation.

> A school nurse was approached by two teachers because of the erratic behavior of one teenage girl. From the information the nurse collected, she suspected the possibility of some form of substance abuse. Before taking any further action, she reviewed the literature and collected a list of criteria to be used in further evaluating the girl's behavior and appearance. With this information in mind, she planned several observation sessions.

In other instances, the patient and family can confirm or negate certain possible problems.

> One nurse working with a Southern family who had moved to a Northern industrial area was very concerned with the dynamics between the young mother and father. By the nurse's standards, the husband's behavior was irresponsible, self-centered, and neglectful of the wife and children. She suspected that the mother was very dissatisfied with the marriage. On talking with the mother to validate the problem, she was surprised to learn that the mother considered her mate to be nearly an ideal husband and father and believed she was much more fortunate to have her husband than the husbands of many of her friends.

Of course, there are situations in which a legitimate problem does exist which the nurse should consider even though the patient remains unaware of it. But the nurse should remember the old surgical axiom, "It is difficult to improve the asymptomatic patient."

Other possible problems may only be validated or negated by referring to others. For example, a nurse may believe that a certain change is occurring in a patient's physical condition which requires expertise outside the realm of nursing. She can report her assessment to the appropriate resource, the physician, for confirmation.

It is possible that the nurse may find only partial support, in which case she must make a judgment as to whether or not the problem exists based on the evidence she has and proceed from there. All problems which have been confirmed can be noted in a problem list which is useful for later reference.

It should be mentioned that the nurse may uncover problems which are not hers to solve. Nurses may never become masters in specific recognized areas until they decide that they are not masters of everything. Problems which are within the realm of another discipline should be referred if possible.[22] Learning what problems one is capable of solving and what problems one is not is a continual process.

## Problems Are Organized into a Nursing Diagnosis

Although there has been much written about the area of nursing diagnosis, varying opinions persist about what it is. A nursing diagnosis is actually similar to an hypothesis. An hypothesis can be defined as an educated guess, and this is also true of a nursing diagnosis because it represents the nurse's hunch as to what is occurring in a specific situation. Diagnosing is the process which results in a summarization of the problems identified by the assessment into a concise statement or statements as a nursing diagnosis. The diagnosis indicates the situations related to the patient or family which require nursing action.[9]

It may be appropriate to define a nursing diagnosis by first exploring what it is not. First of all, it is not synonymous with the medical diagnosis, although the medical diagnosis may be part of the nursing diagnosis. The nursing diagnosis is more likely determined by the entire needs of the patient and not necessarily just the physical condition.[31] The nursing diagnosis is not likely to be a medical test or a medical treatment. Neither is it the presence of an appliance or piece of equipment. Furthermore, it is usually not useful to resort to one word conceptual labels such as "hostility" or "disoriented" as these do not provide sufficient definition or information about the assessment.[13] Finally, a nursing diagnosis does not state a specific nursing action.[11]

A nursing diagnosis can reflect either the problems of the patient or family which come under the responsibility of the nurse as delegated to her by medicine or be related to her independent areas of practice. It is understandable that there will likely be considerable overlap between nursing diagnoses and the concerns of other health team members.[22] These other health team members might be social workers, physicians, dieticians, psychiatrists, child life workers, or others.

Sufficient information should be given in the statement of the diagnosis to indicate as many of the following as possible and appropriate:

1. The nature of the nursing problem.
2. The possible cause of the problem if known and if relevant.
3. The extent of the problem.
4. How the problem is affecting the patient or family.
5. How long the problem has existed.
6. The symptoms of the problem.

Not all of these are necessary or possible in every situation. One may not know the cause of a situation and it may not even be relevant. For example, a mother was grieving over a stillbirth. The nursing problem was the mother's grief and not the cause of the stillbirth. The nursing diagnosis should be fitted specifically to each patient and family but not so general as to fit several other patients.

It is essential that nursing diagnoses be stated in terms which are recognizable by other nurses and subject to few interpretations. This helps to insure that others who contact the patient or family will logically and accurately comprehend the diagnosis. Thus, nursing diagnoses should be based on the presence of certain understood criteria or symptoms which are generally accepted by others as relevant to the diagnosis.[11]

Below are some examples of nursing diagnoses which have been stated by nurses in various settings. These illustrate that there is no one way a nursing diagnosis must be stated.

1. Acute severe anxiety due to recent knowledge of a possible threatening fatal illness—breast cancer.
2. Mild depression possibly caused by a grossly infected abdominal incision which the patient fears may cause prolonged hospitalization and loss of income.
3. Persistent marital conflict over wife's desire to limit family size and husband's reluctance to use birth control measure resulting in a strain in sexual relations.
4. Fatigue and irritability possibly due to chronic iron deficiency anemia.
5. Recent complete immobility due to application of a body cast.

For any one patient or family the nurse may need to state more than one diagnosis depending on the extent of problems present.

Being able to arrive at a nursing diagnosis is an ability important to the future of nursing practice. When nurses are able to state clearly and concisely their impressions regarding a patient situation based on an analysis of evidence, they are communicating to others that nursing has a legitimate body of knowledge, area of practice, and focus for functioning.

Diagnostic categories and syndromes may eventually be developed which standardize diagnoses.[10]

## Resources of the Patient or Family Are Identified

Another important but often overlooked aspect of assessment involves listing the resources of the patient or family. Resources can be thought of as abilities, strengths, supports, materials, and so forth. The nurse identifies resources in much the same ways as she identifies problems. The patient is a particularly important source of information on resources. The listing of resources is invaluable when the nurse begins the planning phase of the problem solving process as will be seen.

The resources one nurse identified, related to an elderly couple she cared for, are described below:

1.  Husband and wife communicate to each other clearly.
2.  Adequate financial resources are available.
3.  The couple have many friends and neighbors with whom they socialize frequently.
4.  Both husband and wife are concerned with their health and eat sensibly and take walks almost every day for exercise.

Identifying resources is helpful in reminding the nurse to focus on more than just problems.

The skills needed by the nurse in the assessment stage may involve perception, observation, communication, analysis, synthesis, inference, interpretation, and diagnosis.[6,12,20,30] Each step in this phase is highly dependent for success on the presence and use of cognitive knowledge by the nurse. This point cannot be overemphasized.

In a sense, the assessment phase of the problem solving process is never finished but continues as long as the patient interaction does. However, there is usually a point where for one reason or another the nurse has identified a problem and proceeds to the planning phase. Further data may later alter her assessment, however.

It should not be forgotten that the patient and family members are not merely passively providing information to the nurse at this stage but are themselves assessing the nurse— how she interacts, communicates, and reacts.[27] Therefore, it should be stressed that this phase of the problem solving process also frequently serves as the beginning phase of the helping relationship and the nurse must interrelate her action in these two areas.

Mistakes which can be made at this point which lead to an inadequate or inaccurate assessment include failure to include all relevant data, interpreting the data incorrectly, supplying an incorrect meaning to the data, allowing biases to influence collection and interpretation of information, and improperly assuming or dismissing the significance of an aspect of the situation.[3,14]

At this point before proceeding to the planning phase, the nurse can in general evaluate the appropriateness of the assessment phase. She could be particularly interested in determining whether the nursing diagnosis she has made is logical and appropriate, given the raw data she began with, and whether all important discrepancies in the data are accounted for.

In summary, the assessment phase of the nursing process usually begins with the collection of a focused comprehensive assessment and continues with the nurse examining all the data she has available, identifying all the possible problems, validating or negating the presence of each problem, and then summarizing all of her information into the statement of a nursing diagnosis which defines what she has determined. Lastly, the strengths of the patient or family are determined and listed.

## Planning

The planning phase of the problem solving process begins after the assessment is completed or enough data has been collected and analyzed to warrant proceedings. It involves the following steps.

1. Any needs for nursing action are determined.
2. Priorities for nursing action are established.
3. The objectives of nursing action are stated.
4. Possible actions are listed and evaluated.
5. Ways to implement the selected actions are developed.

### Any Needs for Nursing Action Are Determined by Correlating Problems with Resources

The first step in the planning phase is to determine if nursing action is needed for any given problem. It does not necessarily follow that if the patient or family has a problem, nursing intervention is needed. Nor is it true that major problems need intervention while minor ones do not.

The following are all possible decisions:

1. No problems exist and, therefore, no nursing intervention is needed.
2. A major or minor problem exists but nursing intervention is not needed.
   a. The patient or family has the resources to adequately cope with the problem.
   b. The problem is likely to resolve itself without outside intervention.
   c. The problem is not appropriate for nursing intervention and other resources should be sought.
3. A major problem exists and nursing intervention is needed.
   a. The resources of the family appear inadequate to resolve the problem.
   b. The family is coping well presently but their resources are likely to be eventually depleted.
   c. The patient and family are unaware of or denying the problem.
   d. The problem is likely to be prolonged and permanent without intervention.
4. A minor problem exists and nursing intervention is needed.
   a. The resources of the family are likely to be depleted in the future and coping reduced.
   b. The problem is likely to become more significant in the future.[13,30]

The nurse arrives at her decision of whether or not to plan intervention by looking critically at the problem, the resources of the family, and a judgment about what may happen to both in the future.

Nancy was an unwed mother who was keeping her newborn infant. The nurse working with Nancy in the postpartum unit wondered whether further intervention was needed with Nancy in the form of a community visiting nurse referral. To make her decision she considered Nancy's health status, age, maturity, ability to seek out help, knowledge of child care, financial resources, supportive relationships, growth and developmental tasks, and future goals. She also considered the baby's health status and behavioral characteristics. Lastly, the nurse reflected on what might happen to both the problems typically associated with being a single mother and Nancy's and the baby's resources in the future. In Nancy's particular situation, the nurse decided that a referral was not needed.

A careful consideration of this step can increase the efficiency of nursing care delivery by reducing instances in which a nurse exerts a large amount of energy and expense in situations where intervention is not needed and also reducing the neglect of situations where intervention was needed but not recognized.

Learning to appropriately weigh the significance of problems against the resources available to the patient or family, and analyzing the likely development of both in the future, is not an automatically acquired ability but can be developed through experience and study.

## Priorities for Action Are Established

In many situations the nurse will identify several problems which require nursing intervention. She must determine where to begin because one cannot usually focus on many problems at once. Thus, establishing which problems have priority is important. The way to start is usually by considering what the patient or family believes to be of the most importance. If the patient, family, and the nurse are focusing their efforts in the same direction, a successful resolution of the problem is more likely than if they are going in opposite directions. The health care system has often been accused of overlooking the necessity of determining the patient's priorities when he seeks health care.

> A mother brought her five-year-old daughter to a community clinic because she was continuously enuretic at night. The physician wanted to remove the child's adenoids, the nurse wanted to test the child's hearing, the dentist wanted to clean the child's teeth, the dietician wanted to put the child on a diet high in iron, and the psychologist wanted to do some psychological testing. After several hours of being sent from one person to another, the mother abruptly left and the professionals individually shook their heads over her unconcern for her child's problems.

In addition, when the nurse starts with what the patient feels is of importance to him, she is likely to gain his confidence. Often when his priority is met, she may then be able to focus the patient on what she believes is significant. It should be mentioned that the patient or family may need some information from the nurse before they are adequately prepared to establish priorities.[14] For example, the patient may not realize the significance of a situation until the nurse has provided more information. And there are some situations in which the nurse must determine the priority without input from the patient or family. This might be experienced with an unconscious patient, for example. But generally the patient and family are the most appropriate sources of information on priorities.

As another guide to determining priorities, the nurse might wish to refer to the "Hierarchy of Needs" as developed by Abraham Maslow.[15] Inherent in this hierarchy is the belief that needs can be arranged into classifications and listed in order with the most fundamental needs at the base of the hierarchy and progressing to the most esthetic human needs at the highest point of the hierarchy. This is illustrated in Figure 3-1. The philosophy of the hierarchy suggests that the needs in any particular level must be met with some satisfaction before the needs at the next higher level can be met. In this approach one would rate the priority of the most basic biologic needs highest and the most esthetic needs lowest. Using this scheme, physiologic level needs usually have priority only when they are such that they are threatening or crucial to the survival of an individual.[30] Consider the following use of the hierarchy.

A community health nurse working with the Johansen family developed three nursing diagnoses after a

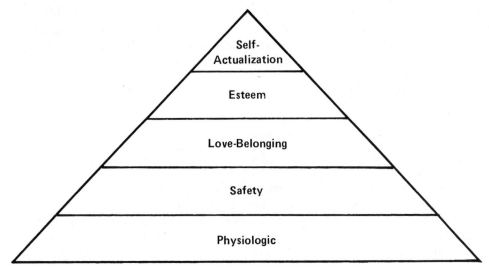

**Figure 3-1.** Maslow's Hierarchy of Needs. (Adapted from Maslow, A. H.: *Motivation and Personality.* Harper and Row, New York, 1954.)

thorough assessment. Using Maslow's hierarchy he arranged them in this order with the diagnosis with the greatest priority first:
1. Failure of the Johansen infant to receive adequate nutrition because his parents are unaware of his needs and he has a weak suck reflex (physiologic level).
2. Structural and electrical hazards in the apartment in which the Johansens live (safety level).
3. Low self-esteem because Ms. Johnsen believes she is failing as a mother due to the fact that her infant is underweight (esteem level).

Referring to the hierarchy may provide a useful starting point for determining priorities but the nurse must recognize that there will be occasions when she must independently make a judgment based on what she interprets to be of utmost importance irrespective of the hierarchy. For example, the nurse working with the Johansen family might have decided the mother's lack of self-esteem was of higher priority because it was reflected in her inability to adequately feed her baby. He would then focus on that problem initially. In this situation, the nurse's initial focus on how to better feed the baby might have made the mother feel even more inadequate.

After priorities are determined, the nurse must usually proceed to problem solve with those diagnoses which are of high priority and reserve those with lower priority for later consideration.

## The Objectives of Nursing Action Are Stated

After selecting the problem with top priority, the nurse establishes objectives to guide the planning. It is helpful to state long term and short term objectives. The long term objectives are usually global and general as compared to the short term objectives. They can be determined by asking, "What should occur after the planned intervention?" For example, the nurse working with the Johansen family stated the following long term objective:

Ms. Johansen will believe that she is an adequate mother.

It is obvious that such a general statement alone is not sufficient to guide the planning of the intervention to be undertaken. More specific, observable, short term objectives are needed. These objectives can be determined by asking, "What will occur if the long term objective is approached or reached?" The short term objectives should be stated in terms of the individual concerned and behaviorally. The nurse in the example given previously stated these short term objectives among others.

> Ms. Johansen will be able to:
> Express satisfaction in how she functions as a mother.
> Give examples of situations with her child in which she believed she functioned appropriately.
> Describe several abilities she has which she believes are related to being an adequate mother.

In some situations, more concrete objectives can be stated.

In the problem solving process, the short term objectives will be used again in the evaluation phase to judge the success of the nursing intervention which was undertaken. For this reason, short term objectives are sometimes referred to as "outcome criteria" because they serve as criteria against which to judge the outcomes of the nursing care given.

Properly stated objectives serve to keep the process focused appropriately. If the objectives are defined too narrowly, the possibilities for intervention may be reduced. For example, one nurse had identified, with a working mother of several very busy teenagers, that a problem existed in providing appropriate well rounded meals for them given their particular tastes, hectic schedules, and the mother's time limitations for shopping, meal planning, and preparation. Extensive snacking, eating out in fast food restaurants, and meals on the run were frequent. When an objective was stated as "The mother will be able to prepare and the children will eat one complete meal each evening" not much progress was made. When a different and broader view was taken of the situation, the objective became, "Each child will have at least one meal each day which contains items from the four basic food groups." Many more options were then apparent and the nurse and mother were then eventually successful in reaching this goal. Another example illustrates this point.

> Mr. Willis was a patient who was to be confined to his home for a lengthy period of recuperation. The nurse who was concerned with the effects of immobility could have stated the objective as, "Ms. Willis will get Mr. Willis out of bed twice each day." In this particular situation, this would have been nearly impossible due to Mr. Willis' size and Ms. Willis' physical limitations. Instead the nurse stated the objective as, "Mr. Willis will not develop any complications associated with immobility." She and Ms. Willis were able to plan many actions towards meeting this objective.

A narrowed objective usually results when one prematurely arrives at a solution to a problem and then uses the solution as the objective. Thus a problem such as "learning prenatal care" is seen as "must attend prenatal classes at General Hospital."

On the other hand, objectives which are too general do not provide adequate direction or reliable evaluation criteria. For example, "Mr. Davis will understand and follow his low sodium diet" is not as helpful for planning or evaluation as objectives such as, "Mr. Davis will keep a log of his food and drink intake for three days and analyze the sodium content."

The nurse may occasionally encounter a situation in which there appear to be only short term goals and no apparent long term objectives. It is worthwhile to search for the long term element inherent in this situation because it may reflect an underlying problem of significance.[30] For example:

> A young woman came to the planned parenthood clinic frequently with vaginitis. Each time, the situation

was seen as a short term situation. One nurse practitioner looked more closely at the situation and proposed a long term objective related to preventing vaginitis as well as treating the current episode.

More information on writing objectives is found in the chapter on the teaching process.

## Possible Actions Are Listed and Evaluated

After the objectives have been developed the nurse determines possible actions to reach the objectives. One valuable way to develop possible actions is by the use of creative or divergent thinking.

Creativity is a concept often misunderstood. It is often assumed that being "creative" is synonymous with engaging in craft or art activities. Actually creativity can be defined as the ability to produce a product which is novel and unusual.[21] Creativity can apply to any individual who is open to what she is experiencing, seeks self-evaluation vs. other-evaluation, and who has the ability to rearrange, flex, reconstruct, or invent elements of a situation.[21] The opposite of creative thinking involves inflexibility, using patterned solutions, having a narrowed perspective, and developing "hardening of the categories." Being creative is not necessarily related to being highly intelligent.[2] Nor does the pursuit of knowledge in the traditional educational process guarantee that one will automatically become more creative. In fact, exposure to the educational system may in some respects decrease creativity.

A nurse who wishes to become creative in planning nursing care may be helped to practice creativity by learning to search for imaginative and unusual ways to think about a problem. Contact with others who are facilitative rather than evaluative can help to increase creative thinking. This may mean avoiding others who "put down" new or divergent ideas. An individual can practice creativity by engaging in cognitive situations where she decides on an unusual solution and then expands on it in detail. Also, one can practice looking for numerous possible options rather than immediate solutions. This helps to reduce prematurely closing off thinking.[13]

How one approaches a problem can increase or decrease creative thinking. Thinking that one knows all of the answers may inhibit seeing a new solution. Searching for more information may expand one's thinking and stimulate new ideas.

Therefore, in order to use one's creative potential to plan nursing actions, it is helpful to begin by first thinking of as many solutions in the form of actions as possible without regard to their actual appropriateness. This freedom allows the creation of novel and unusual solutions. Nursing in some situations is not noted for unlimited creativity.

The patient and family are often an excellent source of possible actions. They should be encouraged to suggest and elaborate on solutions. Their ideas have merit and should be given the utmost consideration in that they are likely to know what will work because they know the situation best. They may also think of creative solutions because their thinking is not limited by nursing routine.

Another technique to help generate solutions is reframing. This involves trying to see the situation from another perspective. First, one determines what preconceived ideas one has about the situation and then how other specific persons might view the situation.[7] An example of reframing is given below.

Missy was young, pregnant, and unwed. The school nurse working with her became increasingly frustrated over Missy's attempts to deny her pregnancy, her unconcern for prenatal care, and her plans to keep her baby and expect her mother to care for the baby. After several weeks of failure with problem solving, the nurse tried reframing. She first realized that she had many biases about how Missy and her mother should be acting in the current situation and listed these. Next she wrote down how the problem might be seen from Missy's viewpoint and her mother's viewpoint. Based on this information, she developed some new actions which eventually were more successful.

Another source of possible nursing actions to lead to the objectives identified involves reproductive problem solving. This requires searching for solutions which have worked in the past in a like or similar problem.[1] Nursing and medical textbooks and journals often contain vast information on actions believed to be successful in specific problems. For example, if a patient has a fever, searching through written information will usually provide a quick and reliable list of possible nursing actions for reducing the fever. Research papers often provide even more reliable problem solutions which may be applicable. Nurses in a specific situation may keep for reference nursing actions for specific problems of a particular patient or family. This can save countless hours of trial and error attempts at solving a problem. Other sources of information are individuals who have gained knowledge or expertise in a particular area.

## Problem Solving Strategies

Another helpful way to generate possible nursing actions may be to refer to a list of problem solving strategies and to determine if there are any new actions suggested by the strategy. The strategies and an example of each are as follows:

1. *Removing the cause of the problem.* If the cause is known, it may be possible to remove it.
   An infected surgical suture accidentally left in an incision was causing an abscess. The nurse removed it.
2. *Minimizing the cause of the problem.* In many situations the cause cannot be eliminated but its effects may be minimized.
   A teenager was troubled and embarrassed by acne. Medical treatment was not able to completely cure the acne. The nurse working with the teenager uncovered several practices which were aggravating the acne. When these were eliminated, the condition was less obvious.
3. *Aiding physiological healing processes.* Often problems can be helped by nursing actions which promote the body's own reparative mechanisms.
   Ms. Wilcox had a painful inflamed episiotomy incision. The nurse used her knowledge of the healing process to plan several measures which helped reduce discomfort as they promoted healing.
4. *Changing or altering the environment.* In some situations, an unfavorable environment can influence a problem. Changing or altering the environment may lead to an improvement.
   Johnny was a hyperactive child who was in the third grade. Although he was on regular medication, his behavior in the classroom disrupted the other students and the teacher frequently. When the school nurse was consulted, she observed in the room for several sessions and then proposed changes in the classroom to reduce the stimulation Johnny was receiving. His behavior did improve.
5. *Altering the sequence of events.* A possible solution to a problem may occur when events in the situation are rearranged.
   Ms. Wheeler was frequently nagging and scolding her children to get them dressed and off to school on time. A nurse suggested she require that all children be fully dressed with coats and books laid out by the door before they could eat breakfast. The problem was quickly solved when the children experienced a few mornings in which they had hunger pangs before lunch time.
6. *Increasing adaptive capacities.* Often the nurse can provide help in the form of promoting her patient's ability to cope.
   Ms. Jacobson had just given birth to a child with Down's syndrome. The nurse visited frequently to listen and to provide support.
7. *Mobilizing resources in the environment.* Often valuable sources of help for a problem exist in the environment. The nurse can often bring the patient or family into contact with these resources or the resources into contact with the family.

A girl from a rural area talked to a nurse about information on birth control. She explained that she was sexually active and did not wish to become pregnant but was afraid to talk to the doctor in her small hometown. The nurse gave her a list of available resources in other more distant towns she could contact.

8. *Altering perceptions of the situation.* Some situations which seem like problems are not when viewed by a different perspective which the nurse may be able to provide.

Ms. Jones came to the community clinic asking for help with her 6-year-old son, Tommy. She described Tommy as bossy, quarrelsome, prone to excessive bragging, and profane. He cheated when he played games if he wasn't winning and resorted to name calling when frustrated by his friends. The nurse provided Ms. Jones with information on the normal behavior of 6-year-old children which corresponded exactly with the troublesome behaviors Tommy was exhibiting. Ms. Jones laughed when she read the information and commented that she guessed Tommy was just a normal little boy.

9. *Providing needed information.* Some problems the nurse encounters may be based on the patient's or family's lack of information. Providing the needed information may eliminate or reduce the problem.

The Sabols had a 4-year-old child with cerebral palsy and slight mental retardation. The mother wished to teach the child to feed himself and to begin bowel training, but all her efforts met with failure. The nurse suggested and demonstrated to the parents techniques of behavior modification and shaping which could be used with their son. After receiving this information the mother was more successful in the training efforts.

By using guidelines such as these problem solving strategies, additional nursing actions may be generated.

After possible actions have been listed, the next step is to evaluate each one. While creative and divergent thinking were needed to devise actions, critical thinking is needed in this step. For each action the nurse should consider:

1. What is the probability that this action would solve the problem?
2. What desired and undesired consequences would likely occur if this action were taken?
3. What expenditures of time, personnel, energy, and resources would be needed? Are these available and expendable?
4. Is this action in line with the philosophy, purposes, and values of this agency?
5. Is this action acceptable with the patient and family?

Those actions which seem appropriate after this scrutiny are then selected to be implemented. It should be remembered that deciding to do nothing at this point is a possible action.

## Ways to Implement the Selected Actions Are Developed

With the best possible solutions selected, the next step is to plan to implement the actions. The plan usually contains:

1. What will be done.
2. How it will be done.
3. Who will be involved.
4. When each step will be taken.

The patient or family will usually play a major role in planning the care. Plans may range from simple to complex. Often the nurse delegates aspects of the plan to others. Again at this point the special strengths and resources of the family should be incorporated into the plan.

The James family had just learned that their 4-year-old daughter had leukemia. They were strongly identified with a fundamentalist religious denomination. The nurse used this knowledge in planning by contacting their minister and providing a Bible at the child's bedside.

The plan developed is often referred to as a nursing care plan and written down where others involved with the patient or family can see it readily such as in a Kardex or posted at the bedside. Often the care plan contains a brief statement of the nursing diagnoses identified, the objectives, and the nursing actions to be taken. The actions to be taken may be referred to as nursing orders in some agencies and may be dated and signed by the nurse writing them. This is believed to reinforce that the actions are serious prescriptions and that those carrying them out are responsible for following them.[5]

The fact that there are frequently situations in health care institutions and agencies in which no legitimate care plans exist for patients may testify to the rarity of deliberative, in-depth problem solving in actual nursing practice. The presence of a care plan for a patient is essential to ensure recognition of nursing actions for a patient or family over and beyond those actions prescribed by physicians. Uniformity of care among professional and non-professional personnel, continuity of care, and the prevention of the casual omission of nursing activities would be facilitated in addition.[25] Care plans which are cross-filed by the patient's name and by the nursing diagnosis could provide a valuable source of information should the same patient later require nursing care again and should another patient or family have a similar diagnosis.

In conclusion, the planning phase of the problem solving process begins after the nursing diagnosis has been stated. It includes determining if intervention is needed given the strengths and resources of the patient and family, stating the objectives to be achieved, and selecting possible actions. It concludes with the statement of a plan to alter the diagnosis. The planning phase of the problem solving process requires relating to others plus skill in determining priorities, creative thinking, and critical thinking. Mistakes which can be made during this phase include ignoring significant problems, pursuing insignificant problems, overlooking high priority needs, stating objectives too broadly or stating narrow restrictive objectives, a lack of creativity in supplying solutions, jumping to a solution too quickly, failure to critically evaluate each solution, faulty planning, failure to communicate the plan, and losing sight of the nursing diagnosis as planning proceeds.

The knowledge base of the nurse based on study and experience is increasingly important in all steps in the planning phase. The nurse with in-depth knowledge of an area will be more adept at evaluating problems, determining priorities, establishing appropriate objectives, generating and evaluating solutions, and planning than will be a nurse who does not understand the variables she is dealing with.

Before proceeding to the next phase, it is useful to first evaluate in general the planning phase in terms of how it correlated with the nursing diagnosis. The nurse does this by asking:

1. Does the plan I have developed appear exactly related to the nursing diagnosis I began with?
2. Can I predict that the plan is likely to work?
3. Is the plan reasonable in this situation?

## Intervention

The intervention phase begins after the plan is formulated and encompasses all those activities called for in the plan plus the collection of relevant evaluative data. How long intervention lasts is dependent on the situation and the objectives. Usually intervention is undertaken until the objectives are accomplished or until it becomes evident that the objectives are not being reached.

Once the plan is put into effect, the nurse does not merely sit back and wait. She has many plan maintenance chores. If she is the one carrying out the plan, she continually evaluates what she is doing and the responses that are occurring. If the patient or family or other health personnel are involved, she has a role in encouraging them, coordinating the efforts of all interveners, monitoring progress, and correcting faulty interpretations of the plan if necessary.

It should be remembered that planning cannot always be perfect. No one can accurately predict the future or judge the psychological and physical reactions of all individuals. Even the best made plans may appear inappropriate in the actual situation. For these reasons, the intervention phase must be seen as a flexible period when alterations based on serious reflection can be made.

During the intervention phase the nurse again assumes data collection activities or delegates them to others. The data to be collected relate to the criteria or objectives which were established during the planning phase. Thus if a goal was, "The baby will gain four ounces per week," the data to be collected include the baby's weight. If the objective was, "Ms. Kelly will state that she is no longer depressed," the data to be collected would be any statements Ms. Kelly makes related to her mood. It is important to collect data broadly enough to permit full assessment of the situation and not just to verify what one hopes to see.

> A nurse worked with an elderly bedfast patient with a decubitus ulcer in his sacral area. Intervention was undertaken to heal the ulcer by a plan of frequent positioning changes. If narrow data had been collected in this situation, it would have shown only that the sacral decubitus was healed but the collection of broad data reflected not only healing of the sacral ulcer but the resultant breakdown of another area.

Skills needed in this phase may include assessment, management, communication, helping, and technical skills. Mistakes which can be made include abandoning a plan too quickly, altering a plan too frequently, failing to recognize a plan which is not working appropriately, and failing to collect sufficient broad evaluative data. The knowledge base of the nurse is important in that it influences how expert application of the plan and collection of data will be.

Once again, before proceeding to the next phase, the nurse evaluates this phase for internal consistency. Was the plan carried out directly related to the nursing diagnosis and was the action taken consistent with the plan previously developed?

## Evaluation

Finally, the nurse, the patient, the family, and others involved are ready to evaluate the effectiveness of the action taken. This is done by comparing the evaluative data collected during the intervention phase with the objectives established in the planning phase. For example, if an objective was to obtain a new properly fitting prosthesis for a youth who had outgrown his old one and the evaluative data show that a new one has been obtained, then the nurse can conclude that the objective was met. If an objective was to help a patient lose 20 pounds and the evaluative data show her weight to have decreased from an initial 163 pounds to 148, the nurse and patient can conclude that the goal was met partially—in this case 75 percent. Hopefully, the majority of the objectives will have been met. Some objectives will have been met only partially and some objectives may prove to have been unmeasurable or inappropriate.

Evaluation at this stage is much easier if the nurse stated appropriate objectives to begin with. For goals which were vague such as, "The patient will gain a better self-concept as a person," she will now find herself forced into vague evaluative statements in return such as, "I think he has." Had she stated, "Mr. Wayne will begin personal grooming activities such as shaving and combing his hair without reminders from others," she will be able to now state whether he does or not. Another most significant evaluative criterion is how satisfied the patient or family is with what has occurred.

If the objectives have been satisfactorily met, the nurse and patient and family now return to consider the nursing diagnosis with the next highest priority if there is one. Or it may be possible that new data of significance have been gained and the nurse returns to the assessment phase. In any event, the problem solving process is likely to begin a new cycle.

If the goals have not been satisfactorily met, the nurse and patient reexamine each phase in reverse order. Was the plan carried out as intended? Was the plan logical? Was the nursing diagnosis correct? Was enough initial assessment data collected? When the point of difficulty is discovered, the nurse and patient begin again from there and correct the faulty step.

## VARIATIONS IN THE USE OF THE PROBLEM SOLVING PROCESS

So far, the problem solving process has been described in painstaking detail. One may well be wondering, "Do I have to go through all of that every time I make a decision?" Obviously, the answer is "No." Great detail was presented to fully define the process. Often the nurse must move through the process much more quickly but the essential pattern remains the same—she looks for information, decides what is wrong, plans a remedy, carries out her plan, and checks to see if the remedy worked to correct the problem. She attempts to use as many of the steps of the process as are feasible in the situation. Continually skipping steps can lead to mediocre or poor nursing care. For example, skipping the assessment phase can lead to missing or misinterpreting problems. Failing to plan before intervening can cause the overuse of routine solutions and inappropriate plans. Skipping the intervention phase can result in no change in the patient's or family's condition. A failure to evaluate may result in a lack of feedback to reinforce appropriate care or extinguish inappropriate care activities.

The process was presented as if each phase occurred in time independently from the others. In practice, phases overlap considerably. The nurse may begin planning and intervening immediately after observing only one piece of data and without a complete assessment. This might be the case if the one piece of data signaled a life threatening problem—lack of respirations, for example. Flow between phases and steps is not only possible, but desirable. For example, a nurse might obtain new information about a problem while intervening. She would revise her plan and intervention correspondingly rather than ignore the information. Thus, phases are in essence continuous without real boundaries, but movement overall is in the direction of assessment to planning to intervention to evaluation.

When time is limited and auxiliary personnel are available, the nurse would probably do the assessment and planning but may delegate the intervention and possibly evaluation to others.

Further, the process was presented as if only one priority need could be dealt with at once. Experience will enable the nurse to concentrate on several problems with a patient or family at once—each possibly in a separate phase of resolution.

## FACILITATING PATIENTS' AND FAMILIES' EFFORTS AT PROBLEM SOLVING

Throughout the use of the problem solving process, emphasis has been put on involvement of the patient and family. Actually, the nurse should strive for more than just involvement. She wishes to actually facilitate use of the problem-solving process by individuals and to teach those she works with to use the process themselves without her help. Below is an example of how a nurse helped a patient to problem solve.

> Mr. Kochne was faced with a difficult situation. His wife had just died after a long illness. He was very capable of caring for himself but wondered if staying alone in his apartment was his best option. The nurse first asked questions to clarify more fully the situation. Later she said, "Now that we have looked at the situation, let's discuss what you would ideally like to have in your living situation." After that discussion she said, "Now that you know what you would like most, what do you think are some options open to you? What have you considered so far?" Later she asked, "Of all of these which we have listed, which ones seem the most appropriate to try?" Next they discussed, "What are you going to do now?" and still later the nurse discussed with Mr. Kochne how the option he had chosen was fulfilling the criteria she had written down when they discussed his ideal living situation. At this time she explained to Mr. Kochne that she had helped him problem solve and the steps they had taken. She suggested that he could use the same steps whenever he had an important decision to make.

When the nurse teaches patients to problem solve she gives them a powerful tool which they can use independently.[10] In some situations this may be done informally and in others more formally with the nurse labeling the steps and phases. Note that in this situation the nurse did not solve the problem for Mr. Kochne but helped him reach his own solutions as he learned the problem solving process.

Facilitating the patient in learning to recognize and solve problems and in reaching his own solutions is an extremely important technique in nursing. The solutions so reached are almost invariably of more appropriateness than the solutions imposed on the patient or family by others. Facilitating the patient's solution of his problems means that the nurse is working with the patient rather than acting for him arbitrarily. It implies the philosophy that the person involved knows what is best for him in his particular situation and at that particular time and that the nurse's role is to help him identify it.

It is important especially to facilitate children's efforts at problem solving. The nurse does this by guiding the child through the stages appropriately for his age and letting him develop skill in solving his own problems. It is helpful to teach parents this function because they may be inadvertently overlooking chances to help their children learn to problem solve. The parent learns to respond with, "What do you think you could do?" rather than "Why don't you . . ." and "How do you think that worked out?" rather than "I think that you . . ." Valuable learning occurs when parents allow the child to experience the consequences of his solutions.

Ms. Wells discussed with 9-year-old Bobby that sometime during the morning he was to pick the green beans in the family garden. Bobby decided that he would do it later in the morning and went out to play with a friend. At lunchtime the beans were still not picked. When Bobby came in to eat lunch with the family he found that his place at the table was not set. He had chosen to wait until then to pick the beans and he had to endure the consequences of his choice—being tired and hungry while he worked. Two days later when Ms. Wells again told Bobby to pick the beans during the morning, he picked them right away.

## THE NURSE AND PROBLEM SOLVING

Problem solving has been discussed previously only as it relates to solving patient's problems, but the nurse can use the problem solving process with problems she faces personally. The following are suggestions for problem solving related to oneself adapted for use by a nurse.[19]

1. It is important first that the nurse learn to recognize when she has a problem and attack it immediately. Often supportive others may give implicit or explicit messages that a problem exists.
2. In planning, it is helpful if the nurse knows what she values because one's values influence the meaning and importance of the problem and the actions to be taken.[30] Information on values clarification is often found in nursing journals and courses.
3. Female nurses have often been conditioned by social upbringing to establish priorities in terms of concern for approval by others. A more mature view is to consider one's priorities in terms of her own needs as well as its relation to the needs of significant others.
4. When planning action, it is often helpful to make decisions only when the emotion of the immediate situation has cooled. Decisions made in haste and when upset may not be the most appropriate.
5. Have available a contingency plan. The knowledge that there is something else to fall back on may increase one's feeling of security and an alternative plan which is ready for use can reduce anxiety if the first plan falls through.

It would seem that life experiences condition some to frequently problem solve and others to habitually make decisions in other ways. Each nurse should evaluate how likely she is to use the problem solving process in her life versus operating under the influence of the first thought which comes to her mind. She also should know when she is likely to be at her best in making decisions, what circumstances influence her abilities to make decisions, what time of the day seems best, and when she is likely to overestimate or distort problems. With this information she can plan her work to capitalize on her abilities to problem solve. Lastly, the nurse should realize that not deciding about a problem is in itself a solution.

The problem solving process is not a substitute for knowledge. Unfortunately a nurse may feel that expert use of the problem solving process can compensate for a lack of knowledge in any area. She might feel that if she keeps assessing, planning, intervening, and evaluating she can accomplish anything. Trying to use the problem solving process when one does not have information about the specific entity diagnosed is doomed to failure unless luck intervenes. For example, a nurse who does not understand depression is unlikely to notice the complete manifestations of the patient, to plan the appropriate intervention, to properly carry out the plan, or to correctly evaluate the patient's responses. Expert use of the problem solving process, therefore, requires a great amount of knowledge in all phases.

On the other hand, knowledge is not a substitute for problem solving skill. One may possess considerable knowledge about an area and yet not be effective if one cannot use the knowledge through problem solving. Through the use of the problem solving process, knowledge is mobilized and made operational. One occasionally encounters a nurse who has adequate knowledge but does not know how to use it in a specific situation. Thus knowledge and problem solving are inextricably tied together and neither will substitute for the other.

Neither can the problem solving process be considered as a form of nursing research. Research in nursing aims to reveal new information applicable to many situations. The situation studied is closely controlled and the results are evaluated statistically. In problem solving, existing knowledge is applied to solve one problem. The situation is loosely controlled and the results are not evaluated with statistical tests.[28] However, the nurse can certainly use research findings when problem solving if they seem applicable to her situation. Her attempts at solving certain types of problems may well suggest research studies.

The problem solving process is not the only skill the nurse needs to know. As has been mentioned repeatedly, many skills are needed in various phases of the problem solving process. For example, a nurse who cannot effectively communicate with a family and does not actively listen will be unlikely to proceed very far in assessment and problem identification.

## WHERE TO START

Having the content of this chapter will not guarantee that one becomes competent in problem solving. Practice is essential. The nurse might begin by working with a simple problem and following through each phase in a simplified form. Next she can strive for more detail in each phase. Some of the most challenging exercises would be rapid use of the process, using the process in complex situations, and working with more than one problem at a time. Helping patients to problem solve can be integrated into her experiences from the beginning because teaching the process to someone else often helps in learning it. Writing down each phase is time consuming but invaluable as one learns because the written record can be analyzed at a later time.

The nurse who habitually avoids problem solving must learn to pause before acting and remind herself to search for more information, state a diagnosis, establish objectives, consider several alternatives, and so forth. Soon this thinking process will become more automatic.

## SOME SUGGESTIONS FOR SELF-EVALUATION

The following questions are designed to help the nurse evaluate her use of the problem solving process.

### General Considerations

1. Are situations where problem solving should be done identified?
2. Is the patient's use of the problem solving process consistently facilitated?
3. Are patients and families taught the use of the process?
4. Are parents taught to use problem solving with their children?

5. Can the process be used rapidly when necessary without skipping steps?
6. Is the process used flexibly to allow alterations and revisions when necessary?

## Assessment

1. Are the data collected comprehensive and focused?
2. Are suspected problems identified?
3. Are the data analyzed carefully for significant information?
4. Are hypotheses validated by searching for further data?
5. Are nursing diagnoses stated so that they have meaning to others?
6. Are the resources of the family carefully assessed?
7. Does the nurse encourage the patient and family members to contribute fully to this phase?
8. Are personal expectations and personal biases identified to reduce their influence on the assessment?
9. Is the nursing diagnosis logical and related to the data collected?

## Planning

1. Is the need for nursing action established based on the problems and the resources of the family?
2. Are the priorities of the patient or family considered in determining the focus?
3. Are the objectives stated explicitly and as measurably as possible?
4. Are possible actions creatively developed?
5. Are possible actions critically evaluated?
6. Is the plan developed specific and pertinent?
7. Is the plan readily available to relevant others?
8. Are the ideas and judgments of the patient or family made an integral part of the plan?
9. Is the plan directly and logically related to the nursing diagnosis?

## Intervention

1. Is the plan implemented appropriately?
2. Are the results collected thoroughly?
3. Is someone responsible for directing and monitoring the intervention?
4. Is the plan revised if necessary after a fair trial?

## Evaluation

1. Are the results compared with the outcomes established previously?
2. Is the appropriate further action determined?

## AN EXAMPLE OF THE USE OF THE PROBLEM SOLVING PROCESS

The following example illustrates how a nurse used the problem solving process with a family undergoing a crisis. The example illustrates how a nurse combined aspects of crisis intervention with problem solving.

Mr. and Mrs. Dean had been married for 22 years when Mr. Dean asked for a divorce. Mrs. Dean was totally astonished. In the rural farming community where they lived, divorce seldom occurred—at least not to church-going people who had been married as long as they had. Mr. Dean explained that he had been seeing another woman for almost a year and now wanted to marry her. Mrs. Dean was angry, embarrassed, and humiliated. It now seemed that everyone in the community knew about Mr. Dean's affair except her and their children. She did not know what to do.

The Deans had three children. Bobbie was 21 and worked in a bank in the nearest small town. She was planning to be married in a few months to a local boy who was now away at school. John was 19 and in Germany in the Army. Jeb was 17 and a senior at the county high school.

Mr. Dean packed a few belongings and moved out after breaking the news. He returned every day to manage the farm but never entered the house. The nurse became involved when Mrs. Dean called her, after Mr. Dean left, at the physician's office where she worked. Mrs. Dean felt that she could confide in the nurse, who agreed to come to her home that evening.

The nurse provided mainly a ventilation session on this first visit. Mrs. Dean was angry and depressed. Bobbie was confused and beginning to question the concept of marriage. Jeb was torn between his two parents and alternately angry and sympathetic with both. The nurse noticed that the mother was hardly performing any of her usual activities. Bobbie was staying home from work. The nurse suspected that she was afraid to face neighbors and friends at the bank. The nurse helped the three identify and name their feelings and reactions as well as acknowledge that they were in a state of crisis.

The nurse returned two evenings later and led the family in more discussion. More assessment data emerged at this session about the family and its functioning. The main problems identified and validated by the family were the disruption of usual activities and the emotional reaction to the father's departure. The nurse noted the following nursing diagnosis, "Family crisis resulting in disruption of functioning caused by father's desertion of family." The nurse noted that the family had several resources of value at the present time. They were able to verbally express themselves well, they clung together in the situation rather than disintegrating, and all of them were in touch with their reactions and feelings.

The overall objective informally identified for the family was for the crisis to be resolved. They believed that this would be achieved when they could:

1. Return to normal daytime functioning in their usual activities.
2. Sleep well at night.
3. Think about topics other than the father's departure.

The nurse next focused the family on determining what actions could be taken to reduce the crisis. The following were later labeled as actions the family chose to undertake:

1. Jeb wanted to talk to his father. (He was in school when his father visited the farm daily.)
2. Mrs. Dean wanted to begin consultation with a lawyer. She did not wish a divorce and hoped her husband would come back but she believed she should get some legal advice.
3. Mrs. Dean wanted to arrange a conference with the pastor of her church and with Mr. Dean in the hopes that Mr. Dean would change his mind about leaving.
4. Bobbie wanted to call her fiance and have him come home for the weekend.
5. Mrs. Dean wanted to ask some of her husband's best friends to talk to him.

The nurse allowed the family to arrive at the actions they wanted to take and only voiced an opinion when they decided to call John in Germany. She suggested that he be written instead and that they wait a few more days before writing. The family agreed to meet with the nurse again in three days to assess where they were at that time. The nurse's plan included continually providing opportunities for the family members to discuss their feelings. She notified the school nurse about Jeb's situation.

On returning three days later, the nurse found the situation much more confused. Mrs. Dean had an appointment with a lawyer but not for two weeks. In the meantime she had received papers notifying her that Mr. Dean had filed for a divorce. The presence of the papers seemed to her to be concrete proof of her husband's rejection. In addition, she had talked to him about seeing the pastor and he had flatly refused. Jeb had tried to talk to his father on a Saturday morning but his father had avoided any serious discussion. Bobbie was also very upset. Her fiance's visit had not been as consoling as she had hoped. "He thought it was all very funny," she reported. Mrs. Dean had not found the courage to call her husband's friends yet. She had not left the house and had missed church for the first time in several years.

The nurse wisely allowed ventilation. After several hours when the discussion was beginning to die down, the mother observed, "I guess we all thought someone else would come in and everything would be the same again. I guess we have to get out of this mess on our own." Bobbie and Jeb nodded. This seemed to signal a turning point and for the first time the mother and both children acknowledged that maybe the divorce was inevitable and they had best work on accepting the fact. The nurse now led the family in another planning session. Bobbie remarked that she might just as well return to work. "I'm not getting anything done sitting around here." Mrs. Dean referred later to giving the house a good cleaning to get her mind off of her problems. Jeb still seemed hopeful about somehow talking his father into returning.

At this point the mother suggested that it might be easiest for the three of them to do something outside of the house for the first time together and they agreed to go out to dinner in their favorite restaurant later that evening.

The nurse noted some enjoyment of the idea by Mrs. Dean and Bobbie and mild interest by Jeb. Mrs. Dean also stated that she was going to go to get groceries the next morning and discussed how she hoped not to see any of her friends. The nurse had her consider what she might do and say if she did run into any old friends which was very likely. Thus, the actions the family had selected at this time were related to resuming a near normal life cautiously as opposed to the earlier plan which focused on turning around the problem situation.

The nurse returned two nights later to assess what was occurring. Jeb had gone to a school sports activity. Mrs. Dean and Bobbie reported on their ventures back into society. Mrs. Dean had written the son in Germany. The two planned to continue picking up the pieces.

The nurse did not return again for one week. She found the family evidencing improved functioning and helped the family assess how well they were doing on surviving the situation. They all agreed that they were sleeping better, able to focus on outside activities, and approaching somewhat usual functioning in normal activities. The nurse concluded that so far the problem solving had achieved the objectives partially. She believed her interventions could be terminated based on her assessment of the family's abilities. She gave Mrs. Dean the name of a counselor who often worked with women getting a divorce, reminded Jeb of the availability of the school nurse for talking about problems, invited Bobbie to have lunch with her in town whenever she wanted, and assured the family that she would be available again if they needed her.

## SUMMARY

The problem solving process requires use of a wide variety of nursing skills and nursing knowledges. There are four phases in the process. In the assessment phase, problems and resources are identified, analyzed, and clarified. During the planning phase, objectives are established, priorities determined, and actions are proposed, selected, and organized into a plan. The intervention phase involves carrying out the plan and collecting information on its effects. Evaluation is done in the fourth phase and further action is taken as necessary. The nurse can use the problem solving process in situations outside of nursing.

The expert use of the problem solving process in nursing is vitally important in demonstrating that nurses are "thinkers" and not merely "doers." It can lead to the provision of quality, individualized care rather than mediocre, routine care. Consistent use of the problem solving process by nurses reflects that an aspect of nursing involves the identification of nursing problems and the application of nursing knowledge and skill in a systematic, precise manner. Thus, nursing can be considered as a discipline in the health sciences with a legitimate and independent focus.

## REFERENCES

1. Aguilera, D. C., and Messick, J. M.: *Crisis Intervention: Theory and Methodology.* C. V. Mosby, St. Louis, 1978.
2. Aichlmayr, R.: "A need to identify and develop the creative student." J. Nurs. Ed. 8:19, 1969.
3. Aspinall, M. J.: "The why and how of nursing diagnosis." Matern. Child Nurs. J. 2:354, 1977.
4. Boland, M., et al.: "The nursing process: A method to promote health," in Murray, R., et al.: *Nursing Concepts for Health Promotion.* Prentice-Hall, Englewood Cliffs, N.J., 1975.
5. Carlson, S.: "A practical approach to the nursing process." Am. J. Nurs. 72:1589, 1972.
6. Carrieri, V. K., and Sitzman, J.: "Components of the nursing process." Nurs. Clin. North Am. 6:115, 1971.
7. Clark, C. C.: "Reframing." Am. J. Nurs. 77:840, 1977.
8. Collins, R. D.: "Problem solving—a tool for patients, too." Am. J. Nurs. 68:1483, 1968.
9. Durand, J., and Prince, R.: "Nursing diagnosis: Process and decision." Nurs. Forum 5:50, 1966.
10. Gebbie, K., and Lavin, M. A.: "Classifying nursing diagnoses." Am. J. Nurs. 74:250, 1974.
11. Gordon, M.: "Nursing diagnoses and the diagnostic process." Am. J. Nurs. 76:1298, 1976.
12. Johnson, M. M., and Davis, M. L.: *Problem Solving in Nursing Practice.* Wm. C. Brown, Dubuque, 1975.
13. Little, D. E., and Carnevali, D. L.: *Nursing Care Planning.* J. B. Lippincott, Philadelphia, 1976.
14. Marriner, A.: *The Nursing Process: A Scientific Approach to Nursing Care.* C. V. Mosby, St. Louis, 1975.
15. Maslow, A. H.: *Motivation and Personality.* Harper and Row, New York, 1954.
16. McCain, R. F.: "Nursing by assessment—not intuition." Am. J. Nurs. 65:82, 1965.

17. McPhetridge, L. M.: "Nursing history: One means to personalize care." Am. J. Nurs. 68:68, 1968.
18. Munley, M. J.: "An evaluation of nursing care by direct observation." Supervisor Nurs. 2:28, 1973.
19. O'Neill, N., and O'Neill, G.: *Shifting Gears*. Avon Books, New York, 1975.
20. Parker, C. J., and Rubin, L. J.: *Process as Content: Curriculum Design and the Application of Knowledge.* Rand McNally and Company, Chicago, 1966.
21. Rogers, C.: *On Becoming a Person.* Houghton Mifflin, Boston, 1961.
22. Rothberg, J. S.: "Why nursing diagnosis?" Am. J. Nurs. 67:1040, 1967.
23. Ryan, B. J.: "Nursing care plans: A systems approach to developing criteria for planning and evaluation." J. Nurs. Admin. 3:50, 1973.
24. Smith, D.: "A clinical nursing tool." Am. J. Nurs. 68:2384, 1968.
25. Stevens, B. J.: "Why won't nurses write nursing care plans?" J. Nurs. Admin. 2:6, 1972.
26. Tayrien, D., and Lipchak, A.: "The single-problem approach." Am. J. Nurs. 67:2523, 1967.
27. Vaughan-Wrobel, B. C., and Henderson, B.: *The Problem-Oriented System In Nursing: A Workbook.* C. V. Mosby, St. Louis, 1976.
28. Wandelt, M.: *Guide for the Beginning Researcher.* Appleton-Century-Crofts, New York, 1970.
29. Wiedenbach, E.: *Clinical Nursing—A Helping Art.* Springer, New York, 1964.
30. Yura, H., and Walsh, M. B.: *The Nursing Process: Assessing, Planning, Implementing, Evaluating.* Appleton-Century-Crofts, New York, 1973.
31. Zimmerman, D. S., and Gohrke, C.: "The goal-directed nursing approach: It does work." Am. J. Nurs. 70:306, 1970.

# BIBLIOGRAPHY

Abdellah, F. G.: "The nature of nursing science." Nurs. Res. 18:390, 1969.
Andreoli, K. G., and Thompson, C. E.: "The nature of science in nursing." Image 9:32, 1977.
Finch, J.: "Systems analysis: A logical approach to professional nursing care." Nurs. Forum 8:176, 1969.
Francis, G. M.: "This thing called problem solving." J. Nurs. Ed. 6:27, 1967.
Fredette, S.: "Problem solving with a difficult patient." Am. J. Nurs. 77:622, 1977.
Geitgey, D. A.: "Self-pacing: a guide to nursing care." Nurs. Outlook 17:48, 1969.
Hodnett, E.: *The Art of Problem Solving.* Harper and Row, New York, 1955.
Kaplan, A.: *The Conduct of Inquiry: Methodology for Behavioral Science.* Chandler Publishing Company, San Francisco, 1964.
Little, D., and Carnevali, D.: "Nursing care plans: Let's be practical about them." Nurs. Forum 6:61, 1967.
Malloy, J. L.: "Taking exception to problem-oriented nursing care." Am. J. Nurs. 76:582, 1976.
Mauksch, I. G., and David, M. L.: "Prescription for survival." Am. J. Nurs. 72:2189, 1972.
Moore, M. A.: "Nursing: A scientific discipline?" Nurs. Forum 7:340, 1978.
Moore, M. A.: "The professional practice of nursing: The knowledge and how it is used." Nurs. Forum 8:361, 1969.
Peplau, H. E.: "Process and concept learning," in Burd, S., and Marshall, M. (eds.): *Some Clinical Approaches to Psychiatric Nursing.* Macmillan, New York, 1970.
Redman, B. K.: *The Process of Patient Teaching in Nursing.* C. V. Mosby, St. Louis, 1976.
Schaefer, J.: "The interrelatedness of decision making and the nursing process." Am. J. Nurs. 74:1852, 1974.
Snyder, J. C., and Wilson, M. F.: "Elements of a psychological assessment." Am. J. Nurs. 77:235, 1977.
Tureman, C. A., and Johnson, P. A.: "Observing and recording behaviors of hospitalized children." J. Assoc. Care Child. Hosp. 6:17, 1977.
Turner, M. N.: "Nursing process: An operational framework for nursing practice," in Hall, J. E., and Weaver, B. R. (eds.): *Nursing of Families in Crisis.* J. B. Lippincott, Philadelphia, 1974.

# CHAPTER 4

# THE TEACHING PROCESS

The nurse has long been considered a member of the team responsible for disseminating health information to people she contacts. It is becoming increasingly recognized that the difference between good health and poor health may well be influenced by learned behavior patterns.[17] Thus, theoretically, one can help individuals to adopt behavior patterns conducive to good health. To actually do this requires a working knowledge of how to teach. This chapter will present information which, when combined with practice, should help the practitioner of nursing to teach with effectiveness. This information is useful when working with patients and also can be used when the nurse teaches other health care workers.

## NURSES AS HEALTH EDUCATORS

Nurses have the potential for being good health information teachers because of some characteristics of their profession. The nurse often spends more time with a patient than many other health team members, thus she has time to assess learning needs and teach. She may be more likely than one who is more specialized to look at the whole person and family. Nursing attempts to focus on promoting wellness so that the nurse may be more cognizant of ways to teach patients to stay well than those who focus more on illness. Because nurses often visit patients in their own homes, they have a more realistic view of what life outside the health agency is like.

Health education should therefore be a natural process for nursing. However, there is reason to believe that nurses do not always use the opportunities they have for teaching. Redman has suggested that this may be because nurses may lack knowledge of how to teach, they may frequently underestimate the patient's teaching needs, they may be confused about their role in teaching, they may have absorbed the attitude of the health care profession in general which evidences a lack of emphasis on health education, and they may be remiss in teaching because few employers have expectations that teaching will be done.[27] To this could be added that nurses may be remiss in using educational opportunities because they do not know what or how to teach and they are not thoroughly convinced of the importance of teaching.

Why should nurses spend time teaching patients? The basic reason is usually given that the nurse strives through patient education to change behavior. The behavior she is trying to change may be as simple as not including a source of vitamin C daily in the diet or as complex as not knowing how to initiate, monitor, and terminate home dialysis. She attempts to promote behaviors which help the patient and family maintain wellness, recover from illness early and without complications, or remedy as much as possible the after-effects of illness.

Although this is the major reason for teaching, there are other reasons. Increasingly, the subject of patients' rights is being identified and stressed. Teaching the patient may assure that his rights are met. The nurse may need to consider teaching needs because the patient has a right to know information about his health or about an illness.

In addition, teaching activities by the nurse may be associated with psychological benefits for the patient so that he feels more confident, informed, secure, and knowledgeable about himself and his health and sure of those who care for him. For example, one nurse taught breathing exercises to a group of patients with chronic obstructive lung disease. She found on evaluation that the patients were pleased with the exercises and believed that they were physically better.[11] This is a legitimate and desirable outcome of teaching.

## LEARNING

There are numerous schools of thought on how individuals learn. Nurses have usually been introduced to several theories related to learning in introductory psychology courses. All theories seem to explain how some aspects of learning occur, but no one theory explains the total learning process. Even though there is much confusion and conflict over learning theories, one cannot avoid teaching until the study of the psychology of learning becomes more exacting, but one must operate on the basis of current thinking. Throughout this chapter guides for teaching will be presented which are believed to be relevant and reliable based on what is now known. This may change as new knowledge becomes available.

The following guides deal with learning in general and how it occurs.

1. *Learning can be conscious or unconscious.* People operate on a number of pieces of information which they know they have learned. For example, one may pass up a certain gasoline station in favor of another because he is consciously aware that the prices in the first are always higher and the service poorer. This represents conscious learning. On the other hand, one frequently has learned information and acts upon the basis of that learning without being aware that the learning has occurred. For example, a person may choose one gasoline station over another because a handsome and charming attendant works there, although the person has no idea at all that this is the reason.

The teacher has to be concerned in any learning situation with both conscious and unconscious learning. Unconscious learning is likely to be a stronger determinant of behavior than conscious learning. If the teacher is trying to impress upon a family the importance of prompt treatment of minor health problems but obviously ignores her own minor health problems, the family may unconsciously learn that what she was trying to teach them is really not that important.

2. *Learning is most efficient when the information presented is meaningful to the learner.*

This guide points out several responsibilities of the teacher. First, if the teacher is to present meaningful content, she must know the learner as well as possible and be familiar with his life stage and life style in particular to know what is likely to be meaningful to him. Second, the teacher should build around what the learner identifies as his own meaningful learning needs. Third, the teacher should select for content only information which would be meaningful to the learner. For example, most patients having an artificial heart valve may be interested in seeing and handling an artificial valve but few would find it meaningful to listen to a scientific paper on the engineering dynamics of heart valves. Last, the teacher should inform the learner of why information she is going to present might be meaningful to him and, therefore, increase his interest. For example, the teacher explaining differences in types of insulin and their duration and peaks of actions to a newly diagnosed patient with diabetes might first indicate to the learner why she is going to present this material, how it relates to when he takes his insulin, and how his diet will correspond to the characteristics of the particular insulin he is taking.

3. *Anxiety can influence learning.* It is generally believed that mild amounts of anxiety facilitate learning because the individual is alerted and responsive. It is believed that higher or lower amounts of anxiety may diminish learning. Therefore, the nurse may need to increase the learner's anxiety if it is insufficient and, at the other extreme, reduce the highly anxious patient's anxiety before he can attend and learn. Increasing and decreasing anxiety levels therapeutically is presented in the chapter on anxiety in the next section of this book. Of course, changing an anxiety state is not always possible and the nurse may have to teach patients who are excessively anxious. She should realize that learning will be slower and more limited.

The learning environment can be instrumental in influencing the amount of anxiety the learner experiences. An environment which appears threatening to the learner increases anxiety. An environment which is devoid of threat may lead to excessive relaxation and inefficient learning. The environment which focuses the learner's attention on what is to be learned and requires an appropriate amount of mastery combined with concern for the learner should result in mild anxiety and more certain learning.

Another factor related to anxiety is the difficulty of the learning tasks. Learning tasks which are too easy can lead to relaxation and inefficient learning. Learning tasks which are too difficult can lead to heightened anxiety and frustration and thus diminish learning. The nurse must continually evaluate the appropriateness of the learning tasks for each learner. Mild anxiety is likely when the learner is aware that a new behavior is needed and that he will be supported in learning the behavior.

# TEACHING

All too often the word "teacher" brings to mind the thought of an authority figure who tells others what they should know and uses various methods such as tests and grades to be sure that they have learned it. The learner is visualized as passive and childlike with little knowledge about what he needs to know and whose main function is to absorb. Fortunately, this conception, which could be thought of in the terminology of transactional analysis[15] as a parent-child interaction, is being replaced with a teaching model which is more adult-adult in configuration. In Table 4-1 certain aspects of the teaching process are presented, comparing the all too familiar parent-child model with the adult-adult model.

There are several advantages to the adult-adult model for both the teacher and the

**TABLE 4-1.** Different teaching processes compared

| Characteristic | Parent-child teaching model | Adult-adult teaching model |
|---|---|---|
| Content selection | Teacher determines what learner needs to know | Learner helps determine learning needs |
| Status | Teacher is of higher worth as a person than the learner | Both are seen as of equal worth |
| Predominant teaching methods | Teacher lectures, dictates, advises | Teacher and learner discuss, consult, explore |
| Use of power | Teacher controls learning | Teacher guides learning |
| Evaluation | Done by teacher | Joint responsibility of teacher and learner |
| Responsibility for learning | Rests with the learner | Rests with the teacher and learner jointly |
| Infallibility | Teacher is always right | Teacher may be wrong as he is human |
| Wisdom | Teacher knows the most | Learner may know more than teacher about some things |
| Direction of learning | Student learns from teacher | Teacher and learner may learn from each other |
| Prescription of behavior | Teacher presents rules learner must follow | Learner and teacher derive guides to behavior |
| Goal | Teacher presents everything learner will need to know | Teacher guides learner in developing a life-long process for learning |

learner. The teacher who is functioning as an adult and therefore processing information is likely to present information different from parent-type information. Information taught from the adult ego state is likely to be related to use of knowledge and problem solving while parent-type information may be rules, regulations, prejudices, "shoulds," and "oughts."

There are advantages for the learner in the adult-adult teaching model in that he is better able to remember and use information when he is in his adult state than when forced into his child state. Learning will be thought of as a pleasant task which does not necessarily result in a lower sense of self-esteem. In the child state, the learner's self-esteem is likely to be threatened and learning occurs to please the teacher rather than the self.

The nurse who wishes to accomplish the most optimal learning would be well advised to practice maintaining an adult-adult relationship with the learners she contacts and focus her teaching in this manner. This may not always be easy because teachers tend to "teach as they were taught" and unfortunately most individuals have experienced predominantly parent-child teaching. In addition, learners may expect to continue this pattern and they may find it difficult to adapt to the adult role rather than the child role. If the teacher remains consistently in the adult role, the learner may move to the adult role also. It may be a unique experience for him to learn as an adult rather than as a child.

The preceding discussion of adult-adult teaching does not exclude using the adult-adult teaching model with children. It is a widespread trend in elementary and secondary education systems to treat the learner more as an adult and less like a child. Therefore, the nurse working with children and adolescents will find that the methods of adult-adult teaching apply equally well to children, adolescents, and adults.

# THE STEPS IN THE TEACHING PROCESS

There are many conceptualizations in the literature of the steps in the teaching process. The steps to be presented—assessment, planning, intervention, and evaluation—were chosen to parallel those of the problem solving process which has already been discussed. It should be remembered that individuals learn continuously and not just during a formal teaching process, but using the teaching process in a planned manner can lead to more predictable results than might occur if one left learning open to chance.

## Assessment

In general, assessment in the teaching process focuses on two areas. The teacher first of all identifies learning needs and, secondly, specific relevant characteristics of the learner.

### LEARNING NEEDS

Learning needs can be identified by the learner, inferred from his behavior, or anticipated because of his situation.[27,34] When the patient identifies a learning need, he may search out a source of information. For example:

> Mrs. Jasper has been told at the clinic that her two young children have mild iron deficiency anemia. She asks the nurse how she can learn about increasing dietary sources of iron in her meals.

Needs which are inferred from the behavior of another are usually somewhat more difficult to identify.

> Ms. Johansen has come to the abortion clinic for termination of an early pregnancy for the third time in 2 years. The nurse considers that a possible learning need for Ms. Johansen may be information about birth control measures.

Another source of learning needs involves recognizing anticipatory learning needs related to a patient's particular health situation. Nursing literature frequently suggests to practitioners learning needs of patients with different conditions. For example, it is commonly stated in nursing texts that patients with asthma can benefit from being taught about their disease, treatment, medications, and so forth. Needs also are identified for other aspects of the patient's life besides illnesses. For example, it is recommended in nursing texts that the new mother may need information on bathing the baby, formula preparation, dressing the baby, and so forth. In the example of Mrs. Jasper, the nurse might have found in a textbook that for any child diagnosed with iron deficiency anemia, the caretaker may need to learn about dietary treatment. In addition, because iron medication might be prescribed, the nurse would anticipate that most individuals would need to have certain information about giving the medication, safety precautions, and some possible side effects. Thus, many learning needs may be assumed by knowing the situation of the patient or family.

Using all three of these sources to assess learning needs will increase the comprehensiveness of the nurse's assessment. For example:

Julie was a six-year-old whom the nurse was going to follow in the home. Julie had just been diagnosed as having rheumatic fever. In the first visit the nurse collected some data about the family and identified several learning needs for the family in general and Julie in particular. For example, Julie was the oldest child and would begin school the next fall, so the family might need to learn about some special factors related to school entry. In addition, Julie's mother was able to identify several learning needs that she had, most of which were related to Julie's condition. The nurse had already listed learning needs which she knew were usually relevant for any family who has a child with rheumatic fever. All of these were compiled into a list of potential learning needs for Julie and her family to be validated by them.

In evaluating the identified needs, several things are important to remember. (1) The needs identified by the learner should usually have the highest priority. These will be the most meaningful to the learner and satisfaction of them may enable the learner to more successfully turn his attention to other learning needs. The teaching should not stop at this point, however, because the learner is not always in a position to realize what other learning needs he may have and the teacher has a responsibility to suggest those she feels are valid learning needs. (2) Learning needs identified by the use of a list of anticipated learning needs related to a specific situation and needs identified by the nurse which were not stated by the learner should be carefully validated with the learner to make sure they are relevant to the learner and his unique situation. It is almost impossible to teach someone something when he does not think he needs to learn it.

## CHARACTERISTICS OF THE LEARNER

Two particular characteristics of the learner need to be examined in the assessment stage. They are readiness and motivation.

### Readiness

Assessing readiness, simply stated, is assessing if the learner is ready to learn. Readiness is important to consider in that it relates to the timing of learning opportunities. To determine readiness the nurse assesses whether the learner has the physical and emotional maturity to profit from the learning experience and whether it is an appropriate time for the learning to occur. A three-year-old is not ready physically or emotionally to give his own allergy injections. He does not have the intellectual or emotional maturity to do so. The patient who has just suffered a myocardial infarction is not usually ready to talk about rehabilitation. He is mostly concerned with survival.

Learners who are ready to learn something behave very differently from those who are not. The learner who is ready to learn about care of his amputation stump may begin to watch as the nurse provides the care, ask questions about what she is doing, make suggestions, and participate by holding supplies. The nurse will need to ascertain what behaviors the patient is likely to show when he is ready to learn and watch for these. Such behaviors might include:

1. Searching for information or reading articles on a subject.
2. Talking to others about the subject.
3. Gradual participation.
4. Increased interest.

Signs that the learner is not ready include:

1. Avoiding the situation or the topic.
2. Thinking that someone else will take care of the problem for him.
3. Somatic symptoms which "prevent" his attention such as headaches, upset stomach, or gas pains.[19]

The nurse may be able to facilitate intellectual readiness by gently calling attention to a learning need. This might be done by asking the patient questions, leaving information for the patient to read, or pointing out a learning opportunity. She may even be forced to teach when the patient has not demonstrated readiness and she must realize in these situations that learning is hampered. For a few individuals, readiness may not occur until the learner is forced to experience the consequences of his lack of knowledge.

Tommy, aged 15, paid little attention as the nurse talked about his diabetic diet. He was confident that his mother would handle all the details and he probably thought that in reality he could still eat as he pleased. After Tommy had been home for a few weeks he was brought to the Emergency Room in diabetic acidosis. He was very annoyed that he had to be admitted. After the acute period was over, the nurse asked Tommy if he was interested in learning how he might be able to prevent readmission in the future. When she began teaching about the diet, Tommy paid attention. His experience had prepared him for learning.

## Motivation

While readiness relates to whether the learner is ready or not to learn, motivation refers to whether or not the learner wants to learn. Generally, motivation is highest when the learner is ready, recognizes the learning need, and sees the content as meaningful. Motivation can be increased by allowing the learner to select the topic and by making the content meaningful to him. This type of motivation which arises from within the learner is described as internal motivation and is usually associated with optimal learning and retenion.

External motivation arises from outside of the individual and is usually created by the teacher. Methods may include threats, testing, bribes, praise, and honor. Some methods can be somewhat positive incentives and somewhat negative incentives such as examinations. Some motivators may work for some people and not for others. External motivation is less reliable than internal motivation because it is believed that the learner who learns to meet his own needs does so more effectively than one who learns to meet criteria imposed upon him by another. Positive measures of external motivation such as praise and rewards seem more effective at eliciting increased learning than negative measures or reinforcement such as criticism and threats. There may be differences between males and females in this regard, however, because it has been found that boys who are told they are performing poorly in a cognitive task tend to try harder while girls tend to give up. This is believed to be related to differences in expectations towards males and females.[10]

In reality, an individual probably has some sources of both internal and external motivation operating in each learning situation. He may desire to learn the content and he may also wish to please or impress the teacher or others, such as his family or other learners in the situation. The nurse can assess what seems to be motivating for each learner. The student who is self-motivated is identifiable by the fact that he often takes independent responsibility for his learning and does more than required. The learner who is externally motivated may seek feedback more often and feel more compelled to stress to others his knowledge to receive reinforcement from them or to assure himself that he knows more than they do.

The nurse who assesses the learner's motivation may be able to increase it appropriately. Internal motivation can be increased by helping the learner to see the relevance and importance of what he is to learn, presenting the learning situation as pleasant and enjoyable and not as frustrating, and concentrating on allowing the learner self-direction. External motivation is probably most effective when it is of the positive reinforcement type and when it is done sincerely. Negative reinforcement may be motivating when it explains how to correct what was wrong and gives encouragement. In some situations the nurse may need to artificially build in motivation. This is often done by increasing the learner's anxiety slightly. She might say, "This gingivitis isn't causing you any problems right now but if untreated it could lead to . . ." In situations where the patient has no symptoms, motivation to change behavior can be difficult. For example, patients with essential hypertension may be asymptomatic and, therefore, negligent in taking their antihypertensive medications.[24] Recently an advertising campaign has encouraged hypertensive patients to take their medications for the "others" in their life as a source of motivation.

Motivation and readiness are two sides of the same coin. Tommy, in the example above, not only gained in readiness to learn about his diet but also became more motivated. However, readiness can occur without motivation as when the patient is physically recovered and ready to learn about home care but not motivated. Motivation can occur without readiness as when a woman desires to obtain an effective method of birth control but is already pregnant. Obviously, teaching is most effective when the two occur together so that the patient is ready to learn and wants to learn.

## Other Characteristics

In addition to readiness and motivation, the teacher who knows the learner as an individual may be more effective. Age, religion, social-cultural factors, and life experiences all influence learning. The patient whose life is most like the nurse's will be the easiest for her to teach and she will have progressively more difficulty teaching patients whose background and life style differ markedly from hers. Learning about others who are different from her may increase her effectiveness, however. Contrary to popular belief, educational level does not have a marked influence on learning. Remember that educational level is not synonymous with intelligence. Several studies have shown that learning of several kinds was not influenced by educational level of the participants.[25] The person with a doctorate in physics and the farmer who dropped out of high school may learn equally well. The nurse may need to remind herself that those who have advanced education have not cornered the market on intellect or learning ability. They may, however, be expert test takers. Of course, some areas they have studied may make for more application to what they are learning.

## ESTABLISHING PRIORITIES

Not infrequently nurses do not have the time they might wish to teach patients. Thus it is imperative that the nurse establish priorities among the learning needs she has identified.

The learner is the best source for determining priorities. What does he see as his most pressing need for information? Also, Maslow's Hierarchy of Needs can be used to determine priorities as explained in Chapter 3.

## Planning

After the teacher has determined and validated the learning needs with the learner, and assessed his readiness, motivation and other characteristics, she can plan the teaching which is to occur. This will involve consideration of several areas.

## TYPES OF CONTENT

The teacher will find that she is often teaching many kinds of knowledges or skills. Understanding what these types of content are will help in planning aspects of the teaching situation.

Some information which she teaches has to do with knowledge such as why a medicine should be taken or how breast feeding may benefit a baby. This type of learning is referred to as *cognitive* learning since it involves such things as remembering, thinking, applying, analyzing, and evaluating.

*Affective* learning, on the other hand, has to do with attitudes, emotions, and values. Although it seems questionable, teachers try to influence the learner's attitudes and values as they teach. For example, a nurse working with the mother of a handicapped child may be trying to promote the attitude that optimal development of the child is desirable and possible. The nurse working with a patient who feels discouraged and victimized by society may want to promote the attitude that the individual can change things and improve his life by learning certain processes.

Another type of learning is the learning of manual skills. This is *psychomotor* learning. The family member learning to change an indwelling Foley catheter or the patient learning to irrigate his colostomy are learning psychomotor skills.

In addition to cognitive, affective, and psychomotor learning, some would suggest that there is another form of learning called process learning.[32] Process learning involves learning how to apply a cognitive process to a situation. This teaches one how to define problems, consider alternatives, and select actions. The emphasis is on the process and not the decision reached. The teacher guides the learner to learn and use the process rather than memorize answers.[36] For example, many patients with diabetes are taught the process of insulin dosage adjustment based on their activities and other factors. A mother might be taught some aspects of the therapeutic communication process to use with a child she is having trouble communicating with. Increasing emphasis is being placed on the value of teaching processes because they provide the learner with a valuable tool to apply to many situations.

Obviously all of these forms of learning are not mutually exclusive. The person performing the psychomotor skill of temperature taking needs certain cognitive knowledges about temperatures to make the procedure meaningful and useful. Similarly, an increase in cognitive learning may be necessary before affective learning can occur. For example, an individual who hears or reads information about homosexuality as a normal variation of sexual expression may then change his attitude about homosexuals. Process learning is very dependent on cognitive learning because the application of knowledge is an inherent part of the use of any process. For example, one who tries to apply the process of teaching must have adequate knowledge about what he is teaching.

It is essential for the teacher to analyze the learner's needs and determine what types of learning she will be presenting because this will influence the methods she selects. Considering these four areas of possible content will increase the comprehensiveness of the teaching experience.

Mary was preparing to teach John about diabetes. She identified his cognitive learning needs such as information about the disease process, characteristics of insulin, diet, and health promotion. Next she identified affective learning she hoped John would gain such as believing that having diabetes need interfere little with his life and that careful management would benefit him the most. Psychomotor skills she identified which needed to be taught included insulin injection, site selection, and urine testing. Understanding about these involved additional cognitive content. Process learning she planned to include concerned decision making about insulin dosage and when to call the physician.

## DEVELOPING OBJECTIVES

After the learning needs of the patient or family have been determined and the types of content needed, it is helpful to translate them into learning objectives. For example, Mary decided that one thing John needed to learn was about the diabetic exchange diet. She then wrote this need as several specific objectives which gave direction to what she would teach. Objectives serve a number of purposes. First, they serve as a reminder that the focus of the teaching is on the learner and his behavior as a result of the learning experienced. Second, they provide a framework for determining content and learning experiences. Third, they provide guidelines to use in evaluating the results of the teaching experience. For example, the nurse preparing to teach John wrote:

John will be able to explain why he should not use a heating device such as a heating pad or hot water bottle next to his skin.

This objective reminds the teacher that the focus of what she will teach is on what John will be able to do afterwards. It indicates the information she is to teach—the danger of using excessive temperatures when the skin has diminished sensation. Also, the objective indicates how to evaluate whether or not John learned the information—he will "explain."

To be most effective, objectives should contain the following characteristics:[27]

1. They should be written in terms of what the learner is to do and not in terms of what the teacher is to teach. ("The learner will be able to" is assumed to precede each objective.)

Identify appropriate and inappropriate sites for insulin injection on his body.

Not: The teacher will demonstrate appropriate sites for insulin injection.

2. Objectives should describe an action or behavior which will occur, which can be observed, and which is subject to few interpretations.

Classify foods into the appropriate categories in the diabetic exchange diet.

Not: Understand the diabetic exchange diet.

3. Objectives should state only one behavior per objective so that it is possible to judge each behavior separately.

> Correctly perform the procedure of urine testing.
>
> Explain what actions he should take based on each possible result.
>
> Not: Correctly perform urine testing and explain what the results mean.

4. Objectives should be realistic and achievable in the situation.[18] It does little good to write objectives which are too far above or beneath the capabilities of the learner or the possibilities of the situation.

5. Objectives should focus on the results to be achieved and not the process used to reach the results.[4]

> Select foods daily which fulfill the requirements for a balanced diet.
>
> Not: Use the four basic food groups chart.

6. Objectives may indicate the circumstances under which the behavior is to occur.

> Call Dr. Fry if the tests for urinary glucose are not in the normal range for three progressive days.

Some objectives may contain an indication of the successful level of performance.

> Correctly list at least five symptoms of hypoglycemia.

Even more specific are objectives which state a time requirement.

> Answer correctly 75 percent of the questions on the test six months after the completion of the class.

Obviously, objectives can be very precise as:

> Prepare the insulin bottle for needle insertion.
>
> Draw up the correct amount of air into the syringe.
>
> Insert the needle into the insulin bottle without contamination of the needle or the bottle top.

Or more global as in:

> Draw up the correct dosage of insulin using sterile technique.

Very precise objectives have their advantages in that they minutely specify what the learner is to do and therefore what is to be taught. Realistically, however, writing precise detailed objectives can take immense amounts of time and become a ritual in itself. Usually some "middle of the road" approach is taken. There is also a modified objective technique which indicates in a main objective what the goal is and then uses points under the objective to encompass details. This might appear as:

> Correctly prepare insulin for administration.
>    Sterile technique
>    Correct dosage
>    Equalize pressure in bottle . . .

There are many points of view about how detailed and specific objectives are to be. In reality they are tools for the learner's and the teacher's benefit and they should be specific enough to serve that purpose to the satisfaction of both. Writing objectives is a means to an end and not the end in itself. If the teacher has the time, specific precise objectives have never harmed anyone.

Objectives related to affective learning are more difficult to write than are some others because they deal with abstractions which are difficult to state behaviorally and to evaluate. Generally, it is helpful for the teacher to write affective objectives although she cannot definitely be sure they have been achieved. At least having them written will remind her of what affective learnings she hopes to achieve. Mary wrote objectives related to affective learning including the following:

Follow his prescribed diet in spite of temptations.

Test his urine and record the results twice a day regardless of conflicts and other difficulties.

State that having diabetes will require little change in his usual athletic activities.

Mary knew that her evaluation of these would be dependent more on what John told her than anything else and what John told her may or may not be reflective of his actual attitudes.

When the nurse will be working with an individual or family for a lengthy period of time, it is appropriate for the teacher to write short term objectives which she hopes will be achieved by the end of the teaching experience and also to write long term objectives. Long term objectives are written first and lend a conceptual direction to her work with the individual or family. Long and short term objectives should agree with each other. One nurse wrote the following long term and short term objectives for a mother and father who asked for birth control information. Notice how the two are complementary.

Long term objective:
Become pregnant in the future if and when desired.

Short term objectives:
Describe the advantages and disadvantages of several birth control methods.

Select a method which is acceptable to both of them.

Use the method effectively.

## FINDING AND CHOOSING CONTENT

After the teacher has written objectives, it becomes evident what is to be taught. Getting the content to teach is then the next step. In many situations the nurse will need to go beyond the knowledge she presently has to obtain content.

There are several sources which can be used in obtaining content. Much of what needs to be taught may be found in various written sources such as books, journals, and pamphlets. Another way to obtain content might be through attending a conference, class, or other educational program. Another source of content is to seek out and interview individuals who may know the content. For example, a nurse working in the home with a patient with an ileostomy might learn much information efficiently by arranging to consult with the "ostomy" nurse in a nearby hospital. Another good way to learn about specific experiences is to go through the experience or to watch another experience the situation. For example, the nurse who is going to teach a prenatal class in the community would benefit from visiting the clinic, labor, postpartum, and nursery areas of the hospitals where her patients are to be hospitalized. It is amazing how many nurses attempt to prepare patients for procedures and events which they themselves have never seen.

The nurse cannot then take all the information she has obtained from written materials, educational programs, resource individuals, or personal experience and give it all to the patient. It must be carefully evaluated and compiled. The nurse may have collected extraneous and confusing material which would not be meaningful to the patient or family. Much of the content may be repetitious, but this can be beneficial because repetition aids in learning if used with care. The final content selected is compared continuously with the objectives to make sure that all the objectives will be covered and that no content is included which does not fit the objectives. This is not to say that objectives can never be added, deleted, or altered. After preparing the content the nurse may discover that an area which should be included in the patient teaching has been overlooked and an objective can be written and added which covers the area. Similarly, the teacher may discover as she prepares the content that an area she had planned to teach is not appropriate and that objective can be eliminated. Other objectives may need revision. For example, Mary had planned an objective for John:

Explain why insulin should be kept in the refrigerator.

After preparing for the teaching sessions, she discovered that in her locality endocrinologists were no longer advising patients to refrigerate their insulin. She then revised the objective to deal with newer storage ideas.

Audiovisual aids and content which are to be used in the teaching should be carefully evaluated to make sure that they are appropriate, understandable, and serve the purposes for which they are intended. It is often valuable to have another person look at the A-V aid and comment on its clarity. In this way aspects of the material which were not noticed initially can be surveyed. A-V aids do not always accomplish what one thinks they will. As some authors commented, "Birth films may miscarry."[21]

The importance of searching for appropriate content cannot be too heavily emphasized. A nurse cannot expect the knowledges she graduates with to be all that she will ever need to know in order to adequately teach others. Nurses need resources which they are continually using to update and expand their knowledge base. Without specific and relevant content, the use of the teaching process is a wasted effort. All too often nurses expect that knowing how to teach will compensate for knowing when and what to teach. Rather, the teaching process is only a vehicle to allow for the dissemination of knowledge from one person to another in order to produce behavior change. It is not a substitute for knowledge.

## SELECTION OF TEACHING METHODS

After one has identified the objectives and the content, teaching methods must be selected by which the content will be presented to the learner.

Some general guides which the nurse-teacher might find helpful in selecting methods will be discussed.

1. *Methods which promote the learner's involvement in the learning tasks produce the*

*most certain learning.* Keeping the learner involved can be done by providing him with opportunities to search out the content such as reading a programmed instruction booklet or talking with someone. Asking the learner questions, planning discussion in the learning situation, and having the learner teach someone else will promote activity and involvement. Active involvement in learning seems to promote retention. People remember very little of what they hear, more of what they hear and see, still more of what they hear, see, and talk about, and the most about what they hear, see, talk about, and participate in.

2. *Some methods are more appropriate for different types of learning than others.* Psychomotor learning requires that the learner see what skill he is to perform and practice the skill repeatedly with feedback. One particularly effective technique is parallel demonstration in which the teacher and the learner have identical equipment. The teacher performs one step of the skill while the learner watches her and then immediately repeats the step with his equipment while the teacher watches him. This provides immediate feedback.

Cognitive learning requires that the learner be able to understand content which may be presented in readings, lectures, seminars, films, and so forth. All opportunities possible should be used to facilitate the participation of the learner. It is desirable to aim for application of concepts and not merely the memorization of facts.

Affective learning is difficult to plan. There are several suggested ways to facilitate affective learning. One is to expose the learner to another individual who evidences the desired attitude or value in his behavior. This someone else might actually be the teacher. The teacher who wants the learner to value health habits such as a well balanced diet would want to set an example herself. It is difficult to teach someone the value of not smoking if the teacher smokes heavily. The old axiom, "The best way to teach your values to your children is to live by them" applies equally well to teachers and learners as well as parents and children.

Exposure to others besides the teacher with a desirable value can be planned.[27] For example, one might introduce a patient who has recently had a mastectomy to another woman who has also had a mastectomy and evidences that she has learned to accept her body image. Other teaching methods which may promote affective learning include seminars and discussions. Recently simulation games have been designed to promote attitude and value clarification. They seem to be advantageous in that they are enjoyable and useful at the same time.[6]

Process learning is very difficult and requires mastery of cognitive content as well as skill in using a process. Actual or simulated situations are needed to give the learner practice in applying the process.

There are many methods which have not been mentioned which can be used to teach different types of content. The important thing to realize is that a teacher doesn't have to rely on one method to teach everything, nor should she. Some methods work well for some types of content but work poorly if at all for teaching other types of content. Psychomotor learning in a lecture format is very inefficient. Cognitive learning in a discussion group is not highly effective but affective learning may occur readily. Methods must be evaluated in terms of their expense and time consumption. No one would suggest that individuals who want to learn a low calorie diet should experimentally derive caloric values for foods in the laboratory. A list of calorie values will usually suffice. Experience and experimentation will enable the teacher to refine her methods and can provide variety for the teacher because there are several ways to teach anything.

3. *Not all learners will learn by the same methods.* As if life for the teacher was not complicated enough, it is becoming increasingly apparent that learners differ considerably

in how they learn. A few individuals can absorb auditory information readily. Others cannot understand most things until they see them visually. These two groups are sometimes referred to as "auditory learners" and "visual learners." Another group of learners cannot learn much from what they see or hear but only from what they experience. Colloquially, these learners are often referred to as those who have to learn "the hard way." A learner like this may never understand why his colostomy should be irrigated until he ignores the procedure and experiences the consequences. There may be those who cannot learn something no matter how hard the teacher tries. Not all teaching endeavors will meet with 100 percent success.

It should be obvious that sensitivity to the learner's characteristics and flexibility in using methods can increase effectiveness. Since very few are true auditory learners, all methods should be supplemented by as much visual stimuli as possible. For most learners, then, a picture is indeed worth a thousand words. This should also suggest why written instructions or guidelines are so invaluable to learners. This area has received some attention in nursing but more could be done. Writing down what the patient needs to know not only allows for visual learning but allows the patient to refer to the material again if forgetting occurs—and it does frequently.

It can be seen why much attention is being given to using many methodologies to teach the same content. For example, the nurse teaching prenatal breathing exercises might want to describe them, show a film of someone performing them, demonstrate them one by one, and have the learners practice them and discuss them. She could then distribute an information sheet for each learner to use at home. This approach of using many methods for one content is called a multimedia approach or multisensorial approach and should promote learning.

4. *Methods which provide for transfer are desirable.* When a teacher is presenting content, she is hoping that the material will be used not only in the learning environment but also outside of the learning setting. This use of information in another situation is referred to as transfer. Transfer is not automatic but must be planned for. There are several things the teacher can do to increase the likelihood of transfer. First, she can have the learner discuss how he might use what he has learned outside of the learning situation. When would it be appropriate? What particular complicating factors might be present? Practice might be beneficial in preparing for transfer. For example, the parents of a child with cystic fibrosis who will perform postural drainage and clean respiratory equipment at home can practice with the equipment in the hospital and discuss what will be different at home. Even more effective would be to plan a situation in which the learner is encouraged to actually use his knowledge or skills in another situation. For example, the patient in the hospital learning a diabetic diet could go to the cafeteria for meals and select his diet there because this would simulate choosing a proper diet from various alternatives.

## SEQUENCING THE LEARNING EXPERIENCE

There are several guides the nurse can use in providing a sequence to the content and educational experiences she is planning.

1. *Material which progresses from what is known to the learner to what is unknown is more comprehensible.* The teacher can start with something the learner is familiar with to explain something. For example, a school nurse wanted to teach a group of teenage girls about weight control. This is how she introduced the subject.

> The human body is in some ways like a car. The gasoline we put in the car determines how far the car can go. The same is true of the body . . .

The nurse who wants to start with what is known to the patient cannot always assume what the patient knows. She may need to ask questions first to assess the knowledge that the learner has about an area. This can be done formally through giving a pretest prior to teaching. Studying the results of the pretest can save the nurse and the learner both a lot of time in some situations. It is very frustrating for a learner when others assume he knows things he does not know and very boring to be told things he does already know. For example, one nurse answered a patient's questions about the solutions being used for her perineal preparation before delivery by explaining that they were "special liquids to chase all the germs away before the baby came." She later found out to her grave embarrassment that the patient had a Ph.D. in bacteriology and was involved in research related to asepsis of the skin.

2. *Content which is likely to provoke anxiety may be best taught first.*

> When Mrs. Hadley learned that her husband had pernicious anemia she knew that she would have to learn to give him vitamin $B_{12}$ injections. The office nurse began the teaching program with Mr. and Mrs. Hadley and covered the disease characteristics in the first session. In the second session she discussed general health promotion and began teaching Mrs. Hadley injection technique. In the third session Mrs. Hadley gave Mr. Hadley his injection and was quite relieved and proud of herself. She told the nurse, "Now that we've got that out of the way, why don't you tell me about all the rest of that stuff again."

Clearly, Mrs. Hadley had been so anxious about giving the injection that she had heard little else before then.

Determining what is anxiety provoking can best be done by asking the learner. Then this content can be covered as early as possible. Anxiety may be expected related to learning painful procedures or content related to sex, death, personal beliefs, and extensive change in behavior. One nurse taught venipuncture first to patients who were learning self-dialysis because the patients were the most anxious over it. [12]

3. *Teach the routine first, then the variations.* It is very confusing to a learner to have the teacher present all the variations as the usual is being presented. In general, it is most helpful to present the common picture or routine and, after it is understood, add variations. For example, in teaching a diabetic exchange diet, foods which are exact exchanges in one category could be presented and worked with. Then when the concept is understood, foods which involve more than one exchange group can be discussed. A patient learning care of his amputation stump could learn about normal care, then what to do if complications develop.

## THE TEACHING PLAN

Now that planning has been done for what is to be taught, the nurse has developed a teaching plan of sorts and she might profit by summarizing all her information into a formal plan which she can possibly take to the teaching situations. This can be done in various ways. The form to be suggested is only one of many. The plan will contain a copy of all of the content to be taught in some instances but usually it contains only an outline of content to prod the teacher's memory while she teaches. An example of parts of a teaching plan is shown opposite.

*Date:* November 19        *Topic:* Dental Hygiene

*Time:* 10:15–11:15        *Learners:* Second Graders

*Materials needed:* Film: "Brush, Brush, Brush"
     Large demonstration tooth
     Large demonstration toothbrush
     Toothbrush and toothpaste for each child
     Color tablets for each child
     Posters: "Dental Health," "The Proper Way to Brush," "What is a Cavity?"
     Small hand mirrors for each child
     Paper cups for each child
     Set of demonstration teeth and toothbrush

*Objectives:* The student will be able to:
     State why he should brush his teeth.
     State when teeth should be brushed.
     Brush teeth correctly and thoroughly.
     Identify where he may not be adequately brushing by use of color tablets.
     Brush teeth in the morning before school for one week.

| Schedule | Content | Method |
|---|---|---|
| 10:15 | Introduce topic | Lecture |
| | Count how many brushed teeth before school | Pretest |
| | Introduce and show film | Film |
| 10:25 | Discuss film | Discussion |
| 10:30 | Pass out mirrors, have children look at teeth | Lecture— |
| | Talk about teeth surfaces | discussion |
| 10:40 | Pass out toothbrushes and paste | Supervised |
| | One-half class to sinks to brush, one-half look at posters and | practice |
| | demonstration teeth | Independent |
| | | learning |
| 10:55 | Switch activities | |
| 11:05 | Summarize, answer questions | Repetition |
| | Check objectives 1 and 2 | Learner |
| | | involvement |

*Evaluation of learning:* Come to class the next morning and count how many report that they brushed teeth. Check again one week later. If majority are not brushing, repeat content via another method.

## Intervention

When the teacher has identified what the learner needs to know, collected information, and planned the teaching experience, actually carrying out the teaching is the next step. There are a few guides to teaching which are relevant to this step in the teaching process.

1. *The pace and the length of the teaching sessions can affect effective learning.* There are no general guidelines to state how much material should be covered and how long a session should last. It seems that the beginning teacher invariably attempts to teach too long and to cover too much. A good motto would be to "teach less and teach it better." In

lesson plans that are used over and over, one frequently keeps adding "essential" content and experiences but seldom removes anything. Obviously this contributes to cluttered confusion for the student.

The best way to gauge how fast to teach and how long is to watch the learner carefully. Frequent checks on his comprehension will indicate when material is being presented too quickly or when he has tuned out the teacher because he has reached the end of his absorptive powers. The learner will give subtle or obvious clues when he has had enough. The old axiom, "The mind can only absorb what the seat can endure" is still valid today. Sessions can sometimes be longer if activities are incorporated which provide for a change of pace or movement. Placing breaks within the session also can compensate for longer time periods. While attention spans vary considerably among individuals, most individuals need a break or change of pace in the session after about 30 to 45 minutes. As a rule, men have developed longer attention spans than women. This may be due to the fact that many women perform more repetitious, monotonous, interruptable work which contributes little to the development of attention span. This may change with changing women's roles, however.

Another way to provide flexibility within the teaching session is to arrange the teaching plan so that some activities can be shortened or eliminated if time is running out. This is more acceptable than only teaching the first half of the content and forever feeling frustrated about not teaching the last half. Every teaching plan should have a time built in for questions and to take advantage of learners' responses.

2. *Letting the learner discover the content increases effectiveness.* Almost all teaching can be done in a way that builds in an active role for the learner. Learning which occurs in this way is believed to be highly effective. This is facilitated by using methods which play on the learner's natural interest and curiosity. Learning does not only occur within the teaching session so the methodology can include independent activities by the learner. Ideas are remembered longer than facts.[27] This suggests that activities which enable the learner to work with the content are more beneficial than methods which stress memorization. It is also helpful to provide opportunities for the learner to connect what he is learning with what he already knows. These interconnections reinforce learning and retention.

3. *Characteristics of the environment can influence the learning situation.* This suggestion seems so obvious that it is often overlooked. An environment can detract from learning or enhance learning. Uncomfortable chairs, interruptions, an uncomfortable room temperature, nonrelevant clutter, and distracting noises and sights could hamper the most superb lesson plan. The following are some of the factors in the environment which the teacher should check before the teaching session:

| | | |
|---|---|---|
| Lighting | Sound | Equipment |
| Temperature | Distractions | Supplies |
| Seating | Visibility | Displays |

Although these may seem most relevant to classroom teaching, these factors are relevant when teaching is done at a patient's bedside or in his home.

Ways to use the environment to advantage include planning it to focus attention on what is to be learned through displays, posters, a collection of materials, a list of additional resources, or a model. While the environment is important, a lavish, expensive, and decorative environment does not in itself lead to learning.

4. *The timing of the learning experience can be influential for learning.* It has already been stated that the teaching should occur when the learner is ready and motivated. There are other variables to consider such as the timing of the teaching experience. The hospitalized patient probably will not be interested in learning about his home care during visiting hours. One educational effort designed to orient new patients to the hospital through the use of closed circuit television had to be rescheduled to a time when the patients were not watching their daily soap operas.[1] A home visit teaching session at 4:30 may interfere with usual family activities in some families. A group teaching program designed for young mothers during the day would have to provide for child care before many mothers could attend and avoid the hours when children were coming home from school. While timing factors seem obvious, they are sometimes ignored with less than desirable results. One obstetrics department planned for new mothers to gather in the lounge for coffee and discussion after breakfast. The mothers were reluctant to miss their physicians' morning rounds which occurred at that time.

Learners cannot concentrate as well when they are in pain, anxious over something which is to occur, or preoccupied with other matters. It is believed that learning is probably decreased during acute phases of an illness.[23] Children do not want to listen when they think it is play time. The learner is often the best source of determining the best time to teach.

Timing with children who are being told about upcoming events is especially important. The child should be told about an event long enough beforehand to mobilize his defenses to cope but not long enough to allow for exorbitant fantasies to develop. This might mean that the toddler should be taught general information just before an event, the preschool-aged child a few hours before, and the school-aged child a day or so before. These guidelines may be adapted depending on the particular child.

5. *The teacher creates the atmosphere during the teaching experience.* While the teacher is directing the learning experience, she is revealing much about herself as a person. This information she is revealing contributes to a certain atmosphere in the teaching situation. Anyone who has ever had the opportunity to move from classroom to classroom in a school situation was probably struck by how quickly one senses a certain atmosphere in each classroom. Some classrooms seem stiff, rigid, and formal, others may be confusing and chaotic, still others warm and supportive of the students. While the learners contribute to the atmosphere, certain characteristics of the teacher are believed to be of most significance. Effective learning is believed to be promoted by an atmosphere in the classroom which reflects that the teacher:

1. Is well informed about the subject and interested in it.
2. Is in tune with the learners and has accurate perceptions about their behavior.
3. Is aware of her own behavior and motives.
4. Understands how individuals learn.
5. Uses effective methods to teach.
6. Uses her unique "self" as part of the teaching method.[7,16]

It is probable that these factors are also important at the bedside or in the home. These qualities contribute to an atmosphere where learners ask questions, feel comfortable, know what is expected of them, feel positive about themselves, contribute their ideas, and are therefore free to think and learn. Unfortunately, no one can exactly tell how a teacher can develop these qualities.

One may teach for many reasons and these will usually be clear to the learner. Some may want to teach so that others will realize how brilliant they are and what amazing knowledge they possess. Others may teach because they are forced to. Some teach in ways to guarantee that learners will like them and meet their needs for acceptance and reinforcement as a worthwhile human being. This may not be in the best interest of the learners. Teaching should never be evaluated wholly on the basis of which teacher is the most popular with students. The teacher should arrange to meet her needs elsewhere because teaching is a similar process to the helping process in that the nurse meets the patient's needs but does not expect the patient to meet her needs as might occur in a social relationship. The teacher should reflect on her motive for teaching honestly.

It is helpful in some instances for the teacher to perform the patient's physical care as she may be better accepted as a teacher if she demonstrates interest in the patient first.[19] The nurse who gives primary care will know the learner's needs better as well.

6. *Inappropriate vocabulary can be a barrier to learning.* The teacher who has functioned for any length of time in the health care system has absorbed a highly technical vocabulary which she uses automatically and which most patients do not understand. Many terms which nurses use commonly have been found to be largely misunderstood by patients, such as ambulate, void, force fluids, and "NPO."[8] Other words are subject to other meanings such as dye and stretcher. One patient announced that he was going to sue the hospital because he had overheard the physician telling someone that he had a "staff" infection. Many times our abbreviations are the worst offenders. Learners often do not know what is meant by the ER, the OR, the Del Room, or the PAR. One lady in California was told by a visiting nurse that her child's lungs sounded very congested and she should take him in to the OPD. The mother expressed amazement but the nurse assured her that it was important. The mother had her doubts but she took the child to the Oakland Police Department.

It is very difficult to become aware of how contaminated one's vocabulary is with medical and nursing terminology but the area deserves serious consideration by every teacher. Sometimes a friend who is not in a health related area can look over planned content and point out unclear terms.

7. *The use of advanced organizers can aid retention.* Advanced organizers indicate to the learner what he is going to hear and thus provide structure to aid his comprehension of the material.[27] For example, the nurse could say, "Today I thought we might talk about the baby's frequent ear infections, what might be causing them, and what you might be able to do to help avoid them." Another example might be, "Before you leave the clinic I want to talk to you about this medication you are to take and about what you can do at home to carry out the exercises Dr. Sampson was talking about." Material can then be presented under the organizing statements given.

8. *Repetition strengthens learning.* Repetition for the learner's benefit can be incorporated in several ways. Presenting a subject by several methods and approaching from various angles aids repetition. Summarizing provides another chance for repeating the essential points as does starting one learning session by reviewing the last. Merely repeating the same thing over and over can be monotonous and should be avoided.

9. *The teacher's appearance is relevant to the learning experience.* While it may seem obvious, the appearance of the teacher is influential consciously and unconsciously on the learner.[40] This does not mean that every teacher must be a raving beauty in designer fashions, but that any extremes of appearance can detract from the learner's attention. She should look appropriately dressed, neat, well groomed, and use gestures and mannerisms which do not in themselves become distracting. Since people naturally judge others

considerably on their appearance, the nurse should reflect on how she dresses and behaves and what this may indicate to the learner. While the teacher may not be concerned
with clothing and "artificial trappings," others may decide her worth as a teacher based on
her appearance. This may not be the way one wishes people were but it is the way things
are. An overweight teacher talking about exercise and proper diet is less than effective.
Watching a videotape of one's teaching session can help increase awareness of how one
appears to the learner.

10. *Letting the learner progress at his own rate can facilitate learning.* Not all individuals
learn at the same speed. The nurse can let the learner determine how fast he can go.
Understanding a few things well is probably more beneficial than understanding a lot of
things poorly. Many devices such as programmed instruction and computer-assisted instruction build in flexibility for the learner. Having the content subdivided into what information is essential and what is extra is useful because the more rapid learner can progress
with extra content while the more deliberate learner studies the essential.

11. *Reinforcement or feedback should be built into the teaching process.* Learning is
believed to be enhanced when the learner is immediately informed that he has performed
correctly or what he could do to correct a response.[33] This can be done through continual
encouragement to the learner: "That's a good question," "I'm glad you mentioned that,"
"You've got the right idea," "Yes." In groups learners often support each other with
reinforcement. Because some forms of instruction lend themselves to more rapid reinforcement than others, methods should be chosen which provide for reinforcement.

12. *Recording the teaching done is beneficial.* If teaching is a relevant part of nursing
practice, then it should be recorded. This might be on the usual nursing notes, the care
plan, or on part of the patient's record set aside for teaching notes. The record should
contain the teaching needs identified, the plan to meet them, the teaching provided and
date, and an evaluation of the results. This enables the other members of the health team
to complement the activities of each other and would provide for a different person to
continue the teaching if necessary.

## Evaluation

If teaching is done infrequently in nursing, evaluation of the teaching done is even less
frequent. Partly this is true because teaching is often done on the spur of the moment as
the last thing before the patient or the nurse leaves so that there is not time for evaluation.
Another reason may be that nurses may expect patients to remember everything they tell
them so they see no need for evaluation. Or it may be that nurse-teachers don't know how
to evaluate the teaching they have done.

The following guides contain general information the nurse can use in evaluating the
learning which has occurred as a result of her teaching.

1. *Forgetting is a natural human occurrence and must be anticipated.* Learners do not
remember 100 percent of what they are taught. It has been estimated that one year after
something is taught most individuals remember only 10 percent of the content. Whether
this is true or not, forgetting is a part of the life of a learner. Material which has been
forgotten can be retaught with efforts directed at increasing the meaning of the material to
the learner, increasing its association with remembered material, and applying it more
concretely to the individual's life. Another solution is to encourage the learner to write
down and keep available information which he continually forgets but frequently needs.

Mr. Jenkins had glaucoma, arthritis, hypertension, and angina. He had so many oral medications and eye-drops they occupied an entire bureau drawer. Each medication had been given him by a different doctor and he was desperately confused about them. Some were to be taken daily, others every other day. Some were before meals and others after meals. Some were to be taken 15 minutes after each other. Some could be taken only when he needed them. The nurse discovered that he took them faithfully some days and forgot them the next. He took some of them for the wrong reasons and at the wrong times. The nurse made a large chart with information about each drug. A sample pill or an empty eyedrop bottle was taped to each description. Next the patient and the nurse constructed a perpetual calendar-type chart showing when each medication was to be taken. A separate sheet was used for each month for checking off each day when the medications were taken. Within a few weeks Mr. Jenkins' blood pressure was stabilized, his arthritis was in remission, and he reported that he felt better than he had in years.

Discharge instructions are an example of material which the patient may easily forget and should be written down.

2. *The learning experience should be evaluated by both the learner and the teacher.* It is important for the teacher and the learner to evaluate the learning experience. Informally, the learner may comment on what was helpful, significant, stimulating, or not so. The teacher may make notes as to what she feels worked well or needs revision in the future. More objective information can be obtained by using forms for evaluation which the learner can return anonymously. Having others sit in on the teaching situation and comment can also be illuminating. Videotapes of a teaching session can provide valuable insights for the teacher. One should remember that the enthusiasm or lack of enthusiasm for the teacher or the learning situation is not the most relevant criterion for evaluation. One needs to know if the learner learned what he was supposed to learn. The learner may have relished the session and adored the teacher but learned little, or he may not have enjoyed the session or the teacher but learned a lot. Usually, the two are correlated in that when one enjoys the learning situation one also learns.

3. *Evaluation of learning requires use of the objectives.* In order to evaluate a teaching experience, one needs to again consider the objectives which specify what the learner should be able to do because of the learning experience he has had. Psychomotor content which deals with learning skill and objectives such as "the learner will perform . . ." can be evaluated by watching the learner perform the skill. Often this is enhanced by preparing a checklist from the objectives which can be filled out while the learner performs the skill. This can pinpoint what steps were correctly performed and where reteaching is needed. For example:

A nurse taught Mr. Feldon range of motion exercises to do with his 15-month-old child with cerebral palsy. She demonstrated the exercises and they practiced together several times. When the nurse wanted to see how Mr. Feldon was doing one week later, she prepared a checklist from the objectives. Some of the items on the checklist were:
　　＿＿＿ Stabilizes the knee when performing internal and external rotation of the hip joint.
　　＿＿＿ Carries out each movement only to the point of resistance.
　　＿＿＿ Uses smooth, even manipulation.
　　＿＿＿ Repeats each movement three times.
　　＿＿＿ Each movement is carried out in its entirety.

Cognitive learning can be evaluated by many methods. Testing is one of the more familiar methods to most individuals. Written paper and pencil tests have their limitations, however, which the teacher must take into account. Good questions are hard to write. A learner's performance is affected by more than his knowledge and may reflect how well he is feeling, how interested he is in performing well, and how good he is at taking tests—a definite skill. The questions asked may not adequately test what he has learned either. Paper and pencil tests are handy when teaching large groups and when it would be difficult to talk individually with each student. Often cognitive learning is tested by asking questions verbally of the learner to see if he can state the content. It is useless to ask "Do you understand?" but more relevant to ask a specific question.[19] Oral quizzing has as many limitations as written testing methods do. Checklists can be used to evaluate cognitive learning. The nurse included for Mr. Feldon:

_____ When asked, can explain why range of motion is beneficial.

It is not safe to assume that what has been learned at the end of the session will be remembered forever. One can call the patient several days or weeks later to check on his retention. One nurse followed up on classes for patients with diabetes by sending out questionnaires one year later.[29] Evaluating a child's grasp of cognitive information may be difficult. One can sometimes watch their play and see incorporation of what they have been taught.[31]

Affective learning is difficult to evaluate and is usually done by observing the behavior of the learner and inferring from his behavior or verbal comments whether or not he has incorporated the value or attitude specified in the objective into a personal value. There are difficulties involved in making that assumption, however.

A nurse had taught Mrs. Jason how to count calories so she could reduce caloric intake to lose weight. She noticed on her next home visit that Mrs. Jason was indeed eating a low calorie lunch. Was Mrs. Jason committed to the diet and losing weight or had she rapidly hidden the potato chips and Coke when she saw the nurse coming? Or maybe she could find nothing else in the house to eat.

Asking the learner how he feels about the value or attitude may reveal his attitude but there is the danger that the learner may tell the teacher what she wants to hear regardless of what he really thinks and does. Nevertheless, an attempt to evaluate affective learning, even if subject to error, is better than no attempt at all. Increasing the observations and the number of observers may lead to more reliability in evaluating affective objectives.[18]

Process learning can be evaluated by waiting until the learner has an opportunity to apply the process and knowledge and checking how he does, or by simulating an appropriate situation and evaluating the learner's performance.

A nurse had taught a couples church group about ways to communicate effectively with their children. Then she roleplayed a child involved in several common situations and had members of the group practice responding.

One head nurse led a seminar for her nursing staff on working with patients who were hostile and angry. The staff thought the information was logical, useful, and easy to apply. When the staff thought the seminar was over, the head nurse then launched into some complaints and aggravations she had related to the staff's work in an increasingly angry and accusing tone. The staff at first forgot all about what they had just learned as they retaliated with anger and hostility. One nurse "caught on" to what the head nurse was doing and soon all the staff had picked up on the hoax the head nurse was perpetrating. The staff agreed that understanding the process was easier than applying it and they needed practice.

As nurses become more accountable for their practice, the evaluation of teaching (and nursing care in general) must move towards the more formal and objective measures of effectiveness. It will not be enough to say, "The learners seemed to enjoy it and I think they got a lot out of it." The teacher will need data on achievement.

Because one's behavior evolves slowly and is motivated by multiple factors, it cannot be changed overnight. Some teachers expect the learner to change behavior as soon as he is presented with an alternative.

> The nurse talked to Mr. and Mrs. Sutton who were having difficulties relating to their 15-year-old daughter. The nurse gave them several pointers on changing their relationship with her. They appeared interested in the changes and agreed to try them out. She was very discouraged to find out a week later that little had changed. The Suttons had spent 15 years forming their relationship with their daughter and it was unrealistic to expect them to significantly alter it in one week.

Behavior change frequently follows a pattern. First the individual may intellectually accept the idea of changing but not be able to change his behavior. This occurs when one knows and believes he should be exercising regularly, for example, but does not do so. Next the individual may occasionally change his behavior but mostly operate with his previous pattern. If behavior change does occur, it will be a gradual process with frequent fluctuations between new and old behavior. The old behavior may eventually win out as when an individual exercises for a while but then quits. If the new behavior does emerge, it will be after considerable time and only when the individual is fully committed to the new behavior. The teacher who understands how slow and difficult behavior change is can help the patient, allow for vacillation, and give encouragement. The individual may need to understand that the slow process is normal because he may find it frustrating not to be able to instantly change his behavior. Consider the patient with a stress-related illness who is told to go home, take it easy, and learn to relax. When he finds that this is very difficult because of his life long patterns of behavior, he becomes more stressed than before. Many health teachers are very prone to tell others what behaviors they should change, such as learning to relax and not worry, not abusing chemical substances, learning to exercise, and losing weight by changing eating habits. Teachers are often less adept at understanding the gradual nature of behavior change and helping the learner through it.

## SPECIAL TEACHING-LEARNING STRATEGIES

### Group Teaching

Although much of the teaching done in nursing is one-to-one, there are many advantages to using groups of learners. The use of groups can be very efficient because time and expense for the teacher can be reduced. Groups also may be enjoyable for the learner who feels a sense of comradship and belonging.[27] Affective objectives may be promoted among group members. While groups are frequently used for prenatal teaching, diabetes education and such, there are probably many more situations in which groups are useful. Whenever the nurse finds that she is repeating the same content to many individuals, there may be a way to organize these learners into groups. Groups have been used with good results to teach patients before surgery where one-to-one teaching was traditionally considered essential.[30] One who uses groups can combine group teaching with one-to-one content so that the best method is used for each objective. For example, a group of mothers learning proper nutrition might also have individual sessions with the teacher to discuss their particular needs.

## Team Teaching

Another variation well worth considering is team teaching. Several health team members might participate in planning and teaching learners as a team with each contributing to the teaching according to her particular interests and abilities. Allowing for specialization by teachers in addition to a team approach might increase effectiveness. For example, on a medical-surgical hospital unit each nurse originally taught preoperative heart surgery patients all areas of content. Gradually a team approach emerged so that several nurses made the teaching plan and one nurse taught one aspect and other nurses taught other areas. Careful coordination is essential in team teaching so that all teachers relate to and build on each other's content.

## Contracting for Learning

A new and growing area involves contracting with learners for meeting learning needs. A formal contract is drawn up and signed, specifying the objectives to be reached, the responsibilities of the learner and teacher, a plan, and evaluation criteria. For example, one learner needed to lose 30 pounds and he desired to lose the weight. The nurse and the learner drew up a contract which specified what was to be achieved, what each would do, and the terms under which the contract would be broken. The contract was not used as a weapon held over the learner's head, but rather as an agreement to aid learning.

## Behavior Modification

Since all teaching aims at changing behavior, all teaching involves modifying behavior. All teachers practice behavior modification whether they are consciously aware of it or not. A teacher who smiles or nods when the learner is correct and paying attention or who ignores him or scowls at him if he is inattentive or incorrect is giving reinforcements. Behavior modification often conjures up images of secretive violation of others' rights, of manipulation of behavior, or of animal training.[5] Yet it can be a powerful learning tool and sensitive to the learner's rights if certain guidelines are followed. Behavior modification has been found particularly useful when working with children of limited intelligence because they often lack the normal motivation which leads normal children to learn. An excellent example of the use of behavior modification by the parents of a retarded child is contained in an article by Barnard.[3] The teacher who is not familiar with usual behavior modification techniques will find many source books in the nursing literature such as Loomis and Horsley's *Interpersonal Change.* The following guidelines are suggested to help nurses use behavior modification techniques in learning situations with a clear conscience that the patient's rights are being respected.

1. Avoid the use of adversive stimuli. Use positive reinforcement instead.
2. Use behavior modification for noncontroversial teaching such as teaching a child toilet training and not for producing personality change.
3. If the patient is a young child, let the learner or the parents select the goals of the modification and not the teacher.

4. The learner should participate in developing and approving of the plan.

5. Ignoring offensive behaviors is not the same as ignoring the learner.

6. Evaluate the teacher's motives frequently for using behavior modification. Because teachers are reinforced when the technique works, they may use the technique unnecessarily and compulsively to continue to receive reinforcement.[28,35]

Behavior modification works and produces excellent results. Even if the nurse does not plan to use behavior modification, she should be familiar with the technique and she will become aware of how her behavior serves as reinforcement to learners. Many teachers practice behavior modification without knowing it and in less than desirable ways.

An interesting example demonstrating the combined use of a contract with behavior modification is given in a recent article by Wang and Watson.[39]

## Informal Teaching

Described so far have been predominantly structured formal teaching situations. Much of the teaching a nurse does, however, is informal and less structured. While at first glance this may seem easier, informal teaching is actually more difficult. The teacher must be able to quickly assess a learner's needs, come up with content and a plan, respond to the learner, and evaluate usually on the spot. Informal teaching will only be as effective as the teacher's "walking" knowledge because in many situations there is not an opportunity to consult references or other resources. It stands to reason that one who wants to improve the informal teaching she does should be as knowledgeable about the teaching process as one who engages in predominantly formal teaching. As long as informal teaching is thought of as something anybody can do, it is likely to be of limited quality. The example at the end of this chapter demonstrates how one nurse taught a patient in an informal session.

## Teaching Children

A comprehensive discussion on how to teach children would require several volumes. The nurse who consistently works with children would be well advised to read widely on growth and development of children, educational theory, and cognitive development, and to consult preschool, elementary, and secondary educators and visit their classrooms to gain ideas.

The teaching of children by nurses tends to be neglected. It may be that nurses assume that parents have taught their child about his illness or about a coming event. Another reason for not teaching children is that some nurses may assume that a child cannot understand what is going on so why bother him with details.[37] Another reason is that children may not ask many questions. This may be in part a defense because the child may pretend disinterest in the hopes that the problem will go away.[26] The nurse may find that the child may feign disinterest as she talks with him but may actually be listening very carefully. An increase in anxiety is likely as the child admits to himself what is to come, so the nurse should plan ways to help the child control his anxiety during and after the teaching situation. If he is not being taught by nurses and others, the child may absorb misinformation and misconceptions because the events around him may be more incomprehensible than they would be for an adult. Some brief hints will be given on teaching children of various ages.[13,14,26,37,38] More helpful information is found in a survey text by Petrillo and Sanger.[26] Most of what has been written for nurses about teaching children refers to preparing them for hospitalization and other medical procedures.

## Infants and Toddlers

Teaching an infant or toddler is best done by someone the child knows well—usually a parent. If situations can be anticipated it is best to talk with the parents about how they can prepare the child. Going to the hospital could be presented at home as a game where Teddy Bear packs a suitcase, leaves, and comes back home. Preoperatively, the child can play with the anesthesiology mask. Parents can wear the mask, then the child, then Teddy Bear. Daddy might show the child a doll with stitches and tubes to correspond with what he will experience. The young child is in the stage of sensory motor cognitive development so learning is by activity and exploration. Trips with parents to the intensive care unit or a mock operating room can be planned. One nurse who took children and parents to the intensive care unit preoperatively tried to point out there a picture the child could remember and recognize later. He was also assured that now his parents knew where the intensive care unit was and would be able to find him there. Equipment can be left with the child to handle and play with. The sessions should be short, casual, and right before the coming events. Parents may need considerable encouragement to be honest with their child because they may assume that preparation is upsetting to the child.

## Preschoolers

The preschool child has limited verbal abilities but he can understand much more than he can express. Most of the things described for the younger child are appropriate with the preschooler also. The preschooler can, for example, practice IPPB, coughing, deep breathing, and other pertinent procedures. This age group can play constructively with equipment, bandages, syringes, and dolls to work out fears. This is often best done when the parents are not present because the child may feel inhibited in their presence. Children should not be forced to play with the supplies. Instructions can be given about what part of their body is to be fixed if they are having surgery. A body outline may help. Stress should be placed on reassuring the child that the coming events are not punishment for misdeeds and some would suggest that they need to know that their genital organs will not be harmed. Simple games can be constructively used with this age group to teach cognitive knowledge.

## School-aged Children

In general, school-aged children, like younger children, learn best by playing, manipulating objects, drawing pictures, and such. Their ability to absorb abstract verbal information is limited. Asking the parents what they have previously told the child and what words they have used is likely to make the teaching more understandable. Parents may not know how to teach their child and can benefit by the teacher's guidance or by watching what she does. Parents may interfere if they expect too much from the child, are themselves excessively anxious, or cannot accept the idea that the child needs to know what is to happen. In these cases, the nurse may need to plan separate teaching sessions for children without including the parents and another experience for the parents.

The school-aged child will know more about his body. Teaching outlines to be filled in by the child are helpful. Boys may react negatively to seeing a doll unless it is referred to as a "teaching" doll. Most school-aged children want to know not only what will happen, but why. The school-aged child is very likely to be worried about dying no matter how minor the coming event. He is not likely to mention this verbally. The nurse can provide direct and indirect ways for the school-aged child to express his feelings.

## Adolescents

The teenager may respond better in teaching sessions without his parents present. Although he has much knowledge about his body, he may have some gross misconceptions. The teenager's cognitive abilities are more developed and he can understand abstractions and deal with possibilities and alternatives. Whenever possible, information should be presented in a way which allows the teenager to practice problem solving. This works better than preaching a point. For example, one teacher teaches adolescent women about the use of birth control by presenting them with information on how to go about making decisions about the use of birth control.[36] The teenager can usually read well and absorb written information. Discussion groups have advantages by capitalizing on the security of a peer group and the teen's love of verbalization.

## Teaching the Elderly Individual

It is often assumed that elderly individuals are too old to learn much. There is increasing evidence that older individuals of average health do not decrease in cognitive abilities and even can possibly increase in cognitive functioning during their 60s and 70s. Studies done by researchers who have devoted considerable work to the study of the development of the elderly have found IQ scores and other measures of cognitive ability and flexibility to be maintained or increased in their wide samples of elderly individuals.[2] Unfortunately, the elderly often believe that they are "not as sharp" as they once were because they have absorbed the cultural myth of inevitable intellectual decline in old age. The nurse teaching elderly individuals will have to work against her own and the learner's tendencies to consider the elderly as limited in learning ability. Of course, teaching methods will need to be adapted to visual, hearing, or other possible limitations but expectations can be justifiably held as high for the elderly as for younger adults.

## SOME COMMON DIFFICULTIES

A number of common problems seem to plague nurse-teachers and will be highlighted. First of all, the teacher may have difficulty detecting teaching needs and conclude that there is nothing she need teach the patient. A framework for assessing teaching needs which draws attention to areas to consider for any patient or family might be helpful. The following is only a beginning outline of some needs to consider. Each nurse should develop her own outline similar to this to remind her of assessment areas.

1. General Health Promotion of an Individual
    Diet
    Hygiene
    Rest and relaxation
    Exercise
    Physical development
    Emotional development
    Social development
    Accident prevention
    Community resource awareness
    Health habits
    Immunizations
    Regular health supervision
2. General Health Promotion of a Family
    Husband-wife relationships
    Parent-child relationships
    Birth control
    Financial planning
    Family-community interaction
    Family recreation
    Individual health of family members
    Accomplishment of family developmental tasks
3. Needs Related to a Physical Illness
    Knowledge of condition
    Knowledge of treatment
    Knowledge of medications
    Participation in treatment
    Knowledge of preventive actions

While nurses may believe that the third area is usually considered, few patients in one study cited the nurse as the one who taught them about the medications they were taking. And their knowledge of the medications they were taking was inadequate.[20]

Secondly, teachers often assume that the learner who has had an illness for a period of time knows more about his condition than he actually does.[27] Many opportunities to help individuals and families to live more effectively with various conditions are missed because learning needs are not identified. It is not uncommon to have the patient with a long standing illness comment, "No one ever told me that before" after hearing even fundamental information. Similarly, the patient who has often been hospitalized or had several surgeries is often overlooked.[27] Another group whose learning needs may be missed are health care professionals when they become patients. All of these individuals deserve thorough assessment. More learning needs will be discovered than one imagines.

Thirdly, teaching often tends to be lacking in areas where the roles of the nurse and the physician overlap. The nurse often assumes the physician should teach the patient about his condition, treatment, further care, medications, and so forth. Studies have shown that this information is often not taught even though patients have many questions. In the best interests of the patient, the nurse should check with the physician to see if he is going to do the teaching and if necessary prepare to do so herself. She can have him check the content if she feels unsure of what to teach.

Lastly, teachers often fail to sufficiently elicit questions learners have. One study found that patients had a lot of questions they never asked and a lot of questions which were never answered.[22] Another study indicated that nurses' perceptions of what things patients wanted to know were inaccurate. Patients were mostly interested in broad issues related to their conditions and recovery while nurses thought they cared more about their tests and procedures.[9]

It must be in part that the teacher often does not create an atmosphere conducive to question asking. This may be because she acts as if questions are an interruption, she does not allow time for them, or she gives the impression that the content she has to cover is more important than learners' questions. Other reasons why questions are not asked could be that learners are often hesitant to ask questions because they feel they should know the answer, they are afraid they will appear stupid, they are embarrassed about the subject matter, they have asked questions before and have been brushed off, or they are afraid to learn the answer.[22] A teacher needs to develop ways to facilitate learners' questions. Questions are vitally important to the adult-adult teaching model because they:

1. Show the teacher how the learner is comprehending the information.
2. Indicate where information was not understood.
3. Identify what content should be added.
4. Provide for active involvement by the learner.
5. Indicate that the learner is actively thinking about the content.
6. Add ideas, topics, and points that the teacher did not consider.
7. Aid the learner in making interconnections between what he is learning and what he already knew.

Ways to encourage questions include allowing plenty of time for them, asking for them, and waiting for them to be asked. A teacher might say, "What questions do you have?" rather than, "Are there any questions?" Another important point is to watch the learner for the puzzled expression and ask, "What are you thinking about?" It is a good idea for the teacher to jot down questions learners ask to use in revising her teaching plan. Teachers have been heard to say naively, "They must have understood it because no one had any questions." In truth, a teaching session where the learner never asks a question should be suspect. Asking questions is a high form of mental activity in some respects. The one who reads and hears and then asks good questions is a step beyond the one who merely absorbs what he reads and hears. Teachers may be afraid to allow questions for fear they cannot answer them, but it is easy to say, "I don't know but I will try to find out."

One teacher of patients with diabetes developed an interesting approach to help learners ask questions of a physician. She taught classes for several sessions herself and had the physician attend the last session so that the learners might by then feel secure enough and informed enough to ask him questions.[29] This idea could be adapted to other situations to help patients ask their physician questions because they are often more reluctant to question him than the nurse.

## WHERE TO START

Having read information about the teaching process does not assure that one can expertly perform the process. Practice is needed to polish and perfect teaching skills.

Probably a good place to start learning to teach is by trying short formal teaching sessions to prepare an adult learner for something requiring cognitive learning such as preparation for an x-ray or a trip to a clinic. In this way the content can be prepared ahead of time and evaluated by others and the teacher will not have to think on the spot as much as might occur in an informal situation. The teacher can often observe beforehand what she will be teaching about. The teacher could first talk with some patients and collect their questions and impressions and then use these to develop the content she will teach other patients. Content which is completely written down is usually easiest for the beginning teacher to work from although merely reading it to the learner should be avoided. Since the content is related to cognitive learning, it can be evaluated by asking the learner questions or giving a short quiz. The teacher can repeat the same teaching plan to more patients and each time experiment with different forms of organization, presentation, and methodology. Repeating short sessions several times is sometimes called "mini-teaching" and is especially helpful when videotaped to be studied later. This same lesson plan could then be used in informal situations where the teacher would not have notes.

The next step might be teaching an adult a psychomotor skill plus the related cognitive content. Again this should be repeated with other learners if possible to promote mastery. Evaluation could be by questioning the learner or a quiz and observing the learner perform the skill possibly with a checklist. A good example might be teaching a learner why he should wear ace bandages or occlusive stockings and how to apply them. After the formal method has been practiced, the teacher might try the same subject informally.

Another step might be aimed at affective learning. Still more challenging is teaching a group of learners because one must be able to manage both the teaching and serve as the group leader. Teaching processes would come after sufficient practice has been obtained in the other teaching strategies described. Informal teaching could be strengthened by evaluating what was taught, looking for more content, and planning how the same subject could be better taught again after each informal attempt. Teaching children of various ages might be approached by starting with teenagers because of their more adultlike mental ability and then working with progressively younger children who have less ability to verbalize and whose thinking is more concrete. The ultimate challenge might be planning and conducting a teaching program for groups of learners involving many types of learning objectives such as teaching families to perform home dialysis. Teaching a family requires more skill. Working with learners from other sociocultural groups will be even more difficult. Last of all, various teaching strategies such as behavior modification, programmed instruction, and team teaching could be experimented with.

The nurse who wants to promote teaching and is in a leadership position might find it helpful to assign teaching as a nursing order and require that it be charted since nurses tend to do most consistently those things which must be charted.

## SOME SUGGESTIONS FOR SELF-EVALUATION

The following questions can be used by the nurse to evaluate her use of the teaching process. While evaluation by students and other observers is important, self-evaluation needs to be cultivated as a personal philosophy and as the most valuable form of evaluation.

### General Considerations

1. Is recognition made of the possibility of both conscious and unconscious learning?
2. Is anxiety recognized and controlled?
3. Is the adult-adult teaching model used predominantly?

## Assessment

1. Are learning needs assessed?
2. Are patients facilitated in identifying their own learning needs?
3. Are anticipated learning needs identified?
4. Is the highest priority given to the needs identified by the learner?
5. Are all learning needs validated with the learner?
6. Is readiness determined?
7. Is internal motivation recognized and facilitated?
8. Is positive reinforcement used as external motivation appropriately?

## Planning

1. Are types of content differentiated?
2. Are short term and long term objectives developed?
3. Is content selected appropriate to the learner's needs?
4. Is the learner kept active?
5. Are methods used which logically facilitate content mastery?
6. Are many methods used to increase the possibility that everyone will learn?
7. Is transfer outside the learning experience planned for?
8. Is material presented from the familiar to the unfamiliar?
9. Is anxiety provoking content taught early?
10. Is the usual taught first, then the variation?
11. Is a teaching plan constructed?

## Intervention

1. Are teaching sessions appropriate in length and pace?
2. Are teaching sessions conducted in a way to promote discovery learning?
3. Is the environment considered and planned to facilitate learning?
4. Is the timing of the session well chosen?
5. Is the atmosphere created by the teacher favorable to learning?
6. Is the vocabulary used appropriate?
7. Are advanced organizers used?

## Evaluation

1. Is forgetting anticipated?
2. Is evaluation of the teaching experience done objectively?
3. Is student learning evaluated using the objectives previously established and proper methods?

## Special Strategies

1. Can the teacher apply knowledge of the teaching process to groups?
2. Is team teaching used if appropriate?
3. Does the teacher understand the principles and application of behavior modification?
4. Are children of various ages taught based on their cognitive abilities?
5. Is informal teaching done with the same quality as formal teaching?
6. Are the learning needs of the elderly identified and planned for?

## Overcoming Difficulties

1. Are learning needs assessed for each patient and family thoroughly?
2. Are the learning needs of some individuals repeatedly overlooked?
3. Does the nurse identify areas where teaching may be neglected because of overlapping roles and seek to remedy the situation?
4. Are learners' questions solicited?

## AN EXAMPLE OF THE USE OF THE TEACHING PROCESS

The following example shows how a nurse working in a well baby clinic performed informal teaching in a limited amount of time. The subject was a frequent topic about which the nurse was well prepared to teach.

Ms. Jeffreys had brought her 20-month-old son, Chad, to the community well baby clinic. After the child had been seen by the nurse practitioner, Ms. Jeffreys was experiencing difficulties in getting Chad to leave an electric receptacle alone and put on his clothes instead. In exasperation she sighed, "He won't do anything I say any more. He seems to be getting worse and worse. I don't know what to do with him. Nothing I do will make him obey." The nurse decided to assess further. She asked the mother to describe what kinds of behavior Chad was engaging in. Ms. Jeffreys described things such as running the other way when she called or approached him, tantrums, negativism, and assertion of independence. She next asked Ms. Jeffreys how she responded to these. Ms. Jeffrey's behavior as she described it was not effective or consistent. The nurse found out that the offensive behaviors had been going on for about two months. The nurse asked Ms. Jeffreys if she had ever had much contact with children of this age and she commented that she had not. She asked Ms. Jeffreys why she thought Chad might be acting as he was and Ms. Jeffreys replied that she believed that something must be wrong with him.

The nurse smiled to herself. It sounded like a typical case of a mother unprepared for the inevitable transition of her baby from complacent to a "terrible two." She mentally formulated three objectives. She hoped that Ms. Jeffreys would be able to:

Express her frustrations at coping with her child.

State that Chad's behavior is normal for his age.

Use some consistent alternative approaches to Chad's behavior.

The nurse asked Ms. Jeffreys if she would like to come talk to her in her office for a few minutes about Chad while someone watched him. Chad was soon busy with a volunteer and Ms. Jeffreys was comfortably seated in the nurse's office with a cup of coffee. The nurse first encouraged Ms. Jeffreys to talk about how she felt about coping with Chad. The nurse offered supportive comments as appropriate. Ms. Jeffreys was a concerned mother, but as she was a single mother, she faced many challenges. Next the nurse introduced the subject of the normalness of Chad's behavior. She briefly described simply what Chad was going through in trying to become more assertive and why this was desirable. She also explained his negativism. She mentioned other common behaviors of two-year-olds and Ms. Jeffreys laughed at the perfectness of the description saying, "That's him all right."

Next, the nurse said, "I think since you understand that Chad is doing some of the things because he is normal, we may be able to explore some ways to handle some of the aspects of his behavior which are the most disturbing. Let's talk first about tantrums. Have you thought of any other things you might want to try when he has one?" One by one the nurse and Ms. Jeffreys discussed Chad's new tricks and explored how the mother could react. The nurse encouraged Ms. Jeffreys to come up with her own ideas and occasionally offered her own suggestions. After the major areas were covered, Ms. Jeffreys was quite animated and anxious to try out her new solutions. The nurse gave her the clinic phone number and encouraged her to call when she wanted to talk more. The nurse gave her a small pamphlet explaining growth and development of children from infancy until six years old.

The nurse recorded the teaching she had done in the patient's chart and noted some other teaching needs she had identified. She decided to evaluate her teaching related to the second and third objectives by calling Ms. Jeffreys in a week.

A week later the nurse called Ms. Jeffreys. Ms. Jeffreys reported that things were going much better at home. She had tried a few new approaches to Chad's behavior and was pleased with the results. Tantrums were much less frequent. She reported that in particular the most helpful changes had been seeing that Chad got more sleep and taking him by the hand to help him comply with the directions rather than expecting him to voluntarily comply. She had met another mother in her apartment building and they compared notes on their two-year-olds and found them to be quite similar so she seemed confident that Chad was just "going through a stage." She had questions on toilet training and diet which she asked. The nurse invited Ms. Jeffreys to come to the clinic between Chad's appointments for any other information she wanted or just to talk about anything. Ms. Jeffreys seemed interested in the offer. In addition the nurse told Ms. Jeffreys about a mother's group discussion offered by the county extension home economist. Ms. Jeffreys took the phone number of the home economist's office and stated that she planned to find out about the group.

The nurse concluded that the objectives she had formulated for Ms. Jeffreys related to Chad appeared to have been met. The mother had expressed her feelings about coping with Chad, seemed to know that his behavior was normal, and reported that she was learning to use other methods in a consistent way to cope with him. The nurse had also identified further learning needs for this family and recorded them in Chad's chart for the reference of those who worked with the family.

## SUMMARY

The nurse's ability to identify learning needs of patients and families and teach needed information is one of her most important nursing functions. The use she makes of her knowledge of and skill in the teaching process may well influence the patient's level of wellness.

The teaching process incorporates the stages of assessment, planning, intervention, and evaluation. It can be carried out with individuals or groups and a number of variations are possible such as behavior modification and contractual learning. The teaching a nurse engages in can be formal or informal but hopefully it is based on an adult-adult teaching model rather than the more familiar parent-child teaching model.

Developing competence in use of the teaching process requires practice and experimentation as well as conscientious and continual study by the nurse to improve her knowledge base.

## REFERENCES

1. Ballantyne, D. J.: "CCTV for patients." Am. J. Nurs. 74:263, 1974.
2. Baltes, P. B., and Schaie, K. W.: "Aging and IQ: The myth of the twilight years." Psychol. Today 7:35, 1974.
3. Barnard, K.: "Teaching the retarded child is a family affair." Am. J. Nurs. 68:305, 1968.
4. Cantor, M. M.: "Philosophy, purpose, and objectives: Why do we have them," in Stone, S., et al. (eds.): *Management for Nurses*. C. V. Mosby, St. Louis, 1976.
5. Carruth, B. E.: "Modifying behavior through social learning." Am. J. Nurs. 76:1804, 1976.
6. Clark, C. C.: "Simulation gaming: A new strategy in nursing education." Nurs. Educator 1:4, 1976.
7. Combs, A. W.: *The Professional Education of Teachers*. Allyn and Bacon, Boston, 1965.
8. Cosper, B.: "How well do patients understand hospital jargon?" Am. J. Nurs. 77:1932, 1977.
9. Dodge, J. S.: "What patients should be told: Patients' and nurses' beliefs." Am. J. Nurs. 72:1852, 1972.
10. Dweck, C. S.: "Children's interpretation of evaluative feedback: the effect of social cues on learned helplessness," in Hetherington, E. M., and Parke, R. D. (eds.): *Contemporary Readings in Child Psychology*. McGraw-Hill, New York, 1977.
11. Elwood, E.: "A study of selected physiological responses to breathing exercise practice in patients with chronic pulmonary disease." New York University, doctoral dissertation, Department of Physiology, 1967.
12. Flegle, J. M.: "Teaching self-dialysis to adults in a hospital." Am. J. Nurs. 77:270, 1977.
13. Friedland, J. M.: "Learning behaviors of a preadolescent with diabetes." Am. J. Nurs. 76:59, 1976.
14. Gillon, J.: "Teaching children about heart surgery." Lecture given at Indiana University School of Nursing, Indianapolis, 1973.
15. Harris, T A.: *I'm OK—You're OK: A Practical Guide to Transactional Analysis*. Harper and Row, New York, 1967.
16. Highet, G.: *The Art of Teaching*. Vintage Books, New York, 1950.
17. Hoyman, H. S.: "Models of human nature and their impact on health education." J. Sch. Health 44:374, 1974.
18. Katzell, M. E.: "Evaluation in the affective domain." Presented at the Workshop on Evaluation in the Affective Domain, College of St. Catherine, St. Paul, Minn, 1973.
19. Laird, M.: "Techniques for teaching pre- and postoperative patients." Am. J. Nurs. 75:1338, 1975.
20. Leary, J. A., Vessela, D. M., and Yeaw, E. M.: "Self-administered medications." Am. J. Nurs. 71:1193, 1971.
21. Leppert, P., and Williams, B.: "Birth films may miscarry." Am. J. Nurs. 68:2181, 1968.
22. Linehan, D. T.: "What does the patient want to know?" Am. J. Nurs. 66:1066, 1966.
23. Marriner, A.: *The Nursing Process: A Scientific Approach to Nursing Care*. C. V. Mosby, St. Louis, 1975.
24. Mitchell, E. S.: "Protocol for teaching hypertensive patients." Am. J. Nurs. 77:808, 1977.
25. Nickerson, D.: "Teaching the hospitalized diabetic." Am. J. Nurs. 72:935, 1972.
26. Petrillo, M., and Sanger, S.: *Emotional Care of Hospitalized Children*. J. B. Lippincott, Philadelphia, 1972.
27. Redman, B. K.: *The Process of Patient Teaching in Nursing*. C. V. Mosby, St. Louis, 1976.
28. Roos, P.: "Human rights and behavior modification." Mental Retard. 12:3, 1974.
29. Salzer, J. E.: "Classes to improve diabetic self care." Am. J. Nurs. 75:1324, 1975.
30. Schmitt, F. E., and Powhatan, J. W.: "Psychological preparation of surgical patients." Nurs. Res. 22:108, 1973.
31. Shufer, S.: "Teaching via the play-discussion group." Am. J. Nurs. 77:1960, 1977.

32. Stevens, B. J.: "The teaching-learning process," in *The Nurse As Executive.* Contemporary Publishing, Wakefield, Mass., 1975.
33. Sutterley, D. C., and Donnelly, G. F.: *Perspectives in Human Development.* J. B. Lippincott, Philadelphia, 1973.
34. Talabere, L. R.: "The development and implementation of a cystic fibrosis teaching plan." J. Assoc. Care Child. Hosp. 5:18, 1976.
35. Tarver, J., and Turner, A. J.: "Teaching behavior modification to patients' families." Am. J. Nurs. 74:282, 1974.
36. Taylor, D.: "A new way to teach teens about contraceptives." Matern. Child Nurs. J. 1:378, 1976.
37. Treloar, D. M.: "Ready, set—No: Something is missing from pediatric pre-operative preparation." Matern. Child Nurs. J. 3:50, 1978.
38. Waidley, E.: "Preparing children for radiology procedure." J. Assoc. Care Child. Hosp. 6:6, 1977.
39. Wang, R., and Watson, F.: "Contracting for weight reduction—making the sacrifices worthwhile." Matern. Child Nurs. J. 3:46, 1978.
40. Zentner, J., and Murray, R.: "Health teaching: A basic nursing intervention," in Murray, R., et al.: *Nursing Concepts for Health Promotion.* Prentice-Hall, Englewood Cliffs, N.J., 1975.

## BIBLIOGRAPHY

Beebe, J. E., Pendleton, E. M., and King, E.: "Bench conferences in a large obstetric clinic." Am. J. Nurs. 68:85, 1968.
Healy, K.: "Does preoperative instruction make a difference?" Am. J. Nurs. 68:62, 1968.
Klinzing, D. R., and Klinzing, D. G.: "An evaluation of video-tapes designed to communicate with children about hospitalization, surgery, and casting." J. Assoc. Care Child. Hosp. 4:4, 1976.
Knowles, M. S.: *The Modern Practice of Adult Education.* Association Press, New York, 1970.
Kramer, M.: "Team teaching is more than team planning." Nurs. Outlook 16:51, 1968.
Levine, D., and Wiener, E.: "Let the computer teach it." Am. J. Nurs. 75:1300, 1975.
Loomis, M. E., and Horsley, J. A.: *Interpersonal Change.* McGraw-Hill, New York, 1974.
Manwaring, M.: "What patients need to know about pacemakers." Am. J. Nurs. 77:825, 1977.
Smith, D. M.: "Writing objectives as a nursing practice skill." Am. J. Nurs. 71:319, 1971.
Tollefsrud, V.: "We're for educating our patients." Am. J. Nurs. 56:1009, 1956.
Underwood, P. R.: "Communication through role playing." Am. J. Nurs. 71:1184, 1971.

# CHAPTER 5

## THE LEADERSHIP PROCESS

All of us serve as leaders in some situations and at certain times whether or not we are aware of it. All too often leadership is assumed to be synonymous with formal authority to manage others. If leadership is defined as interpersonal influence, it can be considered independently of management. In fact, management may or may not encompass leadership. Individuals listen to managers because they have formal authority. Individuals listen to leaders because what they say is relevant and logical.[33] In practical terms, the fact that leadership and management are not synonymous means that all individuals, regardless of whether they have formal authority, can exert leadership in certain circumstances if they know how. Often informal leaders have influence equal to or greater than that of formal leaders.

All nurses, regardless of position and setting, need to develop their informal leadership potential. What problems related to the delivery of health care might have already been solved if nursing had more input in the development and administration of health care services? What might clinics, hospitals, and community health agencies be like if nursing wisdom was widely represented? Would a restructuring of the health care system occur with increased emphasis on prevention and health promotion if nurses knew how to develop and use clout? Even more concretely, how might the health and well being of any particular patient, family, or community be affected if nurses were free to assume a forceful and decisive advocacy role in planning and acting rather than the secondary and indirect roles they now assume cautiously?

How a nurse develops her abilities to influence others, therefore, has important implications for her career as a nurse, for her profession, for the health of those she works with, and for communities. This chapter will explore the concept of informal leadership and identify ways for the nurse to analyze and fully utilize her leadership ability even though she is not necessarily in a position of formal leadership. Leadership will not be related to management of others but will be represented as behaviors which a nurse can learn.

### THE LEADERSHIP PROBLEM IN NURSING

There has been much written describing the lack of appropriate leadership in the nursing profession. Nursing leaders are seen as hard to identify and immature in leadership style as

**157**

compared with leaders in other professions. Nursing leaders often are described as administratively oriented individuals who are concerned with rules, orderliness, and close supervision of others.[10,24] The usual administrative style has been described as "management by crisis" which is characterized as attention to the present rather than the future.[10] A more mature form of leadership which is characterized by a person with original and innovative ideas, a change orientation, and a future perspective is believed to be rarely seen.

The profoundness of nursing's leadership problem is attested to by the fact that nursing seldom controls even its own practice.[21,31] Many nurses are not even aware of this fact. And because of the lack of firm and stable leadership, nursing practice frequently falls into fadism.[32] A perusal of back issues of nursing journals shows that nurses often develop a "fad of the year" orientation. One year it was technical education, another year the preparation of nurse clinicians, then a preoccupation with the nurse-practitioner movement. In addition there often seems an incessant campaign to replace nursing terminology with terms borrowed from other fields such as "data base," "component," and "module." Is this because nursing must turn outside of itself for leadership?

There are several reasons suggested for the leadership problem in nursing. Primarily, one must consider the fact that 97 percent of all nurses are women, and women are not socialized in our society to be leaders, but rather followers.[19] Women have traditionally and legally been powerless and exploited by men.[1] In the course of growing up, a female often learns to be dependent, nonassertive, passive, nonambitious, and self-depreciating.[47] If a female does not adopt these attributes she is likely to be scorned as less feminine and as "frustrated" by both males and females. Even the female who enters a baccalaureate nursing program is commonly assumed to be not totally serious about a career but rather improving her chances to meet and marry suitable men.[19] Or she may be learning a skill which she believes will prepare her for motherhood and running a home and be, therefore, something she might fall back on if the future does not work out as intended. This orientation to nursing may not promote serious commitment or interest in leadership.

The nurse who does find herself in a leadership position may feel insecure. If she has leadership strivings she may deny them for they are often considered inappropriate in a female and synonymous with being "mannish" and unattractive.[32] Nor is she likely to see other women who are role models of successful female leaders. She may be criticized, on the one hand, for having traits believed to be "masculine" such as assertiveness and aggressiveness or, on the other hand, criticized for having traits believed to be "feminine" such as indecisiveness and pettiness. To be admired she probably must work twice as effectively and twice as hard as a man in the same position.[19] Both the men and women she works with are often equally negative towards having a female in a leadership position. Effective leadership behaviors such as logical thinking and decisiveness have even been defined as psychologically unhealthy behaviors when they occur in females.[6]

At the same time, men are frequently considered natural leaders. This is shown repeatedly in the rapid rise to power by men in nursing. Even in elections for membership on nursing organization committees where the majority of voters are women, men are often elected more easily than their female opponents regardless of their qualifications. Leadership positions in nursing are already overly represented by men in proportion to their percentage in nursing.[28] Nursing is well on its way to duplicating the characteristic situation present in education where men hold almost all administrative positions and women occupy almost all of the lowest echelon positions.

Obviously the solution to this problem is not to restrict the entrance of men into nursing but to strengthen women nurses' leadership abilities so that they are fairly represented in leadership positions. An appropriate way to do this involves encouraging women to be confident, respectful of themselves and their sex, and self-directive. For those already in nursing who have not been reared with these attributes, developing leadership behaviors will be more challenging. The solution lies with each nurse if she is willing to search for and understand how her socialization has affected her self-esteem and willingness to lead.[19]

Another reason for the lack of leadership experience may be related to nursing's traditional alignment with large agencies or institutions.[10] Nurses rarely are self-employed. This may lead the nurse to direct her loyalties towards her employer and not towards herself and her profession. She may expect her employing institution to look out for her best interests and give little time or thought to them herself. After all, she has often been socialized to find situations where she will be taken care of and will not be dependent on her own initiative. Because she is lulled into a sense of loyalty to and security from her employer, she does not critically evaluate where she or the institution is going and leadership situations may not emerge which test her leadership abilities. In addition, in the many large agencies and organizations where most nurses work, individual initiative becomes less important than team effort. Thus, she is gradually conditioned and rewarded for being a team player and not the coach. It is no secret that physicians and hospital administrators have in many situations exploited health workers who are female.[1]

A further reason for a dearth of identifiable leaders in nursing may be that the nursing profession has long idealized the service aspects of its function.[14] Thus, rather than serving their own best interests, nurses have been busy serving others. The nurse has often been portrayed as a motherly caring individual who puts aside her own needs for the sake of those she serves. Thus to direct attention towards her own needs and those of the profession may seem antithetical to nursing. She might also lose male approval.[14]

In addition, the patterns of education which are used to educate nursing students may contribute to a lack of leadership development. A large number of nurses have been educated outside of legitimate educational settings in a system which is considered frankly inferior.[1] Even education within educational institutions may carry remnants of its hospital based past as demonstrated by an emphasis on neatness, promptness, moral indoctrination, obedience, incessant evaluation conferences, and conformity.[10] Unlike other plans of study, nursing curricula often allow little space for general electives. Within nursing curricula there is seldom room for developing individual interests except for an occasional self-guided experience. Leadership content, when taught, may be closely correlated with team leading, making assignments, conducting team conferences, and management, so that leadership is seen as a particular set of duties and a position rather than as behaviors every nurse can exhibit in any setting. When students are socialized into a role which expects conformity from the beginning, they are unlikely to develop into innovators and leaders upon graduation.[8]

Lastly, the majority of practicing nurses tend to be young, inexperienced, and in their early twenties. Few women demonstrate leadership behaviors until later in their lives when they reach an age of more personal security.[9] Young and inexperienced nurses are not likely to be confident enough to stand up to other more experienced, older, and predominantly male professionals and administrators. It may be tempting, therefore, to deny any leadership strivings and instead identify with the powerful physician, for example, and share his power and prestige through assuming delegated tasks eagerly.[19]

## LEADERSHIP AS A WAY OF LIFE

Leadership in the past has been studied as a compilation of certain personality traits. After a number of studies were compared it became apparent that few traits were consistently found in several studies. Newer sources of information on leadership now focus on leadership as the outcome of certain behaviors exhibited by a person.[33] Leaders can be identified as people who have an exceptional amount of social influence on others.[33] Since human behavior is believed to be largely learned, it follows that leadership behavior can be learned.

## LEADERSHIP BEHAVIORS

Certain behaviors which lead to functioning as a leader can be identified and studied. These will be examined along with suggestions as to how a nurse can incorporate them into her nursing practice and personal life.

### 1. Leaders Develop Good Communication Skills

Leaders are frequently described as communicating clearly.[33] Others understand what they say. Their communications are direct, honest, and open. The chapter on communication contains many suggestions for developing skill in communication when accompanied by practice. Open, honest, clear, and direct communications enable others to trust the leader and more likely guarantee that what she says is perceived accurately.

### 2. Leaders Possess Specific Knowledge and Competence

Leaders tend to be experts in their field.[16] Their competence is evident in their own nursing practice. Others listen to them because it is obvious that they know what they are talking about. If they do not have specific knowledge about a subject, they say so and search out the knowledge.

There is no easy or quick way to develop knowledge and skill. To become an expert, one must pursue a lifelong pattern of study.[16] This requires discipline and perseverance. Extensive reading can be combined with attendance at conferences and lectures and formal coursework. Often arranging observational experiences and talking with others with expertise is helpful. Becoming expert in one subject means that the nurse must make some decisions about what she will concentrate on because one cannot learn about one area in depth if one is trying to learn about every area. The nurse-leader must take personal responsibility for continually developing her knowledge base and skills. The school of nursing she attended cannot teach her everything she will need to know forever, nor will her employer usually provide her with adequate learning opportunities. Studying a subject at one time does not guarantee that the knowledge gained will be adequate or relevant a few years later.

One of the first obstacles to overcome in developing competency is to realize when and where one's competency is less than optimal. In some situations it is easy to drift along without feeling a need to add to one's knowledge. One may collect superficial bits of knowledge which on the surface appear as authentic background. Another problem is one's natural tendency to feel threatened by a lack of knowledge and to build up defenses to deny the need for more knowledge. Thus, when the nurse hears about a new way of doing something which she does not quite comprehend, she may instinctively respond with, "The way I always do that works for me and I'm sticking with it" or "I know they teach all that stuff in school now but this is the real world and not an ivory tower." There are ways to note when one's competency and knowledge are beginning to become obsolete. One can ask oneself:

1. Am I frequently asked questions by students or others that I don't know the answer to?
2. Am I sought out by coworkers and others for advice and suggestions or are others deliberately bypassing me to ask someone else?
3. Am I still regularly reading journal articles in my field of practice or do they seem too complicated, sophisticated, or irrelevant?
4. Am I deliberately avoiding discussions about patient care with physicians or new staff members because they may expose my lack of knowledge?
5. Do I resist attending inservice programs, courses, or conferences because they cost too much, I've heard it all before, or because there is too much trouble finding parking places?[36]

Once she becomes aware of an area where study is needed, the nurse might benefit from formulating a definite plan to increase her knowledge. This would include identifying specifically what she wants to learn about, investigating resources, setting up a time table and plan, and evaluating her progress.

Jane, a new graduate, had worked for a year in a large hospital on a pediatric unit where there were many children having surgical correction of congenital heart defects. She felt she was quite knowledgeable on the subject of open heart surgery and the associated nursing care. One afternoon while she was charting in the nurses station, she overheard a nursing instructor going through a patient's chart with a student. The instructor was questioning the student and explaining to the student the rationale for several treatments and the reasons for some complications after open heart surgery. Jane was amazed at how much new information she was hearing and that the student was able to answer some of the questions that she would not have been able to. She realized that she had fallen into the common trap of operating on superficial knowledge without awareness of where her own inadequacies were. She decided to plan a program of study to improve her knowledge about the care of children having cardiac surgery and she used the instructor as one source of information on material to read. Later after Jane had read considerably on open heart and closed heart surgery, her clinical director arranged for her to observe several times in the operating room. Jane noticed that her care for and observations about patients with cardiac conditions became more specific and definite. She frequently talked with the members of the surgical team about specific observations. Other staff nurses began asking her questions. In a period of a few months the head nurse asked Jane to head a committee to develop a teaching outline for children having cardiac surgery and their parents.

The nurse needs to carefully evaluate the position she is in to determine if her position is providing her with the impetus for continuing to grow in knowledge and skills. One position held for two years may provide two years of growth while another position held for the same length of time may provide one year of growth repeated twice. Changing positions may become warranted when the work has become too routine and the phrase, "We have always done it this way" becomes her byword. Other things which may help prevent a knowledge gap from developing include working towards another degree, belonging to and participating in the activities of a professional nursing organization, and avoiding periods of complete inactivity from nursing.[36] Developing one's sense of professional competence will help increase one's willingness to assume leadership behaviors. This sense of professional self-esteem has long been missing in nursing.[12]

## 3. Leaders Develop Expertise at Problem Solving

Problem solving is one of the major things leaders do. All individuals solve problems daily but leaders solve problems particularly well.[16] They perceive the problem more accurately, gather more complete data, consider more creative alternatives, carry out the plan more carefully, and evaluate more consistently. Information is given in the chapter on the problem solving process to guide the nurse in developing proficiency in problem solving with experience. Leaders realize what decisions they can and should make and which ones they should not make.[16] They realize that failing to decide is a decision.

## 4. Leaders Rely on Others Appropriately

Leaders do not exist in a vacuum. They are leaders only when working with others. Leadership is not synonymous with being known as a "hard worker." Hard workers may or may not be leaders. The leader knows how to inspire and motivate others to quality productive efforts. Part of this may well be because of the example she herself displays. Other aspects of how she motivates others involve relying on the judgments of others who are more knowledgeable about an area than she is. Her sensitivity to others enables her to know what contribution each coworker is capable of so that her efforts can dovetail with theirs.

## 5. Leaders Maintain a Future Orientation

Another behavior which leaders exhibit is being future oriented.[16,33] Leaders see what is ahead or express what they desire to occur and their visions coincide with what the people they work with desire. One way to develop a future perspective is by planning regularly to spend time projecting into the future. The leader periodically sets the concerns of the present aside to consider what is ahead. Attending conferences and professional meetings as well as reading the "news" sections in professional journals also helps as many of these sources call attention to changes occurring or expected to occur in the future.

Keeping the attention attuned to the future is not an easy task. It is very difficult especially when one works under very real pressures in the present. But developing one's ability to consider the future can lead to changes in how the present is perceived and these changes may be highly significant.

> Janice was a community health nurse in a medium sized metropolitan city. She noticed that an increasing number of her new prenatal and child supervision referrals from a large urban hospital were never found at home and were eventually dropped after the customary three attempted visits. She began writing down the numbers of patients who were never contacted. Janice felt that one reason for this high rate of missed referrals was the increasing frequency of women's employment in jobs outside of the home. Janice did some independent study on the area and became interested in exploring the effects of changing women's roles on the area of community health visits as presently practiced. She brought up the subject to her supervisor one day and suggested that the agency might benefit from considering how services might need to be revised in the future to coordinate with changes in society which were occurring. The supervisor had Janice present her data and information at the next staff meeting and the agency began a study of the area.

There are several ways to assess how oriented one is towards the future, present, or past.

1. Have I thought about future problems which will potentially affect my practice area in one year, five years, or ten years?
2. Do I have plans regarding what I would like to see occur in the future in my practice situation?
3. Am I working on projects which are related to future goals as well as present goals?
4. Do I find myself content with the present because so many improvements have been made over the past?
5. Do I seem to be caught by surprise by changes which others knew were coming?
6. Can I visualize a future situation when my practice area would have evolved into something totally different from what presently exists?
7. Do I find that my first thoughts on how to solve a problem often are to do what was always done in the past?
8. Do most changes introduced in my work area seem senseless and a lot of bother?

The ability to consider the future and orient the present towards that vision is an attribute well worth cultivating. At first one may need to plan a specific time to take stock of where one is going and plan goals until futurism becomes an established part of one's behavior. Belonging to a professional nursing organization is helpful in that the leadership of the organization is often attending to events in the future which one may be too busy to observe and reporting about them.

## 6. Leaders Incorporate Expressive Functions into Their Interactions with Others

Expressive functions are those activities in a group which relate to social-emotional aspects.[23] Leaders are described as in touch with their coworkers. They listen actively and validate what they are hearing from others.[33] This is one reason that what the leader suggests and initiates makes sense to her coworkers. Leaders encourage others when they are discouraged. They often exhibit behaviors which tend to unify the work groups.[33] They help individuals adjust to new situations by providing them with helpful information and helping them express their feelings. They notice the efforts of others and offer sincere and spontaneous praise. They provide a supportive and positive influence so that others feel good about themselves and their work. The atmosphere is pleasant and sources of conflict are reduced.[20]

Suggestions on how to relate to others with empathy, acceptance, and a nonjudgmental attitude, for example, are given in the chapter on the helping process. The expressive functions of the leader are the same as the behaviors exhibited in helping encounters and relationships. Thus one who develops expertise in the helping process is also demonstrating behaviors associated with leadership. Some groups need more expressive functioning by a leader than others.[33] It is possible for the nurse-leader to recognize when expressive functions are not being met in the work group and take steps to support group members, decrease conflicts, and increase the pleasant atmosphere.

## 7. Leaders Perform Instrumental Functions Effectively

Instrumental functions are associated with accomplishing the goals of the work group the leader is associated with.[23] They involve the initiation and coordination of actions. Instrumental functions provide for the success of the group and in return elevate group spirits.[33] One way the leader does this is by becoming an initiator herself. She volunteers to perform an activity which will get things started. This may involve calling a meeting, starting a committee, writing a letter, or making an appointment, for example. This attitude can be cultivated by listening and watching for the common situation where someone says, "Someone should do something about this someday" and responding with, "Let's start on it today." These actions delineate and organize the group's work.[20]

Nancy worked as part of the nursing staff in a community health agency which was housed in cramped quarters. One month a secretary who was retiring and moving donated an old small refrigerator to the lounge area. The secretarial staff, who had never used the lounge, began storing their lunches in the refrigerator and eating in the lounge. The nursing staff experienced some annoyance at the presence of many more individuals in the already cramped room. They also felt strained in their conversations about personal and professional matters. The situation persisted for six months with the nursing staff grumbling in private. Each discussion invariably ended with someone commenting that Mrs. Porter, the Director, should be told about the professional staff's discontentment with the situation. One day after the usual disgruntled complaining, Nancy volunteered to talk to Mrs. Porter on behalf of the professional staff. She got a note pad and asked for the points the group would like her to express to Mrs. Porter. Secondly, she asked the group to brainstorm on possible solutions to the problem. Nancy made the appointment to talk to the director after the discussion.

Another instrumental function involves representing the group to others and promoting the group's interests.[33] This may involve telling others what the group is trying to accomplish or speaking up for the group.

Instrumental functions also involve coordination of activity. This requires establishing goals, planning with the work group, evaluating progress, and revising plans when necessary. The amount of coordination of activity which the nurse-leader does depends on the characteristics of the group she is working with and the situation.[20]

Marty is a staff nurse who works in a hospital outpatient unit. Most of the members of her work group are technical nurses with considerable amounts of experience in a traditional clinic role and two new professional nurses with little previous nursing experience. Marty feels the clinic nursing role could be expanded and strengthened from what it now is. The head nurse encourages her efforts. Marty exerts informal leadership which involves considerable initiation of ideas, group representation, and coordination of group activities. Becky, on the other hand, works in another outpatient department where the staff is predominantly experienced professionals. Primary nursing is practiced in this clinic and nurses assume responsibility for teaching and other preventive health care roles and home visits to families by the primary nurse are made when warranted. Although Becky is a supervisor in the clinic, her instrumental role is very subtle compared to the role Marty is playing.

## 8. Leaders Understand the Concept of Leadership Style

Another factor which affects the nurse's functioning is leadership style. Each individual has a leadership style reflective of her personality, experiences as a follower, and socialization.[33] This leads to a wide variety of leadership behavior which might be visualized as existing on a continuum.[34,44]

### Strongly Instrumental

Emphasis clearly on getting tasks accomplished.
Makes decisions independently of the group.
Does not focus on personal reactions of others.

## Somewhat Instrumental

Major emphasis on task accomplishment.
Allows others some role in decision making.
Some sensitivity to and concern for group members.

## Neutral

Equal emphasis on task accomplishment and well being of group members.
Allows others definite role in decision making.
Much sensitivity to group members.

## Somewhat Expressive

Minor interest in task accomplishment.
Allows group freedom in decision making.
Considerable emphasis on group spirit.

## Strongly Expressive

No concern with task accomplishment.
Total unconcern with decision making.
Major emphasis on group solidarity and individual adjustment.

Most individuals tend to function in the middle ranges of this continuum and can shift slightly one way or the other. Very few individuals function on the extremes of this continuum. It is also difficult for individuals to change totally from one end of the continuum to another.[33] There is no right or wrong to any of these styles of leadership, although it is believed that individuals who are strongly instrumental or strongly expressive might be more effective in most situations if they tried to function more in the middle ranges. Balance and sensitivity to the needs of the situation and the other formal or informal leaders present are what is important. All of these styles and the variations in between have their disadvantages and are more appropriate in one situation than another—even the styles in the extremes.[34]

Tanya worked as the charge nurse on nights in a large newborn intensive care unit. The unit was very busy with many critically ill infants and a full capacity. During the night an unexpectedly heavy snowstorm paralyzed the city. Only one of the day staff nurses made it in for the morning shift. Tanya's night staff had been less than usual due to illnesses. The clinical director brought two additional aides to the unit and asked Tanya to carry on as charge nurse until other nurses could be brought in by road crews. After considering how tired her staff was, the capabilities of the nurse who had come in, the lack of knowledge of the two additional aides, and heavy demands of the situation, Tanya adopted a strongly instrumental style. She assumed responsibility for almost all decision making, issued short, clear orders, and established the priority focused on getting all the important care of the infants done. Under her direction the unit functioned efficiently until the usual day staff arrived.

Tom was appointed assistant head nurse on a busy surgical unit in a hospital. The senior staff nurses on the unit were competent, experienced, and responsible leaders who frequently were in conflict with the head nurse. The morale of the staff was low and antagonism and competition among staff factions was growing. Tom concluded that his leadership style should be as strongly expressive as possible so he concentrated on expressive functions such as building a sense of team spirit, offering honest praise and encouragement, and helping individuals work through conflicts. He allowed the senior staff nurse and the head nurse complete decision making freedom.

Both the individuals just described were successful in their particular situations. It is interesting to reflect on what might have happened if Tanya had decided to be strongly humanistic and Tom strongly authoritarian.

In choosing one style over another, the leader reflects then on many things:[44]

1. What is my characteristic style?
2. How much is it possible for me to change my style?
3. What are the competencies and personalities of my work group?
4. What are the demands of the situation?
5. What leadership style do the group members expect and desire?
6. What functions are other formal and informal leaders playing in the situation?

Usually the appropriate style is somewhere near the center of the continuum. Great difficulties can arise when the characteristics of the work group change or the demands of the situation but the leader is unable to change her style appropriately.

Linda was a senior staff nurse on a medical unit in a general hospital. She became convinced of the need for turning part of her work unit into a specialized rehabilitation unit. She was able to win the support of her clinical director and two physicians. She doggedly pursued her goal against generalized resistance from nursing service and the medical staff. The unit eventually became a reality and Linda, while still a staff nurse, played a continuing leadership role in teaching staff nurses rehabilitation techniques, educating physicians in the potential benefits of the unit for their patients, and establishing policies. In a period of months the unit was equipped, staffed, and on the way to being well supported by the medical, nursing, and administrative staffs. However, about this same time, the staff on the new unit and the other hospital personnel complained about repeated difficulties working with Linda. Unfortunately, Linda was not able to modify the hard-driving, "I don't care whose toes I step on," crusading attitude which had led to the development of the unit. And, even though Linda was obviously the most knowledgeable about rehabilitation care, she was bypassed when the unit was enlarged and a separate head nurse was selected.

Another difficult situation involves succeeding a leader who has left behind explicit expectations in the personnel she led. Some individuals like being submissive to a strongly instrumental leader and then vicariously identifying with the leader's strength. This, of course, limits growth by the followers and creates problems for the new leader.[20]

Developing a flexible leadership style then means learning how one functions, developing sensitivity to different situations, and learning to shift styles when appropriate. If a leader finds that she has a very rigid style, there may be another person with whom she may lead who will provide the complementary function to create balance.[33]

## 9. Leaders Understand the System They Work In

One of the most important activities a leader can engage in is learning about the organization she works in.[16] Not learning about the organization in general leads to a very limited perspective and focus. This is commonly seen in nursing where nurses at the lower levels understand little about the organization, but criticize sharply how things are done.[10] One's ability to function, let alone promote change, will be necessarily limited.

A large number of nurses work in bureaucratic organizations. It is popular to blame all the current problems related to the delivery of nursing care on the fact that nurses do work in bureaucracies. Bureaucracies are seen as limiting initiative, preventing quality performance, encouraging dependency, and leading to powerlessness.[18,45] In fact, it would appear that because nurses work in bureaucratic institutions, professional practice cannot exist at all. Whether the bureaucracy limits nursing practice or whether it provides a convenient excuse for less than professional practice remains to be proven. What does seem apparent is that nurses do not function well in bureaucracies. This may be because of their own deficiencies and not necessarily because of inherent limitations of the system. Kramer points out that new graduates lack several important abilities or skills which interfere with their functioning in bureaucratic organizations including self-confidence and the ability to work within restrictions of the system. They experience a lack of role fulfillment wherein the nurse feels unable to perform as prepared to function and still meet the objectives of the organization.[27]

The remedy to this situation may not lie in dissolving all bureaucratic health agencies, as if that were possible, but rather rests with preparing nurses to function within them. It seems unlikely that bureaucracy is on its way out and it may be increasing. Evidence is beginning to be reported that bureaucracies in and of themselves are not all that they have been accused of being. One recent study found that employees at all levels who worked in bureaucracies were more intellectually flexible, receptive to change, self-directive, and open minded than a matched sample of employees in nonbureaucratic settings. Reasons for these differences were felt to be that those employees working in bureaucracies felt more challenged by the complexity of their work and benefited from a feeling of more job security and higher income than nonbureaucratic employees.[26]

What then can be done to help nurses who work in bureaucratic health institutions to reach their potential and function at their maximum? There is not room here to present an entire dissertation on survival in a bureaucracy but an attempt will be made to discuss some relevant points which govern functioning in a bureaucracy of which nurses are often unaware or only vaguely aware.

## THE DECISION-MAKING STRUCTURE

First of all, the nurse needs to understand several things about the health care institution in which she works. Most obvious, perhaps, is the formal organization of the institution. How are departments aligned? Who controls which areas? How many levels of administration are there? In particular, it is helpful to know who is directly, intermediately, and ultimately responsible for nursing.

Next, it is helpful to consider the mission of the organization. Why was the institution created and what purposes does it serve? How does her work unit fit into the overall mission of the institution and what is the mission of her particular unit? In addition, the nurse should understand what her position is. What is she responsible for and what is considered successful performance of her duties? What are the duties of others she will be working with? All of this material is usually available if one knows to ask for it.

More hidden beneath the surface will be other important information which can only be assessed over a period of time. One of these areas involves the reward system of the institution. Rewards are usually at a premium and are competed for among units in the institution. Rewards might be concerned with promotion, staffing, budget, prestige, privileges, or exemption from usual policies. The reward system can influence others whether they are rewarded or not.

> An intensive care unit was opened in a pediatric hospital after the need for such a unit became apparent. A head nurse was hired from a nearby medical center and given a higher salary than was customary for a beginning head nurse. The best staff nurses from other units were offered positions in the new unit. The budget was amply padded to allow new and sophisticated equipment. A small private lounge was provided near the unit for the ICU nurses. This was not the custom on other units. Nurses who worked in the unit who were not needed when the unit's census was low were allowed to take the day off rather than come in and float to another unit as other nurses did. Relations between the nurses on the ICU and the rest of the staff were never good and no one understood why.

In assessing the reward system, one looks to see what rewards are given, for what, who receives them, who gives them, and how fairly they are distributed. The reward system actually confirms the real values of the institution. This information on values is useful to the nurse who wishes to successfully function and influence the system. For example, she might function differently in an institution that rewards individuals for seniority on the job more than for productivity, as opposed to one whose rewards are reversed.

Another more occult aspect to assess relates to the communication within the organization. This refers to who talks to whom and about what. It is assumed that the communications within an organization are somewhat dependent on the formal structure. Thus coworkers talk to each other the most and to those immediately above and below them to a lesser extent. But in addition to the formal structure, communications are influenced by other factors. Prestige influences communication. Nurses are often afraid to talk to physicians. Even a nurse in a supervisory position may feel intimidated by an intern who is administratively much her inferior. Also social relationships such as friendships are important in determining communication channels. Important pieces of information may travel on friendship channels faster than on official channels. Another determinant of communication channels is geographical location. Individuals tend to talk to those whom they find nearby more than those farther away.

The assessing of communication channels guides the nurse in knowing whom to talk to about each particular need. Thus one learns how to collect and transmit information.[4]

Another area to investigate is the policies of the organization. Some will be written, but a large number will be unwritten but just as influential. All organizations also have "tribal customs" which alone account for how things are done.[4] These can be identified and understood.

While looking at aspects of the structure such as formal organization, rewards, policies, job descriptions, and communication patterns may seem of interest but only of slight relevance, it is very important if one desires to function to the maximum in a system.

> Becky had been working as an oncology specialist in a children's hospital. She was adept at working with parents and children, respected highly by the medical oncology team, and had initiated several successful extra programs such as a group for the parents of fatally ill children, a group for fatally ill teenagers, a seminar for parents at the hospital after the death of their children, and a home care project. Becky was unexpectedly offered a position as an oncology nurse in another institution. She accepted the job because she liked the people she met in her interviews, was impressed by the facilities available, and realized that taking the new position would enable her to take graduate work at a nearby university. Seven months later, Becky was near physical collapse, her faith in her abilities shaken, and her employment terminated. She hardly seemed the same person to her old friends. She vowed to never again work in nursing. What had happened in seven months to change Becky's life so dramatically?

First of all, the new position was very different from her old one. She was under the medical oncology team and not nursing administration. She was not expected to engage in any of the activities she had previously assumed but rather to primarily organize and manage the oncology outpatient clinic. Becky had always worked independently and had trouble organizing, directing, and working with a team. Her duties were spelled out in a job description written as part of a grant application but Becky never read it. The new hospital rewarded nurses for following orders more than for personal initiative but Becky never noticed. She tried unsuccessfully to initiate several programs but never cleared them through proper channels first. Many of the nursing hierarchy noticed Becky's plight and tried to be helpful but Becky overloaded them with her pent-up frustrations about her new job and they eventually avoided her. Becky never communicated her distress with the medical director of the grant because she didn't realize this was appropriate. She thought her boss was the head of the oncology department. The nurse who replaced Becky sized up the situation astutely and eventually created the role for herself that Becky had expected to play.

## THE MANAGERIAL TRIAD

Secondly, it is important for the nurse to understand how decisions are made within the institution where she works. All bureaucracies are political structures.[48] This is inevitable whenever there are limited resources and rewards which must be apportioned among many contenders. The major factors in the organization of most health care agencies of importance to a nurse are the administration, the medical staff, and nursing service.[43] However, these three elements of organization do not have equal power. The administrator and his staff have theoretically the greatest power. Their focus is likely to be on rational decision making, the smooth functioning of the organization with high productivity, efficiency, and economy as goals. These values should lead to satisfied physicians, personnel, and patients. The medical staff, while technically of lesser authority than top administration, has a large amount of informal power over administration. Any health care organization must cater to physicians because it is dependent upon their patients for income.[30] And because most health care agencies must compete with other similar agencies for the physician's patients, efforts are made to please him by providing the recognition and services he desires. The physician values quality care for his patients.

The third position in the hierarchy of power of most health agencies is occupied by nursing service. Nursing service is almost always under administration and has historically always been under the dominance of medicine with a few exceptions. Nursing service values efficiency, productivity, economy, quality care, and, as its name implies, service to others including administration, physicians, and patients.

Examining this triad explains why many things often happen as they do in health care institutions. Nursing service is the only member of the top management triad which is truly under another member and it is under both other members.[43] When decisions are made, coalitions must be formed. Nursing service has little chance to successfully oppose anything either other member wants, or to generate support for something they do not want. Administration cannot frequently join with nursing service against the physician faction without danger of alienating the source of its income. The physician faction is unlikely to support nursing service in opposition to administration because this would represent siding with an "inferior" group (nursing) against a "superior" group (administration). Nursing service is also in a weak position to achieve goals which administration or medicine opposes. The result is that the administration-physician coalition usually controls major decision making and nursing service either objects unsuccessfully or concedes to avoid futile battles.[7,43]

The net result of this structure is that nursing service in most situations does not even control nursing practice within any particular institution. It is rather controlled by medicine and administration. The nurse at the patient care end of the nursing service hierarchy may notice this only as the persistent parade of decisions coming down from higher levels which appear as disadvantageous to nursing and sometimes to the patient. She may notice that unlike employees in other departments in the institution, she has three bosses—administration, nursing service, and any physician. This can lead to a squeeze between her professional goals and those of her bosses. This can be painful and disillusioning.[27]

## POWER

This system might be altered if nurses had more power. Nurses have been reluctant to use or even recognize the importance of nursing power. It may well be that our reluctance to develop a nursing power base is responsible for many of the problems of current health care delivery. Because most health care organizations are based on an interaction of three dominant forces as described, a weakening or a deficiency of one element (nursing) may have led to excesses of the other elements (administration and medicine) so that health care agencies may have become efficient organizations where individuals are cured and the physician content but not where health is promoted, the individual is seen as a whole person, and the needs of the community at large are recognized and met.

In order to increase one's power base, the nurse must understand how to develop and use power. The most important determinant of an individual's power base rests on how her competence and expertise are perceived by others.[48] Those who are thought of as highly proficient are granted more informal power. The nurse must not only develop, but continue to exercise competence which others recognize and value. This type of power, that based on reputation, is independent of formal authority.[48] When nurses in an organization at all levels accrue power based on professional competence, each individual nurse and those in managerial positions will increasingly become more powerful and this, in turn, will strengthen nursing's position within the managerial triad. Power is validated by those it serves who see nursing as providing a valuable service.[11] Power should ultimately not come from being grudgingly granted by management but rather from consumer validation. Therefore, nursing would be freed from the dominance of medicine if nurses were able to evidence that their proficiency is genuine but different from and independent of that of medicine. The first step is for each nurse herself to believe that it is.

Developing informal power then rests in the nurse's willingness to undertake a difficult and life long pursuit of knowledge and skill and to demonstrate them to others. One frustrating factor is that in many instances nurses have considerable knowledge and skill but are reluctant to speak out clearly about them and use them.

After informal power is developed, formal power often follows. Formal power is related to one's official position in reference to others.[48] This is seen when promotion of an individual follows proven competence. It is also seen when a new position is created or an old one altered to correspond with the increasing power of the group a person represents. For example, as collegiate nursing programs have proven that they are legitimate academically, departments often become schools and the director a dean. Note, however, that formal power must follow and be based on informal power or the position of authority becomes a sham. If formal power does not follow the increase in informal power, those involved must work to guarantee the formal power. This has been done occasionally in nursing by the use of nursing organizations to collectively support and obtain a higher degree of formal authority in a particular organization. This collective exercise of power, often used as a technique by other groups, is recent in nursing.

The nurse who wishes to improve the power of nursing in her organization, therefore, must start with the assumption that nursing has a lot to offer and by improving her own power base first informally and then formally, if desired. It is essential to never underestimate the value of informal power. The informal power of a nurse may well become equal to or greater than that of other individuals with more formal authority.

As nursing becomes more powerful, it is important to remember that even nursing power must be kept in proportion to the power of others in the managerial triad. One wonders if some community health agencies might suffer from an excess of nursing power with deficiencies of administrative and physician power so that inefficient and costly services are excessive, such as home visits, and no one is ever "cured" but carried actively for years.

Information on these aspects of the structure is essential when a nurse-leader wants to influence the system. This information helps determine in what matters she is likely to be successful and how.

## 10. Leaders Are Successful at Planning Change

The nurse-leader will find herself in situations where she sees problems which are not being attended to. These problems may be as simple as a messy nurses' lounge or as complex as an inefficient system of patient care. Whenever one solves a problem which involves other individuals, some or all of the individuals involved will have to make some changes in behavior. These changes may be as simple as throwing away their empty coffee cups in a wastebasket rather than leaving them on any convenient surface or as complex as learning about and making operational a new form of patient care delivery such as primary nursing. To be effective, the nurse-leader needs to understand how change occurs and what can be done to initiate, promote, or monitor the change occurring. This role is frequently referred to as a change-agent role.

Change is not a rare occurrence in the environment. It can be planned or unplanned. It is commonly stated that all individuals are resistant to change. It is unlikely that this is true. It is probably that one accepts change which seems readily advantageous but resists change which seems disadvantegeous.[37]

A knowledge of the process an individual may go through in adapting to a new idea is helpful when promoting change.[39,41] Because change in the behavior of another implies that one has accepted some different ideas than previously held, change involves adopting new ideas. It is believed that initially intellectual *awareness* of the idea occurs. This stage is followed by a stage of *interest* in the idea. The time lapse between awareness and interest may be quite long. Actually interest may never occur. If interest does occur, the individual may move towards the stage of *evaluation or mental trial*. Still later an *actual trial* may be conducted by the person. Thereafter, *adoption* of the idea as part of the individual's behavior is likely.[39,41] Rejection of the idea may occur at any point. Note that this process moves from intellectual acceptance of an idea to emotional acceptance when the idea becomes part of the behavior. This process may take years or only minutes. Then too, an idea may be accepted intellectually but never completely accepted emotionally.

Joy worked in a Planned Parenthood satellite clinic in a rural area. She understood why young unwed teenagers engaged in sexual activity and she believed that contraception should be easily available as an alternative to unwanted pregnancy. However, she always found herself surprised and perplexed when a teenager she knew personally came to the clinic for contraception. She accepted the idea of premarital relations among teenagers intellectually but not emotionally.

A number of variables have been found to be related to adoption of an idea.[39] The adoption of an idea by peers, especially when they are respected, leads to earlier adoption of the idea by other individuals. The readiness with which an individual adopts a new idea is related to how tenaciously he will continue to accept the idea. Individuals who adopt a new idea very slowly are more likely to give it up easily while those who adopt readily continue with their acceptance longer. The individual's perception of the idea and its advantageousness or disadvantageousness to him personally is more relevant to his adoption of the idea than the actual objective facts. Ideas will be adopted more quickly when they lend themselves to trial and when they are consistent with the individual's present knowledge and experience. One who is interested in promoting a new idea might draw the following guidelines from this knowledge on idea adoption.

1. Individuals should be given time to accept a new idea and a trial if possible should be provided.
2. Don't expect everyone to accept a new idea in the same amount of time or to be equally committed.
3. Selling a few influential group members on an idea first may aid acceptance by a group.
4. Making the idea easy to understand and relevant to the individuals involved should aid adoption.
5. Because intellectual acceptance can occur without emotional acceptance, expect group members to verbalize commitment to an idea before the idea becomes part of their behavior.
6. Finding out how the individuals involved are perceiving the idea is an important part of selling the idea.

Another useful area of knowledge for the change agent is related to methods which can be potentially used to produce change. Strategies which can be used have been divided into three types.[15] One method focuses on a *rational strategy*. In this method the individual is presented with facts and information related to a new form of behavior and it is assumed that he will, in his own best interests, adopt the new behavior. This strategy would be used when one presents another with information on the dangers of cigarette smoking and relies on him to not smoke or to stop smoking. Another method employs a *coercive strategy*. This method can only be used when the change agent has power over the other individual. Coercive techniques usually involve political or economic pressure to change behavior. This method would be used if the tax on cigarettes was doubled or if cigarette smoking was made illegal. The third strategy for producing change is a *value re-education strategy*. This rejects the idea that rational arguments or coercion can alone produce change, holding that the individual must be re-educated in such a way that his attitudes and values change and he is internally motivated to change.

Each of these strategies has its advantages and disadvantages. The rational strategy is easy to employ but does not work with all people or in relation to all situations. The coercive strategy is usually effective although not completely so, but tends to cause resistance and rebellion in the individuals affected. The value re-education strategy is highly effective but takes time to produce change. The importance of this information for the change agent lies in knowing which strategy to use in which situations and how the individuals may react. The rational strategy might work ideally in a situation where the individuals involved are themselves rational in their behavior.

Sue worked in a multidisciplinary community health clinic. She felt that many of the professionals she worked with on her team were unduly prejudiced against working mothers. Since many of the women who used the clinic were working mothers, she believed these attitudes to be transmitted to them. When it was Sue's turn to present the monthly inservice program, she gave a program on current research findings related to the considerable benefits to the family of maternal employment and the irrelevancy of many of the old findings. The professional team members were impressed with the research findings and several confessed that they had been operating on older assumptions which they learned in the past which no longer seem reliable. Several asked for more sources of information. Sue noticed a reduction of judgmental statements afterwards.

The coercive strategy, although unpopular and seemingly harsh, is appropriate when a change must be made quickly and without much hope that the individuals involved can be convinced otherwise of the value of the change.

Joyce was the office nurse in charge of all nurses and aides in a small orthopedic clinic. During the summer two newly hired aides began calling in ill excessively. There had never been a policy on illness before. Joyce talked to the aides on several occasions hoping to appeal to their sense of fairness but the unjustified illnesses resumed shortly after each talk. The other staff members in the clinic were becoming increasingly annoyed. Joyce developed some written policies on staff illnesses and absences, read them to the staff, and posted them. They included sanctions related to loss of pay and eventual termination for repeated absenteeism. The health of the two aides in question improved miraculously.

The two examples above are not meant to imply that all professionals are rational and all aides must be coerced. Rather the situations could have been reversed. The examples do show that the change agent must know the methods, their characteristics, the situation, and the individuals involved when selecting a strategy. The rational strategy and the coercive strategy will probably be used less than the value re-education strategy which is probably the optimal method if circumstances permit. It might be mentioned in passing that small amounts of the rational strategy and the coercive strategy added to the value re-education strategy might be highly effective in reaching the majority of individuals efficiently. The first two strategies may have to suffice until the individuals involved do change their values and attitudes. This is the case with seeking adoption of the maximum 55 miles per hour speed limit on highways. The rational and coercive methods are being used while the nation's drivers are slowly becoming re-educated in their attitudes towards speed.

In addition to understanding how change from intellectual awareness to adoption occurs and methods by which change can be produced, the nurse-leader may find it useful to consider types of acceptance of a change which individuals may evidence.[13,25]

One level of acceptance of a change is *compliance*. The individual involved appears to accept the change but in actuality exhibits the changed behavior only when observed. His acceptance is not based on true commitment but only on the desire to achieve a certain reward or avoid punishment. Should the reward cease or the punishment not occur, the behavior will stop.

The head nurse in a newborn intensive care nursery, after attending a conference, instructed her staff to talk to each infant as they cared for him, rub his skin lightly, and provide other types of sensory stimulation. Millie personally thought the whole idea was ridiculous. She did as instructed but only when the head nurse came into her module.

A second type of acceptance of change is *identification*. In this level of acceptance, the individual carries out the behavior because he identifies with the change agent and wishes to be like her. The behavior occurs with or without surveillance but since it is based on personal liking, it may cease if the relationship changes.

George worked in the same newborn ICN. He was very impressed by the head nurse and believed her to be an excellent nurse. He followed her guidelines for sensory stimulation, although he didn't care about them much. If the head nurse believed in them, he did too. Later he became less respectful of the head nurse who he felt was not assigning his hours fairly. He began to provide sensory stimulation to his patients less frequently.

A third type of acceptance of a change is *internalization*. When one internalizes a change he is personally committed. The behavior occurs consistently and becomes very permanent.

> Christine accepted the head nurse's suggestions on sensory stimulation because it made sense to her and was compatible with material she had read before. She asked the head nurse for more information and devised some new stimulation techniques on her own. When she moved to another area and began working in another newborn ICN, she continued to include sensory stimulation in her care.

The change agent can use this information to determine if acceptance of a change occurs because people feel they must comply, because they like and identify with the change agent personally, or out of true commitment. This knowledge will also help the nurse-leader to predict how permanent the change is likely to be. Although internalization is preferable, there may be situations in which the change agent has to settle for compliance or identification. Putting these types of acceptance of change together may hint at the approach of the change agent who is able to exert the most universal influence: others accept the change because they feel to a degree they should comply, they identify with the change agent personally, and the change is something to which they are committed.

Still another concept useful to the change agent involves analyzing the forces involved in the situation in which change is desired. Lewin has developed a theory to explain why change occurs in some situations and not others. He proposes that in any situation there are two opposing sets of forces. One set of forces, called driving forces, is conducive to change. The other set, the restraining forces, serves to prevent change. Change does not occur when the forces are equal but will occur when the restraining forces are decreased and/or the driving forces are increased.[29]

> Bob frequently drank soft drinks which contained saccharin because he was several pounds overweight. When stories first began to appear about the possible health dangers of saccharin, he switched to sugar sweetened beverages although he dreaded the thought of gaining weight. The stories he heard served as a driving force for a change in dietary habits. The strength of this driving force was strong enough to overcome his dislike of possibly gaining more weight. Soon other stories began to appear in the media which cast doubts on the actual dangers of saccharin. Also he had gained 3 pounds since he began to drink sugar sweetened soft drinks. The restraining force (being overweight) had thus become strengthened and the driving force was getting weaker because of the possible fallacy of the saccharin scare and Bob returned to the use of saccharin. A month later, however, he read an article on the saccharin controversy in *Consumer Reports*. The article was convincing and he again gave up saccharin. In fact, the article he read was for him such a powerful driving force that he continued to avoid saccharin even after gaining 2 more pounds. Another fellow worker read the article but continued to use saccharin.

This example illustrates several additional points about restraining forces and driving forces. Not all forces are equal in strength and forces can change in strength from one time to another. Were Bob to continue gaining weight the change in dietary habits might again be nullified. The forces involved can have a particular meaning to one individual but not another. In addition, not always are all of the driving and restraining forces known.

Using this theoretical formulation, the nurse can analyze the driving and restraining forces in any given situation to determine what is causing change to occur or preventing change from occurring. This is referred to as "force field analysis."

> Bobbie worked in a postpartum unit. She noticed that many parents were discharged who knew little about the care of their baby, his characteristics, and his needs. The nursing staff were not very involved in interactions with the mothers and fathers on the unit, especially related to teaching. A new clinical director had been named who stressed parent teaching and several new baccalaureate graduate nurses had been added to the staff. Still little teaching seemed to be occurring. Bobbie wrote down the following analysis of the situation:

*Situation:*
Parent's learning needs are not being assessed or met.

*Restraining forces:*
Belief in lack of time to spend with patients.
Greater satisfaction derived from socialization with other staff than with parents.
Lack of knowledge by some staff on how and what to teach.
Failure to see needs of parents.
Lack of role models who do teach parents.
Lack of push and sanction from physicians.
Lack of encouragement from head nurse.

*Driving forces:*
Urging of new clinical director to teach parents.
More new nurses prepared for teaching functions.
My example.

Bobbie could easily understand why nothing had changed after writing down her analysis. There were many more restraining forces than driving forces. She could have also rated the strength of each force on a scale of $+$ to $+++$. This helps show which factors are major and which are minor.

After analyzing the situation, the nurse can learn to promote planned change in several situations. First to be considered is how to initiate change when the problem is accepted by others. The actual mechanism used to play and carry out the change is the problem solving process. This is described more fully in an earlier chapter and involves assessing the problem, planning the action, intervening, and evaluating the outcomes. When the group recognizes the problem, the leader guides the group in using the problem solving process to solve the problem they face. This is the easiest situation in which to promote change and the change so produced is likely to be very well accepted by most individuals. In the process of solving the problem, the resistance of members of the work group is reduced and their motivation becomes a most effective driving force.[16,22,42]

> Bobbie mentioned before morning report one day that she noticed many of her parents seemed in need of help with caring for their babies that they weren't getting. She added specific examples of some of the things they didn't seem to know. Other members mentioned that several things which had been done for parents in the past weren't done any more such as bath demonstrations and demonstrations on how to prepare formula. They also talked about one nurse who had breast fed several of her own babies and who used to spend extra time with the breast-feeding mothers. Bobbie asked the head nurse if the staff could have a short team conference at 10:30 that morning to discuss the problem more fully. Shortly before 10:30, Bobbie reminded each staff member and led the group discussion. The problem solving process was on its way and Bobbie called other meetings to continue the process.

In this particular situation the role Bobbie played was easily accomplished. When promoting change in this manner one must be prepared for a different solution to emerge than the one the change agent would have chosen.[42] In the above case that did indeed happen. Bobbie was hoping that each nurse would become more cognizant of parents' needs and take initiative for teaching. However, the postpartum nursing staff decided to free one person who liked to teach at certain times of the day from any patient care assignments so that person could concentrate on interacting with previously selected parents and on teaching. Bobbie had to admit later that this solution worked well in general. As is shown by this example, change is most likely to occur and is easily accomplished when the motivation comes from within the individuals or group and not from outside sources. An increase in driving forces is likely to increase resistance while a decrease in restraining forces seems to lead to increased motivation for change. Also, change is facilitated when the group feels they control the change themselves rather than an outside force.

Unfortunately, change is not always accomplished this easily. One of the most prevalent restraining forces the change agent will encounter is failure to recognize that a problem exists. The change agent can take several steps in this situation.

First, the change agent should check to be sure a problem really does exist which is significant to others. Consultation with an outside resource may be useful. If no one sees a problem but the change agent, it may well be best to stop all efforts at change for the time being. But if there is a legitimate problem, the change agent should look to see why others are not acknowledging its presence. It may be that recognizing the problem is too threatening to the personal security of the individuals involved. Admitting the problem would be more difficult than tolerating the present situation. In some cases, individuals may deny a problem because attempts to solve the problem in the past were unpleasant or unsuccessful. Some may persist in denying a problem because they feel that to recognize the problem would force them into a course of action they do not desire.[39] The solution to these situations lies in finding opportunities to let the individuals involved see the problem for themselves in an environment where they feel secure and free from pressure.

> Gail was a nurse in a community well baby clinic. In the past the nurses assigned to the clinic had taken turns supervising in the playroom the many nonpatient children who came with their mothers to the clinic. No one enjoyed the task and it was gradually adandoned but the unsupervised children were a problem. Gail noticed that no one wanted to discuss the problem in staff meetings and she guessed it was because they feared that they would all have to again assume supervision duties. Some time later one nurse's billfold was stolen. Since children were frequently running around near their offices, it seemed logical to suspect that one might have taken the billfold. Later another child was injured painfully when he got his fingers caught in the back door of the building. Similar incidents occurred for several weeks. Still, no one wanted to talk about the problem. It seemed that the staff was more willing to overlook the problem than to face supervising the children themselves. Gail now decided to change her strategy. Waiting for the staff to recognize the problem was becoming less likely. Her next approach was to think of a solution to the problem which would not involve what had been done in the past so that the staff would be more willing to discuss the problem. One day in staff meeting she suggested that the clinic enlist the aid of teenage volunteers to perform selected little services around the clinic. She named some such as preparing rooms for patients between patients and answering the phone. There was only mild interest in the project. Then she mentioned that the volunteers might also supervise the playroom. What followed was the first detailed discussion of the problem that had occurred. The promise of a more palatable solution had freed the staff to look at the problem.

The nurse may run into situations where the group recognizes the problem but does not wish to do anything about it. If a way can be found to get them working on the problem, their resistance often is converted into a driving force for change.

> There was widespread complaining among the nursing staff of a small health center over assignment of shifts and days of duty. There were rumors that the director of nursing was investigating changing to a system involving a standardized staffing pattern with computer assignment of hours. Fears of that type of impersonal and automated system were frequently expressed. The director established a committee to study the problem of equitably assigned hours. She astutely selected her committee with care so that some of the individuals who would be most resistant to any change in the assignment of hours but who disliked their hours were on the committee. After study of the situation and possible solutions, a standardized staffing system was selected and the staff enthusiastically implemented the system.

Another way to reduce resistance involves education of the individuals concerned. Often resistance is the result of faulty perceptions related to a change.[39]

> The administration of a visiting nurse service agency recognized that they would need to eventually change to a problem-oriented medical record (POMR) system to comply with accreditation standards. Many of the

nurses knew little about the system but had heard that it would involve all new forms. Unfamiliar sounding words like "flow sheet" and "drug profile" seemed unsettling. The consensus was that it sounded like a mass of paperwork from which they had little to gain. The president of the agency arranged a series of field trips for groups of six nurses to study the use of POMR in a nearby visiting nurse service in the state capital. Each field trip was carefully planned to incorporate a short presentation on POMR, time to study the POMRs of a variety of actual patients of the agency, and a luncheon paid for by the agency in one of the city's best restaurants. The nurses who would be expected to object most were incorporated early in the schedule. The staff returned with a much different perception of POMR and more interest since they had seen first-hand how efficient the system was in general.

Resistance, then, can ideally be lessened by arranging for knowledge of the problem to emerge from the group themselves, getting the group involved in solving the problem and controlling the change, and providing for the education of group members about the problem. Once resistance is lessened, problem solving can proceed at a more efficient level.

The following are frequently cited as leading to problems and are best avoided if possible.

1. Forcing too many changes or major changes too quickly. It seems that people need a chance to assimilate a change before embarking on another one. Too much change has been associated with increasing stress and physical illness,. even when the changes are desired and seen as positive.[40]

2. Pushing adoption of a solution instead of allowing the group to solve the problem their own way. It is sometimes tempting for the change agent to jump ahead of the group and arrive at what she believes to be the only or best solution and then push the group to change toward the solution. The group is likely to reject any solution forced on them because they see it rightly as an attempt at manipulation and resistance will increase.

Angela worked at a state veterans' home. It was no secret that the standard of nursing care was low. She read several articles about phenomenal changes being made by nurses in an Iowa veterans' home. She was very excited about making the same changes in her situation and they were certainly needed. She tried to sell others on copying the changes of the other group in eliminating the custodial care being currently provided. She did not focus on problems in the delivery of nursing care in the current situation, but rather on doing what the other staff had done. Her efforts were rejected and, disillusioned and embittered, she resigned unaware that the potential for change did exist in the situation but only when correctly elicited.

3. Pushing for a change seemingly out of concern for the general welfare but also with a covert, personal, less honorable motive. The group will invariably learn the private motive and resist any change because they sense that they are being used to further another's career or they are working mainly toward a situation which personally benefits another. Needless to say, personal motives usually underlie any change, such as reduced work load or greater convenience. But if these motives become stronger or are against the general welfare of the group, resistance is very predictable from the group.[42] A way to guard against this is for the nurse to freely admit what is in the change for her.

4. Failure to inform others who will be affected by the change appropriately.[35] Almost any change in a system will have effects on others not readily apparent. It is necessary to carefully consider who else will be affected by any change and provide ample opportunities to keep them informed about what is occurring. Others who are not adequately informed and who watch a change occur from without may be very suspicious and may develop faulty perceptions which may filter back to the group involved and increase resistance.

5. Failure to allow the group the opportunity to try the change before it becomes permanent. Mental trials and actual trials are an important part of adopting a new idea.[39] An opportunity to try a new idea to see how it works with the option to accept it or return to the previous situation reduces fear and increases security in the face of change. The change agent who is resistant to allowing a trial may be afraid to trust the wisdom of the

group. If the idea is really good, she has little to fear. She must remember that no change is ever absolutely permanent.

6. Trying to accomplish changes that are not desired by or consistent with the beliefs of those in authority.[2] Promoting change in situations like this is indeed similar to beating one's head against a brick wall. The options are to drop the action, wait until the structure changes, or redesign the change to align with the desires and beliefs of administration. Much futile effort is expended otherwise which could be better used to accomplish something administration can support.

7. Failure to follow through appropriately after the change. Planning for a change is rarely perfect. There must be provisions made for mechanisms to monitor the change situation and investigate any resulting problems. After all, the whole thing may have been a poor idea.

> A unit dosage medication system was instituted in a small community hospital. The planning had been done jointly by representatives of nursing, pharmacy, and administration. The committee was dissolved after the system was initiated and no one person was charged with responsibility for the system. Within a few weeks, problems with the system were becoming obvious. Getting *stat* meds promptly from the pharmacy was an impossibility unless nursing units sent a staff member personally to wait for and transport the medication. The pharmacy was unprepared for the large number of "prn" medications which needed to be stored in the med carts and resupplied occasionally but not often. Tensions increased between nursing and pharmacy and no one knew to whom to turn.

As a checklist to guard against these common errors, the nurse who functions as a change agent should ask herself these questions:

1. Are we moving too fast to allow individuals time to assimilate the changes occurring?
2. Is the focus on problems and helping the group solve them or have I already figured out the solution and am selling it to them?
3. Are my motives pure? Have I identified what I stand to personally gain from this change? Am I trying to hide this aspect or am I allowing personal gain to be my primary motivation?
4. Have I informed all others who are watching this change or are affected by it?
5. Has the change situation been approached as tentative or is it presented as inescapable once started?
6. Has the change been cleared by the appropriate hierarchy of administration?
7. Is there a mechanism to evaluate the change and handle any further situations which may occur?

Hopefully, this knowledge about change can be applied to any situation when the leader sees problems. It may help the leader to understand how she and others are reacting when change is occurring. It should be mentioned that all of this information is most relevant to functioning as a change agent not only in the work group but also when promoting change within a family or community.

The leader has much to say about where the change process begins. Usually a point of stress is a good place to start because individuals may be more motivated.[3]

## 11. Leaders Know How to Manage Conflicts

In almost all nursing situations much is demanded of the nurse. She must please many people including administration, the patient, and the physician and sometimes these goals will be contradictory. She must work closely with a large variety of other individuals who vary in background, focus, and orientation. She has high expectations for her own performance. Some amount to conflict and the resulting frustration is inevitable. Conflict is generally viewed in this society as unacceptable and the sign of poor relationships.[22] However, it is doubtful that one can function in this fast paced and complex health care world without experiencing occasional and justifiable conflict. Conflicts occur when the actions of one person interfere with or thwart the actions of another person.[22] How one handles conflict when it occurs is more indicative of mental health than one's total avoidance of conflict. Successful handling of conflict through the suggestions given below can lead to a stronger relationship with the other individual or individuals involved.[22]

It is important for conflicts to be resolved soon after they occur before both individuals or sides involved begin to perceive that their intentions and actions were as pure as the driven snow while the other individual was totally malicious. In order to resolve the conflict it is important to avoid stereotyping the other individual. If one party begins to feel that the other is vindictive and unreasonable, they may indeed become that way. It is most effective to let the individuals involved work out the conflict themselves before involving people higher up the chain of command. Another useful guide is to keep the channels of communication open between the warring parties while expressing hopes that an agreement can be reached. In the end, the parties should feel that they were treated fairly a majority of the time.[33]

When the leader finds herself as one of the members of a conflict, she can apply these suggestions to herself. Specifically, she would try to:

1. Resolve the conflict as soon as possible after it occurs.
2. Refrain from forming unjustified opinions about the other individual but assume him to be just and fair minded.
3. Attempt to solve the conflict herself before consulting her superior.
4. Maintain contact with the other person.
5. Maintain a positive attitude that an agreement is possible.

As most people know, resolving conflicts is not always easy, but letting them continue unresolved can lead to an increasing hardening of positions, threats, continued tensions, and unpleasantness.

## 12. Leaders Provide for Their Personal and Professional Development

So far, the majority of information presented has related to behaviors of the leader in the work environment. It may have sounded as if leaders devote their entire existence to their work, but this is not the case. People who become consumed by their work and have little else in their lives may develop "burnout."[46] One reason leaders may develop burnout is that they may be entrusted with greatly increased responsibilities. Leaders who never learn how to manage a compromise between their work related responsibilities and personal lives may have a glittering career but it may be shortened by burnout. Their personal life may become unsatisfying and actually distracting.

There are several ways to recognize if burnout is occurring:

1. Do I dread going to work? Is any physical illness significant enough to persuade me to stay home or leave work early?
2. Is my productivity decreasing although I seem to be working more hours?
3. Do I almost always need to take work home or do I plan to use some of my weekends or vacation time to catch up on work I couldn't get done otherwise?

4. Have I become a chronic complainer, yet I never take any action related to my complaints?
5. Am I continually looking for conflicts and attacking those in authority?

Before burnout occurs there are things the nurse can do to prevent it. One is to allow the cultivated existence of a life separate from work.[5] Rather than detracting from one's work, a separate life allows one to pursue her work rejuvenated by diversion.[46] The important factor is to achieve a balance. Another way to counteract burnout is by developing a way to increase one's sense of achievement in her work. A suggested way to do this is to spend more time developing objectives or goals for the next day, week, and month. Some of these objectives should be something which will be very stimulating and interesting.[46] Writing objectives lets the nurse direct her work rather than letting the work direct her. The achievement of the objectives gives one a much needed pat on the back.

Another strategy to deal with burnout involves recognizing and coping with professional frustration.[46] Professional frustration occurs when expectations related to one's work are not met. Maybe the supervisior did not notice or comment on an innovative idea one initiated. Maybe a patient failed to deliver the gratitude one was expecting. Whatever the cause, professional frustration can lead to depression or anger and eventually burnout and may spill over into personal life. Symptoms of professional frustration include a trapped feeling such as occurs when one is caught between professional goals and hospital policy or a generalized feeling of frustration without any clearcut reason for its existence.[17] The result is almost always helplessness and an inability to understand or remedy the situation. Several reactions may permeate one's behavior such as aggressive attacks on others, regressive childlike behavior, resignative apathy, or rigid thinking. If one recognizes the symtoms of professional frustration, there are steps which can be taken to lessen its impact:[17]

1. Try to uncover what expectations were not met and why.
2. Determine if the expectations were realistic in the first place.
3. Use the energy produced by the frustration not in depression or anger but to problem solve what can be done about the situation.
4. Develop realistic expectations for the future.

Another useful way to reduce burnout is to approach one's work as a career and not just a job. This involves directing one's own professional life carefully rather than allowing fate or other persons to direct it.[38] Also one should coordinate her personal and professional lives rather than letting one rule over the other. One who approaches nursing as a career should experience burnout less frequently than one who sees nursing as a job because she calls the action rather than simply reacting to it. Table 5-1 outlines some of the differences.

Still another important aspect of personal and professional development involves a personal support system. Everyone needs to talk to someone else sometimes. The accompanying release of feelings and the chance to tell someone else how things are helps the individual involved reach a better understanding of herself and work out solutions to old and new problems. A supportive person can be found at work or outside of work, and may be a spouse, a fellow worker, a parent, or a neighbor. One good way to assure that a supportive network is available is to serve as a support to others when they need support. This increases the likelihood that those one has supported will be available when needed. If a support system does not exist in the environment, one can also turn to a professional counselor.

Other necessary elements to promote one's personal and professional development are more individualized. Some may benefit by pursuing challenging hobbies, reading difficult

**Table 5-1.** Orientation to Nursing

| Career Orientation | Job Orientation |
| --- | --- |
| Realizes that continued pursuit of knowledge and skill is necessary. | Assumes that past training or education is all that will ever be needed. |
| Exceeds employer's expectations. | Does no more than minimal expectations by employer. |
| Strives to establish and meet own goals. | Has no personal goals. |
| Takes initiative and invests personal time and resources into improving competencies. | Expects employer to provide initiative and resources for improving competencies. |
| Plans career to complement personal life and enrich it. | Gives up job which is seen as a conflict with aspects of personal life such as marriage and child rearing. |
| Is willing to practice leadership formally or informally. | Avoids leadership responsibilities. |
| Plans ahead to assure future options and opportunities. | Rides with the tide, focuses on the present. |

books, or planning low keyed vacations.[16] A helpful way to promote mental health is to associate with people one finds interesting and to avoid people one finds annoying.[16] Probably most important of all, one needs to learn about himself.[16] This includes learning what one values, how culture and religion have shaped one's thinking and where one's strengths and weaknesses lie. This self-study can take a lifetime. Knowledge of self is facilitated by exposure to others and to cultures that are different so that one's characteristics are highlighted and challenged.

Another important aspect is to determine in which situation one wishes to be a leader and when one wishes to be a follower. Trying to assume leadership roles in too many places and too much of the time can lead to diffusion of one's effectiveness. Priorities must be established.

Providing for personal and professional development may be the most important, the most difficult, and the most ignored area of leadership.

## 13. Leaders Go in the Right Direction

It should be recognized that all that has been said about informal leadership can be used effectively, but with disastrous results, if one is not headed in the right direction. Consider Hitler's leadership of Germany. Leaders have a great responsibility to continuously ask themselves and others if their goals are honorable and just. Because of their power, they may spread an illness as easily as a cure.[4] For this reason the leader must know herself well and seek out those who disagree as well as those who agree and listen to them all carefully. It is especially important that she listen carefully to the health care consumer if she is to function as his advocate as she leads others.

## WHERE TO START

Reading the preceding material on leadership does not insure that one can function as a leader. Developing leadership behaviors requires continual practice and self-assessment. Most importantly one should begin by evaluating how one's socialization, life experiences, and exposure to role models has developed one's orientation to leadership behaviors. The beginning nurse will have a head start on becoming a leader if she next concentrates specifically on developing her personal competence in one particular area of practice. Becoming proficient in other or larger areas comes next. This knowledge base is very essential and is the keystone of informal leadership and informal power. Next the nurse who develops the processes of problem solving, communication, and helping and applies them to her work situation may find that others begin to view her as a leader. Learning to adopt differing leadership styles can be attempted systematically. Learning instrumental functions can be done initially on a small scale such as by volunteering to start a committee in a small work group and in progressively larger groups or in more complex situations. One should watch for seminars and published information on management techniques to build a knowledge base on instrumental functions. If one gains a position of formal leadership, there are many management behaviors one will need to learn through a study of administration such as delegation and supervision in addition to continuing one's pursuit of competence in leadership behaviors. Learning to promote change can be done first in simple situations and then with more variables. Developing a future orientation must be planned for by frequently setting aside time to look ahead. Similarly one must set aside time to plan for and carry out personal and professional development. Leadership behaviors can be practiced with patients, families, and communities as well as in work situations.

## SOME SUGGESTIONS FOR SELF-EVALUATION

1. Are my communications to others clear and appropriate?
2. Am I able to detect areas where my competencies, knowledges, and skills need improving?
3. Have I established a pattern of continual pursuit of competency and knowledge?
4. Have I learned to use the problem solving process well?
5. Do I appropriately rely on others?
6. Have I developed the ability to regularly focus on and plan for the future?
7. Do I use the helping process with others I work with?
8. Have I learned to exhibit instrumental leadership functions such as initiating and coordinating?
9. Can I recognize my leadership style and adopt a style for a particular situation?
10. Am I able to alter my style when appropriate?
11. Do I continually study the characteristics of the system in which I work and use the knowledge gained to plan how to effectively function?
12. Do I recognize the benefits of improving my power base and the consequences for myself and nursing of neglecting to develop power?
13. Do I understand the change process?
14. Can I promote planned change with sensitivity to my work situation?
15. Can I handle conflicts which occur around me?
16. Do I provide for my personal and professional development?
17. Am I leading in the right direction?
18. Do I use available opportunities to engage in informal leadership?

## AN EXAMPLE OF THE USE OF THE LEADERSHIP PROCESS

The following example illustrates the use of the leadership process in a nursing situation where the nurse who served as a leader had little formal authority. Notice in particular the importance of the nurse's knowledge in exerting influence.

Marge was working for the summer on a medical ward in a small private hospital. Shortly after she began working in the unit, she noticed that the nursing staff who worked days had very little understanding of the behavior of elderly patients who were often ill and afraid. The staff who usually gave most of the direct care to most patients were LPNs and aides because the RNs on the unit were busy just passing the many medications ordered for the patients. Marge was soon aware that the lack of understanding of patients' behavior was very evident in the care the staff gave the patients they were assigned to. Marge noticed that their treatment of some patients was very rude. Out of the room, they often complained about the patients and insinuated that they were mentally ill.

Marge wanted to do something about the situation to establish more understanding and acceptance of patients' behavior among the staff. After watching for a few days, she noticed that one LPN, Joyce, who had worked on the unit for seven years, was particularly influential in establishing how the staff would relate to any given patient. Joyce had considerable informal power among the auxiliary staff. If Joyce pronounced a patient as a problem, everyone else would soon relate to that patient as if he were. Marge noticed that Joyce could give excellent physical care, was very observant, and she could be very helpful to patients she liked. Marge believed that Joyce's negativity relating to some patients was most likely due to the lack of knowledge about certain aspects of human behavior in physical illness. The head nurse was a kind and diplomatic person but was going through a personal crisis and was temporarily distracted from leading her staff. Marge decided to see if she could influence Joyce's behavior towards one specific patient by using her personal informal leadership. She selected Joyce for her experiment in leadership because Joyce seemed to be the informal leader of the auxiliary staff. She also believed that Joyce liked her personally. She next selected a patient. Mr. Hodges was a 68-year-old patient with terminal cancer who Joyce particularly disliked. He had been frequently admitted to the unit. Joyce complained long and loud whenever assigned to him. Even though he seemed to have adequate hearing, Joyce talked very loudly to him and treated him like a child through tone of voice and scolding statements. Joyce also insinuated that he asked for medication, not because he had pain, but because he was addicted. To Marge, Mr. Hodges seemed to be a frightened and lonely person who was very aware of his condition and was not getting any support from his family, physician, or the nursing staff.

Marge began her project by volunteering in report one morning to take care of Mr. Hodges in addition to being team leader. Marge noticed several startled looks around the report table. Apparently no one ever volunteered to care for Mr. Hodges. Marge spent her time with Mr. Hodges learning more about him and she also read his chart thoroughly. Later, she asked Mr. Hodges' physician for more specific information about his illness and located several articles to read so she would have a complete understanding of his physical condition.

After caring for Mr. Hodges for a few days she wrote a few notes on the Kardex which she placed strategically and made very brief so that they would likely be read. She was hoping to initiate some awareness in Joyce that Mr. Hodges was a unique person with reasons for his behavior. She wrote:

Mr. Hodges is aware that his malignancy is untreatable.
He lives between admissions in a nursing home.
He hasn't seen his sons for 2 years.
He fears most of all being alone when he dies.

In addition to these comments on the Kardex, Marge commented occasionally to Joyce and other staff members on Mr. Hodges' physical condition. For example, one day when

Joyce was assigned to Mr. Hodges, Marge remarked as she gave report, "Why don't you come find me when you want to turn Mr. Hodges? His latest X-ray shows that his vertebrae are becoming very deteriorated from the spread of his tumor. Being turned must be very painful for him and should be done slowly and carefully." Joyce seemed to yell much less at Mr. Hodges that day. Marge came in several times during the morning while Joyce was there and talked to Mr. Hodges in the manner that she hoped Joyce would imitate. Mr. Hodges seemed cheerful and animated when she came in.

Another part of Marge's plan involved commenting positively whenever Joyce or anyone else expressed interest or understanding of Mr. Hodges. One afternoon Marge noticed that Joyce checked on Mr. Hodges although she was not assigned to him and without his light being on. Marge thanked her. Joyce began to complain less when she was assigned to Mr. Hodges.

Another aspect of Marge's plan was related to Mr. Hodges' medications. He was receiving among other things a narcotic and asked for it regularly. The team leaders had developed the habit of stalling before giving him his medications to try to increase the length of time between injections. By the time the injection was finally given, Mr. Hodges was usually in severe pain. Larger and larger dosages were gradually being given. Marge had read an article which advocated giving narcotics in smaller dosages and more frequently so that the pain-injection-relief cycle was not continued. She discussed her plan with Mr. Hodges' physician who agreed reluctantly to try the approach and rewrote the medication order. The change was successful within two weeks so that Mr. Hodges got his medication regularly, ceased watching the clock, and the dosage size was gradually reduced until it was half the original dosage. Marge explained the change to Joyce and why it worked as well as why Mr. Hodges needed a narcotic for his particular condition.

Over the period of a month Joyce's behavior towards Mr. Hodges gradually changed. When assigned to him she no longer complained at all. She also began to include personalized comments in the nurse's notes which Marge interpreted to be evidence of her increased sensitivity to Mr. Hodges as a person. She began to read the medical progress notes following Marge's example and asked Marge to explain what the physician had written on one occasion. The reactions of the rest of the staff changed slightly but not as dramatically as Joyce's. When Mr. Hodges became comatose, Joyce seemed honestly sad and remarked once on his amazing ability to survive with such widespread disease. In general, Joyce became less antagonistic towards several other patients.

Encouraged by her success with the past project, Marge turned her efforts of informal leadership towards working with some of the other staff members who were stereotyping patients.

## SUMMARY

Leadership is not a trait one is born with, nor a formal position, but is rather the result of certain learned behaviors which grant the user interpersonal influence. Leadership in nursing has been sparse and possibly immature due to many factors. This may have resulted in decreasing nursing's contribution to the health care system and to individual patients, families, and communities. Developing proficiency in leadership behaviors is not an easy task and requires continual effort. Most importantly, the nurse needs to develop competence and a knowledge base of great depth, increase competence and skill in the use of the problem solving, communication, helping, and change processes, acquire instrumental skills and a future orientation, select leadership styles, and learn to understand the system she works in including the development and use of personal and collective nursing power. In addition the nurse-leader should provide for her own personal and professional development.

# REFERENCES

1. Ashley, J. A.: "Nursing and early feminism." Am. J. Nurs. 75:1465, 1975.
2. Becker, M.: "Hospital system: Conformity or chaos." Presented at the 12th Annual Conference, Association for the Care of Children in Hospitals, Dearborn, Mich., 1977.
3. Benne, K. D., and Birnbaun, M.: "Principles of changing," in Bennis, W. G., Benne, K. D., and Chin, R. (eds.): *The Planning of Change.* Holt, Rinehart and Winston, New York, 1969.
4. Bennis, W. G.: "New patterns of leadership for tomorrows organizations," in Stone, S., et al. (eds.): *Management for Nurses.* C. V. Mosby, St. Louis, 1976.
5. Bindschadler, H. P.: "Dare to be you." Am. J. Nurs. 76:1632, 1976.
6. Broverman, I. K., et al.: "Sex-role stereotypes and clinical judgments of mental health." J. Consult. Clin. Psychol. 34:1, 1970.
7. Caplow, T.: *Two Against One: Coalitions in Triads.* Prentice-Hall, Englewood Cliffs, N. J., 1969.
8. Christman, L. B.: "Leadership is more than rhetoric." Presented at Annual Luncheon, Sigma Theta Tau, Indiana University-Purdue University at Indianapolis, Indianapolis, 1977.
9. Christman, L. B.: "Leadership: Problems and possibilities in nursing." Am. J. Nurs. 72:1449, 1972.
10. Christman, L. B.: "Nursing leadership: Style and substance." Am. J. Nurs. 67:2091, 1967.
11. Cleland, V.: "The professional model." Am. J. Nurs. 75:288, 1975.
12. Diers, D.: "Leadership: Problems and possibilities in nursing." Am. J. Nurs. 72:1447, 1972.
13. Dyer, W. G.: "Planning change in the family," in Reinhardt, A. M., and Quinn, M. D. (eds.): *Family-Centered Community Nursing: A Socio-cultural Framework.* C. V. Mosby, St. Louis, 1973.
14. Fagin, C. M.: "Nurse's rights." Am. J. Nurs. 75:82, 1975.
15. Fischman, S. H. "Change strategies and their application to family planning programs," in Stone, S., et al. (eds.): *Management for Nurses.* C. V. Mosby, St. Louis, 1976.
16. Gortner, S. R.: "Strategies for survival in the practice world." Am. J. Nurs. 77:618, 1977.
17. Gunderson, K., et al.: "How to control professional frustration." Am. J. Nurs. 77:1180, 1977.
18. Haase, P. T.: "Pathways to practice. Part I." Am. J. Nurs. 76:806, 1976.
19. Iafolla, M. A.: "The dilemma of women leaders." Nurs. Forum 4:54, 1965.
20. Jackson, J. M.: "Ways of thinking about leadership," in Stone, S., et al. (eds.): *Management for Nurses.* C. V. Mosby, St. Louis, 1976.
21. Jacox, A. K.: "Who defines and controls nursing practice?" Am. J. Nurs. 69:977, 1969.
22. Johnson, D. W.: *Reaching Out.* Prentice-Hall, Englewood Cliffs, N. J., 1972.
23. Johnson, M. M., and Martin, H. W.: "A sociological analysis of the nurse role," in Skipper, J., and Leonard, R. (eds.): *Social Interaction and Patient Care.* J. B. Lippincott, Philadelphia, 1965.
24. Katz, D., and Kahn, R. L.: *Social Psychology of Organizations.* John Wiley, New York, 1966.
25. Kelman, H. C.: "Processes of opinion change." Public Opinion Quart. 25:57, 1961.
26. Kohn, M. L.: "Benefits of bureaucracy." Human Nature 1:60, 1978.
27. Kramer, M.: "Collegiate graduate nurses in medical center hospitals: Mutual challenge or duel?" Nurs. Res. 18:196, 1969.
28. Levinson, R.: "Sexism in medicine." Am. J. Nurs. 76:426, 1976.
29. Lewin, K.: "Group decision and social change," in Newcomb, T., and Hartley, E. (eds.): *Readings in Social Psychology.* Holt, Rinehart and Winston, New York, 1949.
30. Little, D. E., and Carnevali, D. L.: *Nursing Care Planning.* J. B. Lippincott, Philadelphia, 1976.
31. Maas, M., Specht, J., and Jacox, A.: "Nurse autonomy: Reality not rhetoric." Am. J. Nurs. 75:2201, 1975.
32. McBride, A. B.: "Leadership problems and possibilities in nursing." Am. J. Nurs. 72:1445, 1972.
33. Merton, R. K.: "The social nature of leadership," in Stone, S., et al. (eds.): *Management for Nurses.* C. V. Mosby, St. Louis, 1976.
34. Moe, E. D.: "Patterns of leadership." Unpublished paper. University of Utah, 1963.
35. Mullaly, L. M., and Kervin, M. C.: "Changing the status quo." Matern. Child Nurs. J. 3:75, 1978.
36. Peipgras, R.: "Obsolescence of nursing skills." Am. J. Nurs. 66:1980, 1966.

37. Plachy, R.: "These are elements of decision making," in Stone, S., et al. (eds.): *Management for Nurses.* C. V. Mosby, St. Louis, 1976.
38. Reres, M.: "Assessing growth potential." Am. J. Nurs. 74:670, 1974.
39. Robinson, R. D.: "Toward a conceptualization of leadership for change." Unpublished paper.
40. Rodgers, J. A.: "Theoretical considerations involved in the process of change," in Stone, S., et al. (eds.): *Management for Nurses.* C. V. Mosby, St. Louis, 1976.
41. Rogers, E. M.: *Diffusion of Innovations.* Glencoe Free Press, New York, 1962.
42. Rosenberg, P.: "Dynamics of change." Minnesota Nurs. Accent, Feb. 1969.
43. Sills, G. M.: "Nursing, medicine, and hospital administration." Am. J. Nurs. 76:1432, 1976.
44. Tannenbaum, R., and Schmidt, W. H.: "How to choose a leadership pattern." Harv. Bus. Rev. 36:95, 1958.
45. Theis, C., and Harrington, H.: "Three factors that affect practice: Communication, assignments, attitudes." Am. J. Nurs. 68:1478, 1968.
46. Veninga, R.: "Trust only yourself and other good advice from burnt-out cases." Interview written by Maureen Smith. Update (University of Minnesota) 5:3, 1978.
47. Withers, J.: "Background: Why women are unassertive." Nurs. Digest 6:68, 1978.
48. Zaleznik, A.: "Power and politics in organizational life," in Stone, S., et al. (eds.): *Management for Nurses.* C. V. Mosby, St. Louis, 1976.

## BIBLIOGRAPHY

Archer, S. E.: "Politics and economics: How things really work," in Archer, S. E., and Fleshman, R. (eds.): *Community Health Nursing.* Duxbury Press, North Scituate, Mass., 1975.
Barnard, C.: *The Functions of the Executive.* Harvard University press, Cambridge, Mass., 1938.
Brazil, A.: "An inspiration for all new graduates." Nurs. Digest 3:53, 1975.
Francis, G. M.: "How do I feel about myself." Am. J. Nurs. 67:1244, 1967.
Francis, G. M., and Munjas, B.: *Promoting Psychological Comfort.* Wm. C. Brown, Dubuque, Iowa, 1975.
Goldberg, P.: "Are women prejudiced against women?" Transaction 5:28, 1968.
Haase, P. T.: "Pathways to practice. Part II." Am. J. Nurs. 76:950, 1976.
Kibrick, A.: "Leadership: Problems and possibilities in nursing." Am. J. Nurs. 72:1450, 1972.
Leininger, M.: "Conflict and conflict resolution." Am. J. Nurs. 75:292, 1975.
Maas, M. L.: "Nurse autonomy and accountability in organized nursing services," in Stone, S., et al. (eds.): *Management for Nurses.* C. V. Mosby, St. Louis, 1976.
Malone, M. G.: "The dilemma of a professional in a bureaucracy." Nurs. Forum 3:58, 1964.
Moore, M. A.: "The professional practice of nursing: The knowledge and how it is used." Nurs. Forum 8:361, 1969.
Nelson, L. J.: "The nurse as advocate: For whom?" Am. J. Nurs. 77:851, 1977.
Norris, C. M.: "Delusions that trap nurses—Into dead end alleys away from growth, relevance, and impact on health care." Nurs. Outlook 21:18, 1973.
Shockley, J. S.: "Perspectives in femininity. Implications for nursing." J. Obstet. Gynecol. Neonat. Nurs. 3:36, 1974.
Styles, M., and Gottdank, M.: "Nursing's vulnerability." Am. J. Nurs. 76: 1978, 1976.
Wachter-Shikora, N.: "Scapegoating among professionals: How to avoid scapegoating by using a transactional approach." Am. J. Nurs. 77:408, 1977.
Winstead-Fry, P.: "The need to differentiate a nursing self." Am. J. Nurs. 77:1452, 1977.

# PART 2

## COMMON RESPONSE BEHAVIORS OF PATIENTS AND FAMILIES

This section describes theory and related nursing interventions for five frequent reactions to adverse situations commonly seen in most nursing settings. The responses included are assumed to be occurring at nonpathologic levels. In other words, this section deals with the normal ranges of anxiety, denial, anger, grief, and depression which most mentally healthy individuals experience from time to time and not with behaviors consistent with neurotic or psychotic responses.

In exploring each response behavior artificial separations have been made for the sake of clarity of discussion. The reader should bear in mind that in actuality these behaviors are interrelated and often inseparable. For example, the individual who is grieving is likely to be anxious, angry, and depressed at times. Similarly, an individual who is denying may become anxious and depressed when he develops awareness of reality.

Also for the sake of clarity a deliberate attempt has been made to avoid intricate operational definitions, psychological jargon, and excessive speculation about the childhood psychic origin and manifestations of each response behavior which might result in semantic debates and becoming mired in conflicting theories. Rather an emphasis has been put on understanding each behavior enough to recognize its occurrence and intervene appropriately.

Readers who are interested in more detailed discussions of these response behaviors and their manifestations in individuals at extreme pathologic levels should seek resources beyond the scope of this book.

# CHAPTER 6

# ANXIETY

Anxiety is a normal and common part of the behavior of all individuals from infancy to death. Rarely is one totally free of anxiety. While anxiety is in essence a protective response, its presence can become unhelpful in some situations. The nurse can become proficient at recognizing anxiety in individuals she has contact with and in intervening to increase, decrease, or rechannel anxiety. The nurse herself frequently experiences anxiety and must learn to deal with her anxiety. This chapter will describe how anxiety can be recognized, what the nurse can do to help the anxious patient or family, and how the nurse can learn to recognize and cope with her own anxious feelings. This chapter will focus on the normal levels and types of anxiety that many individuals experience from time to time and not with neurotic or pathologic anxiety.

## REVIEW OF THEORY

As mentioned, anxiety is not an unusual occurrence in an individual's life. Anxiety is usually perceived as a subjective experience which varies for each individual, usually characterized by a vague feeling of uneasiness or dread.[5] The anxious individual appears alert, tense, or excited. He is not always aware that he is anxious because anxiety is often subconscious. Anxiety may exist without any observable signs although this is uncommon. Although one often thinks of anxiety as undesirable, the presence of anxiety is not an indication of mental illness or abnormality.[35] In fact it would be abnormal to be totally without anxiety.

### The Anatomy of Anxiety

There are many complex definitions of anxiety and theoretic representations of how anxiety occurs in the literature. The following represents in a simplified manner a summation of some of the major ideas on the occurrence of anxiety.[17,23,29]

1. The individual is in a steady state.
2. A stressor or threat occurs.
3. Discomfort is experienced consciously or unconsciously as anxiety.
4. Energy results.
5. Control behaviors are used consciously or unconsciously until the energy is consumed.
6. Discomfort is reduced and the individual returns to a steady state.

Anxiety as a process is protective when the threat is realistic and action is needed. Some stressors or threats may lead to disease or even death. If one could not mobilize energy when faced with a realistic danger, life might be short. Unfortunately, the process can occur when the threat is not realistic and the response can be more pronounced than warranted by the threat. These two possible events can then cause problems for the anxious individual.

## Causes of Anxiety

Anxiety is believed to be a learned behavior.[5] Therefore, the events which cause anxiety will be unique to each individual. An event which causes heightened anxiety for one person may not affect another. Some events or situations are predictably likely to lead to increased anxiety in most individuals, however. These events or situations are referred to as stressors or threats. Examples of stressors or threats which are believed to lead to anxiety are described below.

### 1. THREATS TO BIOLOGIC INTEGRITY

Any situation where one's physical self is threatened can cause anxiety.[17,19] An example of this is the dread most people feel when faced with an injection. Other examples include fears of physical violence, fears associated with surgery, fears associated with accidental injury, and fears of death.

### 2. THREATS TO PSYCHOLOGICAL INTEGRITY

When the mental image one has of himself is threatened, anxiety can occur.[17] The dread one has about speaking before a group is related to the fear that one will be judged poorly and thus one's image of oneself is threatened. Similar examples include taking tests, meeting new people, performing new tasks, entering a new situation, and going for an interview. This group of stressors accounts for a large portion of the anxiety one daily experiences.

### 3. FRUSTRATION OF A NEED OR MOTIVE

Anxiety can occur when one cannot meet a motive or need without simultaneously violating another motive or need.[5,19,29,40] This results in a state of frustration or conflict. Thus, anxiety may occur when one wants to buy a new coat but also wishes to save money, or when one desires to talk to a friend after work but also get home early. In these situations either vacillating between choices or choosing one over the other may lead to increased anxiety.

## 4. INABILITY TO CONTROL OR INFLUENCE A MEANINGFUL SITUATION

When one feels helpless or without options in certain situations, anxiety may increase. For example, the individual who is driving to an important job interview and is delayed by a passing train may feel anxiety increasing unbearably as he sits helplessly waiting for the train to pass. Other situations which may lead to a feeling of helplessness and loss of control include having no voice in an important decision or being far away from a family tragedy.

## 5. UNMET BIOLOGIC NEEDS

Biologic needs which are unmet can result in anxiety. For example, hunger, thirst, and the need to urinate when a bathroom is unavailable can increase anxiety. Physical pain is frequently reported as a source of anxiety. The presence of unmet sexual needs is becoming more recognized as a source of anxiety for individuals.

## 6. ASSOCIATION WITH A PREVIOUSLY ANXIETY PRODUCING SITUATION

Consciously or unconsciously, one often remembers situations associated with anxiety quite vividly. Any new situation which simulates the previously threatening situation can lead to increased anxiety even though the present situation is not seen as a threat.[17] For example, entering a dentist's office can revive anxiety associated with an earlier experience with a dentist in many individuals. In these situations, the individual usually becomes anxious without any conscious awareness that the behavior is occurring or any reason why.

## 7. TRANSFERENCE FROM ANOTHER PERSON

Anxiety seems to be particularly contagious. Observing or interacting with an individual who is anxious can lead to a heightened anxiety level for the observer.[29] This may occur without conscious awareness. For example one or two anxious members of a group can increase the anxiety of other group members. These group members who become anxious secondarily may not realize that they have become more anxious or why.

Some references classify threats to bodily integrity as leading to stress and threats to psychological integrity as leading to anxiety.[17] It appears likely that the emotional and physical responses to either threat are simultaneous, interrelated, and inseparable, making it meaningless to differentiate between the two on this basis.[19]

It should be noted that illness can easily involve all of these causes of anxiety.

## Manifestations of Anxiety

Because anxiety is believed to be a learned response and manifested uniquely in each individual, manifestations of anxiety will vary from person to person. In general, however, the person experiencing anxiety usually manifests some classical behaviors.[5,26,32] These will be described as they might be seen in a very anxious individual. Later levels of anxious behavior will be described.

The person who is quite anxious usually appears alert and attentive. His body is held stiffly with muscles taut. He may move quickly and startle readily. His eyes are open wide, dart around quickly, and his pupils are dilated. He usually talks rapidly, loudly, and frequently. He tolerates any lags in conversation poorly and interrupts. He listens little to the other person. He may perspire heavily or appear flushed. Parts of his body may move repetitively and rapidly such as his feet, legs, fingers, hands, or arms. He may grip his hands tightly around something such as the arms of his chair. He may make grimaces or display other facial mannerisms. He may at the same time appear fatigued and tired. In many patients, anxiety is obvious, but in others it is more hidden. The nurse should learn to look for covert signs which are more subtle such as muscular tension. Are the hands relaxed or held tightly closed? Is the lower jaw relaxed or are the teeth clenched? Normally the upper eyelids cover the uppermost quarter of the pupils. If more of the upper part of the pupils is visible it may indicate anxiety. How is the body held? One salient test is to "accidentally" drop something small but noisy near the patient and observe for an exaggerated startle reaction. These tests apply well to the silent, poised individual and the supposedly relaxed, joking individual. In the absence of other manifestations of anxiety, the eyes alone may betray the presence of anxiety.[5] Because anxiety is contagious, one can sometimes assess the presence of high anxiety unaccompanied by usual symptoms by noting when one feels anxious for no apparent reason after talking to another individual.

Internally, anxiety affects many parts of the individual's body by the complex psychophysiologic mechanisms related to the autonomic nervous system. Most notable are the effects on the respiratory, cardiovascular, gastrointestinal, and genitourinary systems. The manifestations are an increased respiratory rate, increased blood pressure, increased heart rate, nausea, vomiting, diarrhea, gastrointestinal distension, pain, anorexia, constipation, "butterflies" in the stomach, increased frequency of urination, impotence, and nonorgasm.[5] There are also changes in the endocrine and metabolic systems.[37]

Of course, not all of these behaviors and physical manifestations will be seen with each anxious person. Some individuals do not readily manifest anxiety in their behavior while others do.

## Levels of Anxiety

An understanding of the characteristics of various levels of anxiety can be useful when the nurse must decide whether or not to intervene to increase or decrease a patient's level of anxiety.

As was mentioned previously, an individual normally experiences some anxiety and it is usually of a mild to moderate amount. A total absence of anxiety would only be expected in one heavily sedated or unconscious. The stages described below represent points on a continuum so that levels between points are possible. This information is drawn from descriptions of anxiety in the literature. [18,29,32,33]

---

## 1. RELAXATION

---

The person in the stage of relaxation feels little anxiety. He has a sense of well being and comfort. This stage might occur after eating a delicious and filling meal, while listening to pleasant music, after engaging in moderate exercise, or after a satisfying sexual experience. This stage often precedes sleep. The individual in this stage is not particularly alert or receptive to new learning. This stage can be somewhat simulated by medication or hypnosis.

---

## 2. MILD ANXIETY

---

When mildly anxious, a person is alert and attentive. His attention is not particularly focused on any one thing so he is in general aware of his surroundings. In this stage problem solving is facilitated because the individual's perception is enhanced, he can consider many variables, and he can arrive quickly at a decision. It is also a good stage for learning to occur. This is the most common level of anxiety for most people. At this level the individual is open to new experiences and motivated.

---

## 3. MODERATE ANXIETY

---

In this stage the individual appears less comfortable than in the two previously described stages. Some signs of anxiety such as excitement, restlessness, or excessive talkativeness are likely to be noticeable in his behavior. More covert signs include frequent urination, diarrhea, a tension headache, or other signs of muscle tension. His attention to the environment will be narrowed although he will be able to attend to a particular if his attention is specifically directed to something by someone. This stage might occur after receiving very good news or a surprise. Problem solving in this stage does occur but it is more rigid and stereotyped, resembling automatic activity. Any activities or skills which the individual has just acquired will not be available to use in problem solving but older patterns of behavior will be used. Self-awareness will be decreased. Learning will be minimal although rote memorization can occur. The individual in this stage frequently states the he feels nervous or excited. Some individuals lead lives of almost continual moderate anxiety. The individual experiencing moderate anxiety or greater amounts is preoccupied with the future and shows an inability to experience fully the here and now.

---

## 4. SEVERE ANXIETY

---

Anxiety at this level is likely to be obvious. The individual paces the floor, his conversation rambles, and he talks constantly. He may engage in repetitive movements of the hands or feet. He appears to be most uncomfortable. Covert signs include anorexia, insomnia, and gastrointestinal malfunction. He cannot do much else. Due to restriction of his perceptual field, he is unaware of his environment except for perhaps one small area he is focusing on in detail. He cannot attent to other aspects of the environment even when his attention is directed to them. The individual in this stage might state that he is upset and "doesn't know what to do." Problem solving does not occur. Learning is impossible. This stage might occur after receiving devastating news or upon learning of a serious problem.

## 5. PANIC

Panic is rarely seen. The individual in panic is for the moment psychotic. He is out of control and runs about wildly until exhausted, or he sits unmovingly. This stage cannot last but a few minutes. The individual in this stage perceives nothing in the environment. Other synonyms of this stage might be "blind rage," "wild terror," or "frozen with fear." This stage could occur after an overwhelmingly frightening experience such as witnessing a disaster.

## *Control Behaviors*

Because anxiety is uncomfortable and produces energy, each individual develops ways to subdue or abate his anxiety.[23,28] Unfortunately, some methods of control can become problematic to one's health. Individuals may at times use a variety of control behaviors although some become more characteristic for each person over time. Control behaviors tend to eventually occur quickly and predictably in stressful situations without conscious awareness.[29] It would appear that control behaviors are to some extent learned from significant others. Thus the daughter faced with some stressor may react with a headache the same as her mother always does. It should be remembered that control behaviors can occur without awareness of the presence of anxiety.[5] In addition, control behaviors characteristically used for mild stressors may not be effective when the individual is faced with a more profound challenge and another behavior may occur. Control behaviors may differ depending upon the cause of the anxiety as well. Thus, threats to bodily integrity may lead to different control behaviors than threats to psychological integrity. Control behaviors have been classified as outward behaviors, inward behaviors, or mixed responses.

## OUTWARD BEHAVIORS

Some individuals readily evidence their anxiety by displaying behaviors which are visible. These behaviors represent attempts to rid themselves of the excess energy produced by anxiety. This method is common. Some outward behaviors are easily recognized and include restlessness, talkativeness, and bodily tension. More disguised outward behaviors to relieve anxiety include slamming a door, kicking the dog, taking a walk, hoeing in the garden, pounding nails with a hammer, eating, and chewing gum vigorously.

## INWARD BEHAVIORS

Inward behaviors can be conscious or unconscious and can be divided between those involving mental activity and those involving somatic activity.

### Mental Activity

Some individuals may withdraw into themselves when anxious. Their outward behavior may give little if any evidence of anxiety. They may become depressed, fantasize, or escape sleep. When faced with a serious threat, they may become immobile. Others may mentally investigate the reasons for their anxiety and plan how to relieve their anxiety. They may repress, sublimate, project, displace, or rationalize away the anxiety they are feeling.

### Somatic Activity

Some individuals do not express in thoughts or behavior any awareness of high anxiety but their body organs are believed to be compensating for the energy of anxiety with altered function. They are likely to develop what have been proposed as "stress" disorders. Examples of these are peptic ulcer, ulcerative colitis, bronchial asthma, essential hypertension, hyperthyroidism, and neurodermatitis.[6] These disorders may become self-perpetuating. For example, the individual who develops an ulcer may become anxious over his stomach pain which exacerbates his gastric acid secretion and further aggravates his pain, resulting in more anxiety and so forth. It is believed that one body system is usually preferred unconsciously by an individual.[17] Therefore, the person who develops colitis is usually not bothered by tension headaches and vice versa. The mechanisms and manifestations of the somatic response to stress are still being investigated and much is currently speculative.

## MIXED RESPONSES

It seems logical to believe that many individuals use a variety of inward and outward behaviors to handle stressors. Thus one individual might typically become talkative, experience some fantasizing, and some somatization.

It has been speculated that some of the behaviors an individual uses to control excessive anxiety are more healthful in the long run than others. Behaviors which deny or suppress the anxiety are believed to be hazardous.[5] Somatic activity obviously has its drawbacks as a method of controlling anxiety. Behaviors which might be more healthful are those which are most likely to lead the individual to discover his anxiety and discharge the energy it produces while at the same time exploring the situation which led to the anxiety. Thus, playing tennis would be therapeutic if the player is at the same time reconstructing and analyzing the anxiety producing situation he experienced but less therapeutic if he is fantasizing. Likewise, talking with someone else to analyze and evaluate one's anxiety can be healthful.[29] This point will be considered in more detail when nursing intervention is discussed.

Control behaviors can become so frequent and pronounced that they not only control anxiety but also come to dominate the life of the individual. His life style may be detrimentally affected because of his control behaviors. For example, the individual who eats when he is anxious may soon find his life dominated by his oral needs and limited because of his obesity. Therefore, it is believed to be healthiest when one uses a variety of control behaviors rather than relying on a few to handle all threats or stressors. Of course, one cannot consciously choose how one will respond to each threat one experiences because most control behaviors are automatic and unconscious. As will be seen, anxiety plays a role in other common responses discussed later in this section such as denial and anger. These responses control the anxiety in a sense by converting it into more tolerable forms.

## Variables Affecting Anxiety

Because anxiety is a unique experience to each individual, many factors related to the stressor can influence how anxiety is experienced.[3,35]

The *strength or intensity of the stressor* which leads to the anxiety is one variable. Few individuals would not react with anxiety to the possibility of an airplane crash.

A situation which involves a *number of threats* can be expected to precipitate more stress than one which does not. Therefore, impending surgery involves a physical and psychological threat and produces anxiety in most individuals.

The *duration of the stressor* can also determine the anxiety produced. Missing work for a week because of illness can provoke more anxiety than missing one afternoon.

Aside from characteristics of the stressor, certain *characteristics of the person* involved affect how anxiety is experienced.[3,5,35,40]

Some individuals are more prone to develop anxiety to one type of threat than to another. Being laughed at by his friends may cause more anxiety in one child while another child dreads going swimming more. Thus, the threat involved and its meaning to the person are individual.

It is becoming apparent that genetic endowment may account for differences in one's tendencies to become anxious. Infants have been shown to react quite individually to stressors shortly after birth.[5] It is possible that the control behaviors one needs to use may be genetically predetermined as well as learned.

Numerous other factors, including culture, education, past experiences, values, and religion can influence how one perceives a threat. An out-of-wedlock pregnancy for a teenager in a religious working class family may evoke more anxiety than the same circumstances for a girl from a family less bound to religious teachings.

Age is also an important determinant of how one experiences anxiety and will be discussed more fully later.

## Chronic Anxiety

In some individuals, high levels of anxiety can occur for days, weeks, or months. This is likely to occur when the person's control behaviors are not effective in coping with a particularly strong or prolonged stressor or when a multitude of stressors occurs at once. The individual experiencing chronic anxiety will usually seek help because of troublesome symptoms such as an inability to relax, sleep, eat, work, or a lack of interest in sex. He may also present with fatigue headaches, gastrointestinal upsets, or "jittery nerves."[5] The fact that the underlying problem is prolonged anxiety can be missed.

Prolonged anxiety can interfere with interpersonal relationships so that an individual may find significant others turning away. This in turn can further escalate his anxiety. Prolonged anxiety interferes, in addition, with learning, memory, concentration, reasoning, psychomotor efficiency, and use of other capacities.[5,11]

Chronically anxious individuals may be placed on medications specifically designed to alleviate anxiety such as minor tranquilizers and barbiturates. For some individuals, the results are very beneficial. Others experience concerns over taking regular medications, develop troubling side effects, and develop dependency and tolerance to the medications. Often the individual whose anxiety is controlled by medications does not receive any nonmedical help for his chronic anxiety. For these reasons, the chemical treatment of anxiety has been described as a curse and a blessing.[42]

If the nurse suspects that a patient has chronic anxiety she should seek help from resources beyond this text.

## *Acute Anxiety Reactions*

It is possible for an individual to experience attacks of anxiety which are acute enough to simulate a heart attack or a seizure. The individual feels acutely ill and is usually concerned about his health status. Common symptoms are cardiac palpitations, dyspnea, and paresthesias. The attacks may be erroneously thought to be due to respiratory or cardiac insufficiency, hyperthyroidism, or drug overdosage or withdrawal. The troublesome physical symptoms and concern over his condition may lead the individual to experience increasing anxiety which can augment and increase the anxiety attacks. The individual is usually totally unaware of any emotional circumstances which could cause the attacks.[5]

The nursing intervention with patients with acute anxiety reactions will not be considered here.

## *Crisis*

A stressor or group of stressors can become so overwhelming to an individual that he cannot adequately cope with them because the threats have become more powerful than his available control behaviors. The individual will become highly anxious, helpless, and disorganized and may have difficulty seeking help. This is referred to as a crisis and will be discussed in a separate chapter.

## *ANXIETY AND THE LIFE CYCLE*

It does not appear that any specific developmental age group has exclusive rights to anxiety. Each step on the developmental ladder has its own unique sources of stressors.

Attempts to avoid excessive anxiety are believed to be major determining facets of personality development as can be seen throughout the following sections.

## Infants

According to most sources, the infant is free from anxiety for several months because he must learn to be anxious. He will have a physical response to stresses such as illness. He experiences tension when his biologic needs are pressing but this is not the same initially as anxiety.[29] Through the processes of learning and ego development, it is believed that he begins to experience "anxiety preparedness" by six to eight months.[4] "Eighth month anxiety," which involves recognition of and fear of strangers, usually is the first evidence of the infant's ability to experience true anxiety. It seems likely that the infant can experience anxiety through transference from another. This is commonly observed when a tense individual tries to feed an infant.[29] The infant eventually appears tense and does not nurse well.

The infant is believed to control anxiety with primarily one behavior: crying. It is possible that apathy and a lack of desire to nurse may also be symptoms of a state of anxiety.[11]

## Toddlers

Increasing life experiences provide the toddler with increasing sources of anxiety. In particular weaning, toilet training, parental limit setting, changes in routines, bodily intrusions, separations, strange situations, masturbation, and rivalry are commonly believed to be anxiety provoking situations or experiences common to most toddlers.[11,36,40] The toddler also may experience anxiety when others are anxious.

The toddler is developing beginning control behaviors and will respond to anxiety less with crying and gradually more with temper tantrums, the use of security techniques or objects, and by projecting aggression onto other things such as animals or the darkness.[11,40]

## Preschoolers

The preschool child commonly experiences many emotions and situations which are believed to have a potential for anxiety. Some of these include sexual curiosity, feelings of aggression, strivings for independence, hostile wishes, sibling rivalry, separations, unfamiliar surroundings, and fears of abandonment, punishment, loss of parental love, and physical injury.[11,31,32,36,40] In many of these situations the preschooler is in conflict between expressing his desires and pleasing the others significant to him.[32]

In this period anxiety, therefore, plays a part in development of a conscience and in role identification.[32] It is believed that parents at this stage in some respects influence how much anxiety a child will later feel as an adult. If they demand more than the child can ever achieve, he may grow up with an internalized conscience which is never satisfied with any achievement. This may lead to continual anxiety. Similarly, it is postulated that parents who pamper and indulge their children may leave them unable to tolerate the normal stresses of later life.[38] The preschooler also readily learns the fears of his parents and some parents unknowingly increase anxiety by using fearful consequences to encourage appropriate behavior.[40] For example the child might be told, "If you aren't good I will leave you," or "If you don't eat like a big girl you'll get sick and have to see the doctor."

Because of his increasing experiences, a lack of knowledge, misinterpretations, and growing cognitive abilities including a powerful imagination, the preschooler can be quite beset with fears and anxiety. Several inward control behaviors can be used by the preschool child with some success including regression, withdrawal, projection, identification with the aggressor, repression, denial, displacement, and sublimation.[36,40] Outward physical control behaviors are readily available due to his increasing physical capabilities. However, these defenses function crudely and anxiety is usually readily discernible to the discriminating observer. The control behaviors will function more effectively as the child matures. The preschool-aged child with restricted physical activity may evidence increased anxiety.

## *School-Aged Children*

The school-aged child encounters an ever increasing world replete with sources of anxiety. In particular the school-aged child is believed to experience anxiety potentially over fears related to school entry, school adjustment, social and intellectual competence, meeting sex role stereotypes, lying and stealing, chores, meeting parental standards, death to himself or family members, and acceptance from peers.[11,21,32,40] Some television programs are believed to be a possible source of anxiety in children due to the vivid portrayals of violence and personal aggression which he may see but which he is not allowed to express. The school-aged child's sources of anxiety are more in line with reality and realistic dangers than those of the younger child.

Control behaviors used by the middle-aged child are more sophisticated versions of those of the younger child with the appearance of the behavior of somatizing.[32] Headaches and stomach aches may become predominant in some children as methods of handling anxiety. Outward control behaviors are often incorporated into sports activities. The physically limited or handicapped child may need other outlets for controlling anxiety. Some have suggested that the pattern of use of control behaviors present in the school years will persist throughout adulthood.

Recently several interested researchers have investigated how children who have had stressful childhoods are doing as adults. The conclusion is emerging that children have a marvelous ability to weather and benefit from early traumatic situations such as divorce or death of parents, parental alcoholism and addiction, hospitalization, or physical abuse. One study found that those individuals who were the emotionally healthiest at age 30 were often individuals with the most "difficult" childhoods. Another study of over 400 prominent Americans concluded that 70 percent of them had childhoods which by our cultural standards would be ranked as unhealthy because of rejection, abandonment, and abuse by parents who were cruel, cold, insane, bizarre, or alcoholic.[18] While such findings do not warrant the planning of stressful childhoods for children, they suggest that some of our ideas about how individuals and particularly children react to stress in life may not be valid in that stress and adversity may quite likely have a strengthening effect on individuals rather than leading to irreparable wear and tear. Because most children adapt well to stress, maybe our efforts should be directed towards assuring that they do so rather than towards making experiences stress free.

## Adolescents

The teenage years are abundantly supplied with anxiety provoking situations. Conflict seems to be the instrument necessary for establishing self-identity.[15] Specific threats concern aggressiveness, competitiveness, peer relationships, heterosexual relationships, emerging sexual drives, strivings for independence, and fears of failure.[11,40,41]

The teenager has well developed inward and outward control behaviors and is likely to use in addition intellectualization and asceticism in which he separates himself from his unacceptable strivings through attempts at purity.[40] Much of the religious fervor and naivete characteristic of some adolescents may be related to this. Acute anxiety reactions not uncommonly occur in adolescence and sometimes in preadolescence. They are uncommon before then. The manifestations of an acute anxiety reaction in a teenager are the same as those for adults.[11]

## Adults

The major anxieties of adults seem to center around personal security, work, marriage, and parenthood. This may sound deceptively simplistic until one reflects on the myriad of threats involved. A complete listing would be impossible but most notable would be anxieties and fears related to competency, interpersonal relationships, competitiveness, self-esteem, identity, money, aging, illness, death, and achievement.

Control behaviors are likely to be those developed during the earlier years. As the demands of life increase, the adult is more and more likely to encounter threats for which he is less prepared. The desire for freedom from anxiety may lead some individuals to a life of safety and rigidity. Expectations one had when younger related to oneself and others as well as life in general may begin to demand alteration.[30]

Control behaviors may become well established and great difficulty may be encountered in attempting to change one's control behaviors.

## Older Adults

Threats for the older adult can center around losing a spouse, personal losses, relinquishing of roles, retirement, and an aging body. Helplessness and dependency, if they occur, can be devastating.[8,16]

Control behaviors related to somatization are believed to be frequently seen in the elderly.[9] Anxiety may occur in a delayed fashion making it difficult to recognize or with less intensity or more intensity than expected.[10] "Free floating" anxiety, so common in younger persons, is believed to be rare in the elderly.[39]

Although one tends to think of anxiety and stress as situations to be avoided and many authorities warn that stress and anxiety take their toll on the spirit and the body, there seems to be little objective proof that people should consciously attempt to avoid anxiety— if that were possible. What is important is how each person interprets and handles stress.

# NURSING INTERVENTION IN ANXIETY

## Primary Prevention of Severe Anxiety in Patients

Since mild to moderate anxiety is a normal occurrence and not necessarily an unhealthy situation, this section will not deal with preventing anxiety *per se* but with preventing excessive anxiety. In addition, in some situations a low level of anxiety is not optimal; therefore, some information will be given on therapeutically raising an individual's anxiety level.

### PREVENTING EXCESSIVE LEVELS OF ANXIETY

Several preventive measures can be taken to prevent moderate, severe, and panic levels of anxiety. First of all, recognizing moderate anxiety in any of its manifestations and focusing on it may prevent escalation. One specific principle of intervention is to make the patient or family member aware of the anxiety and have him confirm that the anxiety does exist.[17,22,29] The nurse can say "You look anxious," "This must be a tense situation for you to be in," or more indirectly, "How have you reacted since learning about your pregnancy?" After the patient acknowledges his anxiety, it often seems more endurable.[25] The vague discomfort he felt now has a name he can grasp. The nurse then helps the patient to discuss his anxiety using careful communication skills. Reassurance is particularly ineffective with someone who is anxious so she should avoid her tendency to offer the well known "everything is going to be all right." The patient may at first deny anxiety because one is frequently unaware of his own anxiety but after talking about how he feels, he may eventually recognize his anxiety. If the patient persists in denial, it is considered best to allow the denial but to continue to facilitate the patient's communication of feelings.

Specific information given to the patient about a situation he is to face may prevent anxiety from escalating.[17] It is often said that man's greatest fear is his fear of the unknown. Thus, the adult or child who is instructed and prepared beforehand for a cystoscopy and has his questions answered clearly may be more likely to remain at lower levels of anxiety than someone unprepared.

The presence of another person when one is anxious may prevent anxiety from increasing.[22] With children, the presence of one or both parents is often helpful. The nurse who stays near and shows her interest may help the patient or family to maintain lower levels of anxiety. Of course, the nurse cannot be continually present with every anxious patient but she may be able to plan ways to provide another human presence when she must leave the patient. One common anxiety provoking situation for many children and adults who are hospitalized is going to the x-ray department. Concerns may already be present over what will occur there and what the x-rays may show. The already present anxiety may be increased when the patient is brought into a dim, strange room with formidable equipment and promptly left alone.

Nonverbal communication is important because the nurse's serene, calm manner is readily communicated. However, if she is tense and anxious this is communicated also. The use of therapeutic planned touch may help prevent heightened anxiety. Holding someone's hand or a pat on the shoulder are examples. Children especially are often comforted by being held or rocked.

Anxiety may be contained when the patient feels secure in his present situation.[22] Measures which are likely to enhance a feeling of safety and security are ones which lead him to expect that he will be frequently and carefully attended to. This includes prompt response to requests and the provision of privacy. Children and teenagers may feel more secure when they know the limits in their situation and discover that they are enforced consistently.[40] Confident caretakers who know what they are doing and do it well can increase the patient's feelings of security because the patient gains a feeling of trust in those around him.[14]

If possible, the patient or family can be helped to explore in some detail what they fear might happen before it happens. Increased anxiety is easier to prevent if one can identify any specific fearful aspect of the future. For example, two patients who are leaving their homes and familiar neighborhoods for nursing homes may both be likely to develop high levels of anxiety but the specific aspects of the move which cause each to be anxious may be entirely different. One may fear most isolation from former neighbors. The other may fear neglect. When specific anxiety producing factors can be identified, nursing intervention can become more effectively focused on those factors. In addition, once the patient puts his fears into words, they may seem less fearful and more controllable. Children may reveal their specific concerns best through play activities and other symbolic methods of expression.

Patients can often identify what measures may help them to maintain control during a stressful situation. Even young children have developed control behaviors or security measures and attachments to objects which well may help to prevent increasing anxiety. Adults too use security measures such as smoking and biting their nails. Patients may be able to suggest other things which they feel would help. One young woman identified that she thought she would get through labor and delivery better if she could keep her glasses on and not have her hands strapped down.

The foregoing information is summarized in Table 6-1.

## PLANNING THERAPEUTIC INCREASES IN ANXIETY

In some situations, the nurse may find it useful to increase a patient's or family's anxiety to a mild level. The patient or family member that is comfortable and relaxed may not use learning opportunities or problem solving opportunities well. In this situation the nurse might wish to point out the realities and personal dangers of the situation to increase the patient's anxiety and facilitate learning. She might say, "When you go home Tuesday you are going to need to do this entirely by yourself," or "Once you get to the health center, a

**Table 6-1.** Possible nursing actions for the primary prevention of excessive levels of anxiety

1. Attempt to have patient or family acknowledge or confirm presence of present anxiety.
2. Prepare patients or families for events ahead.
3. Provide the physical presence of another person.
4. Stay calm, use touch if appropriate.
5. Provide a feeling of security and safety.
6. Explore present fears specifically.
7. Help patient or family identify measures which may reduce anxiety.

lot of people are going to be asking you what you want done and you will have to know by then." A family might be told "She eats at home now and is accepting this diet well, but next week when she starts eating at school and she sees what the other kids are eating, she may begin to feel differently." It is important that the nurse offer a statement of support immediately after each statement designed to increase anxiety. Thus she adds, "So let's have you take the major responsibility for this now and I can stay here with you to help," or "We can talk about this now and plan some alternatives should this become a problem." In no instance should the nurse attempt to raise the patient's anxiety and then abandon the patient. Supportive statements also reflect favorable results which may occur.

> Mr. Jacks was scheduled for minor vascular surgery. He ignored the nurse's efforts at preoperative teaching and appeared unconcerned. The nurse told him, "You are going to have some uncomfortable periods after the surgery. We will have many ways to help you and when it's all over, you should have far fewer problems with your legs."

This balance between fear promoting and supportive statements has been found to be appropriate with patients facing surgery. In one study, patients with moderate anxiety fared better postoperatively than those with either slight or severe anxiety.[20] It may be that "worry work" is therapeutic. Because of this possibility, nurses should seriously evaluate the practice of giving optional sedative medications to patients facing stressors or threats.

In conclusion, it appears that a nurse may desire to increase anxiety in some situations because anxiety causes a mobilization of resources which can be beneficial for the patient or family if the anxiety is kept to moderate levels. There is much to be learned about this area. Information on therapeutically increasing anxiety is summarized in Table 6-2.

**Table 6-2.** Possible nursing actions for increasing anxiety to facilitate learning or problem solving

1. Point out a danger or problematic situation ahead.
2. Immediately offer support and help in facing the situation.
3. Possibly suggest the positive results which may occur.

## Secondary Prevention of Severe Anxiety

When the nurse detects a high level of anxiety, she should determine if it should be reduced. In general, all anxiety should be reduced which is greater than a moderate level. Reducing severe anxiety will be discussed under tertiary prevention. If anxiety is at a moderate level, the nurse must decide whether the individual or family is benefiting from the anxiety. If the anxiety is motivating the patient or family to constructively work on their problems, she should probably not interfere. If, on the other hand, the anxiety is being used in ways which are not constructive, it may be wise to attempt to reduce the anxiety. To determine this the nurse looks for several manifestations. First, the individual might be controlling his anxiety in ways which tend to remove him from sources of help. Examples of behaviors which in a sense move others away include withdrawal, depression, irritability, arguing, and complaining. Secondly, if the individual is expressing his anxiety through somatic symptoms, it is probably indicated to attempt to reduce his level of anxiety.[17] Somatic expressions of anxiety are believed to cause more problems than they solve. Thirdly, moderate anxiety should be reduced if his control behaviors are no longer serving a purpose but have become a greater burden to the individual than the anxiety.[5] For example:

> A college student used escape sleeping when anxious and initially handled anxiety related to course work by taking short naps. As final examinations approached and anxiety increased, the longer and more frequent naps seriously interfered with class attendance and study time. Thus, the control behavior had begun to contribute more to the problem and had become less effective as a solution.

Lastly, moderate anxiety which appears to be increasing should probably be reduced.

The nursing literature suggests several specific measures the nurse can use to reduce moderate anxiety. The first priority in secondary prevention of severe anxiety is to detect heightened anxiety which should be reduced quickly and to act to reduce it immediately.

Some measures which have been previously described for preventing the escalation of anxiety are very useful in reducing anxiety as well. Confirming anxiety is very important in secondary prevention as well as primary prevention. Many patients will likely deny that they are anxious at first but will later express that they are. Acknowledging that they are anxious is in itself somewhat therapeutic because the patient may then have a verbal label to attach to the discomfort he has been vaguely aware of. What can be named can usually be more easily coped with. It may be appropriate for the nurse to offer understanding at this point. She might say, "I can understand why you are feeling so tense." This allows the patient to accept what he is feeling. One frequently feels that they should not ever let anything bother them. Thus, one can become increasingly anxious over being anxious. Learning that someone else believes that one's anxiety is justified and acceptable can result in a diminished level of anxiety. Children may not acknowledge their anxiety verbally but only indirectly, such as through drawings or other play activities.

When talking with the patient or family about their anxiety, it is possible to be the most helpful if the patient or family member can specifically pinpoint what they are anxious about.[14] This is not easy to do or always possible. The nurse may find that more directive communication techniques are needed when trying to determine specific sources of anxiety. She might say, "What specifically about coming here to the clinic makes you anxious?" or "What do you think worries you the most about your son's diagnosis?" If the patient is able to pinpoint the cause of his anxiety, he may feel less anxious immediately and the nurse may be able to use the information to guide specific intervention. For example:

> One teenage patient decided that what he dreaded most about getting his yearly school athletic physical was having his blood pressure checked. After the nurse questioned him further she found that specifically the sensation of having his arm constricted was uncomfortable and that he feared his arm might pop like a balloon. The nurse decided to teach him more about the procedure. They talked about his fear, she explained the procedure thoroughly, and answered his questions. When she took his blood pressure, she allowed him to pump up the cuff himself and listen to the Korotkoff sounds. The reading was the lowest reading they had ever gotten in the office.

Another way to reduce the patient's anxiety once he has acknowledged its presence is to help the patient use the energy created by the anxiety to explore the situation.[1,29] He should be helped to explore what behaviors he is currently using as control behaviors. Next he can be helped to reflect on what happened before he became anxious and possibly what threat or stressor led to the anxiety. Then he may be guided to consider the reality of the threat and why it occurred. This problem solving approach may provide the patient with a learning experience and a way to deal with anxiety in the future. The nurse working with a very anxious patient may find it helpful to use short, direct statements because of the patient's difficulty in attending to the environment. She should concentrate on her role as a listener and avoid the temptation to offer her own explanations. The patient is unlikely to be able to concentrate on them. Children may explore their anxiety through the use of play materials, story telling, or through drawing pictures.

In many cases, anxiety is "free floating." That is, the patient is anxious without being able to indicate any specific reasons why. Although it is not possible to determine why the person is anxious, nonspecific interventions can be carried out to reduce anxiety.[17] These interventions focus on providing the individual with activities to use up the energy produced by anxiety. One such activity is talking. Although the individual cannot discuss reasons for his anxiety, he can be listened to as he discusses anything he wishes to talk about. The nurse uses nondirective communication techniques to facilitate his verbal expressions. Groups of people often spontaneously engage in "anxious socializing" to relieve free-floating anxiety. For example, this is often seen in students before an examination. Other individuals relieve the energy or anxiety by crying. The nurse may provide the patient with opportunities or permission to cry: "You look as though you are close to tears," "Go ahead and cry if you feel like it," "Here are some tissues." Walking is another way to dispel the energy of anxiety. The individual may need a suggestion to engage in this behavior.

The presence of another person who is relatively calm may decrease an individual's anxiety, as may the use of touch as discussed previously.

Because security is the antithesis of anxiety, the provision of a secure environment is doubly important with the moderately anxious patient or family. Often increasing the patient's sense of trust in those present in the environment through increasing contact and promptness in responding to demands will alone significantly reduce anxiety. Physical comfort is important and should be promoted with skillful nursing care. Patients and families who are given information and who are made to feel in control of their destiny may become more secure, especially children.

In some situations, the nurse may be able to encourage the patient to use control behaviors. This may not be the best time for an individual to try to give up smoking if he uses his cigarettes to meet oral needs. The nonsmoker or one who must quit may meet oral needs through munching on raw vegetables, popcorn, or peanuts. Fidgety hands can be kept busy through craft projects such as origami, needlework, or working picture puzzles. Children often instinctively use control behaviors if the nurse plans their availability. Often, the patient can be helped to remember earlier effective control behaviors which are appropriate such as piano playing or painting. Walking and other forms of physical activity are effective control behaviors for many individuals. If the patient is engaging in a control behavior such as pacing, she should allow him to continue despite her impulse to quiet the behavior. She can walk with the patient who is pacing and still carry on a conversation. These activities keep the body busy and disperse the energy of anxiety but allow the mind to do "worry work." The patient's attention is usually so consumed by his anxiety that the nurse needs not only to suggest the activity but also to help the patient to engage in it.[17]

The nurse should remember that the adult or child who uses somatic symptoms as control behaviors may not appear excessively anxious. Some special nursing measures may help him reduce his anxiety level.[17] The nurse should promptly respond to his physical complaints and use her medically related knowledge of his physical condition to alleviate as much discomfort as possible. Concern over unmet physical needs can increase anxiety, secondarily further aggravate symptoms, and result in more anxiety. Even if the basis of the condition is suspected to be psychosomatic, the symptoms are very real and not just imagined. The patient with an ulcer believed to be caused by stress has a real ulcer. The nurse should not dwell on the condition, however, as this might reinforce the patient's symptoms.

After relief of discomfort, the patient with somatic control behaviors may respond to other methods already discussed to control anxiety. In addition he may respond to diversion. Diversion which takes the form of physical activity is doubly effective. Promoting interpersonal contact between the patient and others is another effective form of diversion because loneliness and depersonalization are known to increase anxiety. Periods of diversion should probably be balanced with periods of inactivity which allow the patient time to worry.

Planned desensitization of a threat may be useful in secondary intervention.[22] First one must identify the specific anxiety provoking threat in a situation and then plan experiences combining increasing exposure to the threat with positive rewards.

Denise was an 11-year-old girl who was extremely afraid of dentists. Mary learned of Denise's fear when making a home visit to Denise's family. She discovered that Denise had not been to the dentist for four years and needed a checkup. She reported that going to the dentist resulted in a state of acute anxiety. Denise would become physically ill for a week before the appointment. Mary talked with Denise about decreasing her fears of the dentist and the two of them developed a plan based on Denise's hierarchy of fear related to the dentist. The hierarchy they developed from lowest level to highest level of anxiety was:

1. Thinking about the dentist
2. Making and appointment with the dentist
3. Seeing the dentist's office building
4. Entering the waiting room
5. Entering the dentist's chair
6. Seeing the dentist
7. Hearing the sound of the equipment

Next Mary discovered that one of Denise's favorite foods was guacamole dip with taco chips. They developed a plan in which Denise would progress up the hierarchy pairing each step with eating guacamole and taco chips. Each step was planned for Saturday mornings and repeated until the step could be taken with minimal anxiety. Denise agreed to not have guacamole at any other time. Mary contacted the dentist so that Denise could come to the office as part of the desensitization. Denise's desensitization took about three months after which she had her teeth checked with relatively little anxiety.

It may be possible for a patient to persist with anxious behavior because he has been rewarded and reinforced for doing so. In this case the nurse might find planned desensitization a valuable nursing action.

The nursing actions related to secondary prevention are summarized in Table 6-3.

**Table 6-3.** Possible nursing actions for reducing moderate levels of anxiety

1. Act quickly to recognize and reduce anxiety.
2. Attempt to have patient or family acknowledge or confirm presence of anxiety.
3. Try to pinpoint the anxiety producing event and reduce its significance.
4. Use the energy of anxiety to explore the anxiety producing situation if possible.
5. Provide or encourage activities to use up energy of free-floating anxiety such as talking, crying, or walking.
6. Provide the presence of another calm person and use touch if appropriate.
7. Increase feelings of security and control.
8. Encourage use of control behaviors.
9. Promote physical comfort and provide diversion for those who use somatic control behaviors.
10. Use planned desensitization.

## Tertiary Prevention in Severe Anxiety

Panic is a very dangerous state because the patient may easily hurt himself or others. The management of a patient in a true panic state is beyond the scope of this book. The nurse should consider the patient in panic as a psychiatric emergency and immediately get help while protecting the patient from harming himself or others. Severe anxiety is also a dangerous situation because it is believed that it can easily develop into a panic state. Fortunately, severe anxiety, like panic, is not a common state but quick action by the nurse is needed if it should occur.

The child or adult with extreme anxiety is not processing information with much success so the nurse will need to be very direct and authoritarian. It is recommended that she speak in a soft, calm, and commanding tone and make short clear demands.[22] She might say, "Stay in this room" or "I am here with you now." The environment should be made as nonstimulating as possible. Turning off the television, closing the door, sitting as quietly as possible, and closing the drapes are all measures to curtail stimulation. Another alternative is to take the patient to a bland environment.

Next the nurse should provide activity. If the patient is pacing as a control behavior, forcing the patient to sit down may increase the patient's anxiety. She should not tell the patient to be quiet as talking may be a viable control behavior. She may want to help the person engage in some suitable repetitive activity. She could say, "Walk with me" or "Chew this gum." Such activities can help release some of the energy mobilized by the anxiety. The severely anxious patient should never be left alone.

It is advisable to encourage verbal activity. This is not the time to try to focus the patient on determining what caused the severe anxiety. She should let the patient control the subject. The nurse should try to attend to the patient's conversation and limit her comments as much as possible. This is not a time to ask the patient questions.[22] She may find herself shouting at the patient or talking loudly but she should strive to keep her voice moderately soft and calm.

Injectable sedatives may be warranted. The nurse can aid their effectiveness by adding the suggestion that "This will help you to feel more comfortable." The patient may likely misinterpret what the nurse is doing.

The patient may experience pronounced physical symptoms such as heart palpitations and fear that he is going to have a heart attack or die. The nurse should attend to his symptoms carefully. Usually severe anxiety will abate after a period of time if it does not progress to panic.

Patients who have experienced severe anxiety will usually not later recall the episode or may recall it only partially. Attempts to think about the period of time may lead to increased anxiety. It is felt by some that the patient can later learn from the situation and should integrate the near panic or panic episode.[13] The nurse attempting to help the patient recall what happened can bring up the subject and ask the patient for information and details about the situation. The patient's anxiety may increase and he may change the subject but may discuss the situation more later. This process may take many periods of discussion.

Judy worked in a rehabilitation center for children. One of her patients was four-year-old Paula who was convalescing from severe and extensive burns. Paula's mother, Mrs. Green, visited regularly. The mother was believed to be adjusting poorly to Paula's condition and the other events which occurred at the same time as the accident which resulted in Paula's burns. Paula's mother and father had gone for a weekend to their cabin in a remote wooded area. After arriving at the cabin late at night, Mrs. Green had gone back to the car to carry in supplies while Mr. Green lighted a small gas stove. The stove had exploded and the entire cabin had burned down. Both the father and Paula's brother died. Judy had often wondered what Mrs. Green did in the situation being miles away from any source of help late at night with her husband and children in a burning cabin. Mrs. Green had never specifically discussed the accident with any of the staff. Judy decided to explore the area in the hopes that Mrs. Green's adjustment to her life situation might be aided by integrating this situation from the past.

Each time Mrs. Green visited, Judy used all possible opportunities to establish a helping relationship. After a few weeks Judy asked Mrs. Green what she remembered about the accident. Mrs. Green replied, "Hardly anything" and changed the subject. Several days later Mrs. Green began spontaneously to talk about the accident. What she said was very global and sketchy. When Judy asked a specific question Mrs. Green again changed the subject. After that almost each time she visited, Mrs. Green talked with Judy a little more about the accident. Judy offered comments of support regarding how difficult the situation must have been. Slowly Mrs. Green began to talk more and more about the accident which had become a preoccupation much as many women are preoccupied with their labor and delivery experience. Many feelings of guilt, depression, anger, and sorrow were expressed. Judy continued to offer acceptance and listened. Mrs. Green expressed amazement several times about how bothered she still was by the accident which she thought she had forgotten about. There remained several areas related to the accident which Mrs. Green never discussed. During this time, Mrs. Green began to gain more interest in Paula's rehabilitation and acceptance of her slow progress. After Paula was discharged Judy found out that Mrs. Green had been taking Thorazine since the accident and had discontinued its use just before Paula came home.

Tertiary nursing intervention is summarized in Table 6-4.

**Table 6-4.** Possible nursing actions for reducing severe levels of anxiety

1. Act quickly to prevent panic.
2. Speak with soft, concise, commanding statements.
3. Provide a low stimulus environment.
4. Provide activity.
5. Remain with patient.
6. Keep the patient talking.
7. Consider sedatives if panic seems likely.
8. Respond to physical symptoms.
9. Provide opportunities later to recall and integrate near-panic episode.

# THE NURSE AND ANXIETY

Anxiety would appear to be a frequent occurrence for a nurse. Many factors have been identified which are seen as contributing to anxiety in nursing practice.

First of all, anxiety present in patients, families, and health team members is readily communicated to the nurse. This occurs even if the anxiety is hidden.[22]

Other aspects related to nursing practice in various settings which may occur and be anxiety provoking include:

1. Performing painful or embarrassing procedures with children and adults such as giving injections and enemas.
2. Performing tasks which may be unpleasant for the nurse such as changing infected dressings, irrigating a decubitus ulcer, or removing a fecal impaction.
3. Coping with mechanical equipment which is complex.
4. Functioning in a limited amount of cluttered space.
5. Having abrupt contact sporadically with a large number of individuals with specific interests and focuses (health team members, families, administrators, and patients).
6. Trying to be objective and detached and at the same time being subjective and involved.

7. Being pressed for use of knowledge and judgments sometimes beyond her base of knowledge.
8. Living with her expectations and that of others to never make an error.
9. Functioning rapidly in critical situations.
10. Living with the reality of overwhelming tragedy, catastrophic illness, and death.
11. Coping with inconvenient and demoralizing working conditions and policies such as rotating shifts, floating, and working holidays and weekends.
12. Accepting demands without the right to question from superiors and physicians.
13. Feeling hopeless and helpless in the face of a costly, inefficient, crisis focused health care system.
14. Trying to cope with incompetence in others which sometimes leads to hazards to oneself and patients. [24,34]

These factors can and do contribute to considerable anxiety. This anxiety may manifest itself in behaviors such as hostility, irritability, constant complaining, apprehension, negativistic attitudes, frequent somatic complaints, physical illnesses, anger, or withdrawal. [7,24] These are hardly desired states for interacting with others. One study demonstrated that environmental stress can affect the performance of nurses. It was speculated that chronic stress which forced rapid problem solving without adequate time could lead to stereotyped and unimaginative behavioral responses to situations by nurses. [12]

Obviously, the nurse needs information on dealing with her own anxiety if she is to be effective with patients. Mild anxiety probably is desirable and may enhance nursing practice. Higher levels of anxiety can be less desirable. The nurse can use some specific techniques to prevent or reduce high levels of anxiety. Much of what has been discussed in relation to the patient and family is also applicable to the nurse. Specifically, the nurse can:

1. Learn to recognize threats and stressors including environmental ones which cause her to become anxious and determine if they can be altered.
2. Learn to recognize when she is anxious.
3. Identify how she controls anxiety.
4. Seek supports in her environment.
5. Identify how she responds to anxious patients.
6. Use situations of heightened anxiety as learning experiences by searching for the cause of her anxiety, how she is controlling it, and how to dissipate it. This is often best done with another person present to listen and reflect.
7. Use desensitization techniques to reduce anxiety in situations which predictably lead to anxiety.
8. Learn techniques of relaxation to combat stress which she can use when away from work and at work. Exercise is relaxing for some. [27] Music is well known as promoting relaxation. Recently increasing attention is being focused on the effectiveness of evoking a "relaxation response" as a technique for relaxation. [2] Frequent and completely absorbing diversional activities may be valuable.

One interesting and usually effective method the nurse can use when she feels anxious about a present or future situation is designed to help identify the threat involved and to appraise it realistically. When the nurse is faced with a situation about which she is anxious, she asks herself, "What is the worst possible thing that can happen?" followed by "How likely is this to occur?" and "What if it does occur?" For example:

Nancy was feeling anxious over taking a new job she wanted but which would demand more from her. She asked herself what was the worst that could happen and decided that her most specific fear was that she wouldn't be able to perform as expected and would be fired. Once she had identified her worst fear she realized it wasn't very realistic. She was qualified for the job and had tackled difficult experiences before and succeeded. Next she asked herself how terrible would it be if her worst fear did come true. She recognized that being fired from her new job would certainly not be the end of the world as she had many other options. Nancy had to go through this process several times but eventually felt much less anxious about her new job.

This technique reduces vague feelings of anxiety into specific fears which can then be examined in terms of their probability and consequence. In most situations the specific fears become much less threatening when placed in perspective. This technique can be used with and taught to patients.

Depression often compounds anxiety when one feels that one has failed in a past situation. This feeling of failure may occur because of unrealistic expectations. A variation of the previous technique which may help uncover these expectations may be helpful. When the nurse feels depressed and anxious over something she can try to determine what she feels she failed in by asking, "In what way did I fail?" followed by "What expectations of myself did I have?" and "How realistic were they?"

> Marty had had a very bad day at work and felt anxious and secondarily depressed all evening. She tried to reflect on what situations had occurred during the day in which she felt she had failed. One specific thing which came to mind was an incident occurring in the morning when an uncooperative four-year-old patient had bitten her finger intentionally when she was suctioning him. She had become very angry and scolded the patient harshly. She realized that this particular child annoyed her considerably. She felt angry because she was always assigned to him and she felt guilty over disliking the child and her actions toward him. When she faced what her expectations were of herself she decided that she expected herself to never lose her temper and to like every patient and their family. She quickly realized that this was unrealistic and that losing her temper when bitten was understandable. She decided that she had possibly provoked the child's behavior by her approach to him and this was something she should work on. Thus her anxiety was relieved and replaced by motivation to work on her relationship with the patient.

When the nurse finds herself becoming anxious while with a patient she can do several things. First she should acknowledge her anxiety to herself. Next she can try to determine why she feels anxious and if there is anything she can do to control her anxiety. If her anxiety is increasing and if it is likely to be detrimental to the patient, it may be appropriate to leave the situation until she can function more adequately. However, many nurses will encounter situations where this is not possible and must function as effectively as possible while trying consciously to remain calm. Needless to say, this is not an easy task. The nurse who continuously finds herself faced with overwhelming anxiety and who cannot adapt well to this type of demand should recognize the need to find a situation in which she can more effectively function.

## A TOOL FOR ASSESSMENT AND EVALUATION

The tool presented in Table 6-5 can be used to determine if a patient's or family member's anxiety is interfering with their functioning and is a threat to their level of wellness. When behaviors which are "less optimal" dominate an individual's functioning, a high risk situation exists.

This tool may also be used by the nurse to evaluate the effects of nursing intervention on the patient. If nursing action is effective, the patient should demonstrate predominantly "more optimal" functioning.

The information in this tool is based on clinical observations and the literature.[3,5,17,22,32]

## AN EXAMPLE OF NURSING INTERVENTION IN ANXIETY

The following example illustrates how one nurse responded to an anxious patient. The assessment, planning, intervention, and evaluation in this situation had to be done quite quickly as will be seen.

**Table 6-5.** Assessment and evaluation tool

| Behavior | More optimal response | Less optimal response |
| --- | --- | --- |
| Relationships with others | Not affected | Anxiety moves person away from others |
| Choice of control behaviors | Expresses anxiety outwardly | Converts anxiety into bodily symptoms |
| Comfort level | Tolerates anxiety | Very uncomfortable |
| Interference with usual life style | Minimal | Maximal |
| Pattern of control behaviors | Uses several behaviors | Persistence of one control behavior |
| Manifestations | Increased urination, perspiration, diarrhea, tenseness, restlessness | Palpitations, agitation, tachycardia, tremors, dyspnea, confusion |
| Intensity | Only major events lead to severe anxiety | Minor events lead to severe anxiety |
| Duration | Anxiety abates when stressor is reduced | Anxiety lasts after stressor is reduced |
| Mode of verbal expression | Constructive talking | Arguing, complaining, attacking |
| Effectiveness of control behavior | Usually effective | Becoming problematic of themselves |
| Time focus | Can comprehend the present | Overwhelmed by the future |
| Use of energy | Mobilizing | Immobilizing |

Kathy was a 16-year-old patient who was admitted to the labor and delivery unit in early labor. Kathy was brought to the hospital by her older sister who left promptly after she was admitted. The nurse who admitted Kathy wrote in the admission note that she appeared frightened and unprepared for delivery. She tried to spend extra time with Kathy and explain what was occurring as clearly as possible. Kathy's labor progressed normally.

When Jackie came on duty several hours later, Kathy was having progressively stronger contractions and had been given some medication for pain. Jackie noticed when she first saw Kathy that she did indeed appear frightened. She lay quietly in bed but her eyes never missed any activity in the room. Her hands tightly gripped the side rails.

Jackie decided that since Kathy might soon be in even more stressful circumstances she should concentrate on attempts to keep Kathy's anxiety at the present level or to lower it. After Jackie had talked with Kathy for a few minutes, she decided that Kathy was even more anxious than she had thought. She asked Kathy if she was feeling anxious and Kathy replied "Yes" with a nervous laugh. As Jackie talked with her more, she discovered that Kathy had received a considerable amount of information about the negative side of delivering a baby from friends and relatives. She was hopeful that she would be put to sleep and wouldn't wake up until it was "all over" although she expressed fears over being put to sleep. Specifically she was concerned that she might be "torn up inside" by the baby's birth because she felt she was very small to have a baby.

Jackie felt overwhelmed as she listened to Kathy talk of other misconceptions and fears. Jackie knew she had very little time and a large challenge. It seemed most appropriate to plan on staying with Kathy and to continue to facilitate her conversation because it appeared that one way Kathy handled anxiety was through talking. Jackie attended carefully as she listened to Kathy and expressed acceptance of her fears. She knew that she didn't have time to attempt to correct misconceptions or teach great amounts of information at this stage, nor could Kathy absorb much information now due to her anxiety. Jackie noted that in addition to talking, Kathy pressed her hands together tightly and gritted her teeth frequently. She wore glasses and Jackie found out that she had limited vision without them.

Jackie focused on keeping herself and the environment as calm as possible. She closed the door into the hall and placed a note on the door which said, "Quiet Please." The volume on the monitors being used was reduced. She tried to give Kathy short and explicit information on what she was doing. She told Kathy that she would be with her throughout the next several hours. She tried to give brief descriptions of what would happen next immediately before each event took place. She eliminated unnecessary discussions which were often used with patients who needed diversion such as "Do you want a boy or a girl?"and "What names have you picked out?" She paid meticulous attention to the physical aspects of Kathy's care because she knew that physical discomfort could compound anxiety. For example, she provided relaxing backrubs and a cool cloth for Kathy's forehead.

Jackie noticed that Kathy's anxiety increased noticeably as the contractions became stronger so she asked Kathy to watch the clock and count the seconds out loud during each contraction. This activity seemed to provide some diversion.

When it was time to take Kathy to the delivery room, Jackie explained that it was time to deliver the baby and deliberately and calmly initiated the transfer. In the delivery room she left Kathy's hands free so she could continue to press them together if she wanted to. She also left Kathy's glasses on because she felt that removing them might be very frightening to Kathy. Jackie also signaled another nurse who was available to perform the delivery room duties so that she could devote her full attention to Kathy. Three "observers" appeared to watch the delivery and Jackie persuaded them to choose another delivery. Jackie encouraged Kathy to continue talking, but Kathy was becoming quieter.She continued to keep Kathy informed in simple statements on what was happening. Jackie knew that Kathy would not be given a general anesthetic due to anesthesiologist's policies but she had decided not to tell her this before, due to Kathy's previous hope to be put to sleep, and instead waited until it was time to give the anesthesia. As this was being done she told Kathy, "Dr. Roberts is going to take care of your discomfort now."

As activity in the room increased, Kathy became increasingly more silent. Her eyes were open wide and darting around the room. Kathy's attention began to focus on the mirror which showed her perineal area. She did not appear to be listening to Jackie who was trying to succinctly describe what she was seeing. Kathy began to breathe very rapidly and strained to see in the mirror. She began screaming "I'm bleeding. The baby is tearing me!" Jackie felt herself become quite anxious as she watched Kathy. Jackie took a long slow breath and felt somewhat calmer. She stood closer to Kathy and talked quietly near her ear. "This is normal. You are not tearing." The presence of a calm quiet voice seemed to help Kathy gain some control. Kathy began to cry and Jackie handed her tissues and encouraged her to cry.

As the baby's head appeared, Kathy again strained forward. "He's blue! There is something wrong with the baby!" Jackie again talked quietly. "He will become pink as he breathes. He is supposed to be this blue." The baby was delivered and let out a vigorous cry. Kathy began to cry again. Jackie wiped her tears and said, "Go ahead and cry." Kathy continued to strain forward periodically and express grave concern over each new event. Each time Jackie would take a deep breath until her voice was calm and then give a short explanation softly in Kathy's ear.

Kathy did not show any interest in seeing the baby immediately but continued to focus on her fears that she was being torn. Jackie waved the assisting nurse away when she started to bring the baby. She felt it best to wait until Kathy's attention could be diverted from her concerns about herself. After the delivery of the placenta and the beginning of the suturing, Kathy at last began to relinquish her exclusive focus on the mirror. The physician assured her that she had come through the delivery in excellent shape and had no tears at all. Kathy began to look around the room to find the baby. Jackie had the baby brought to her. Kathy reached out to hold the baby. Kathy began to cry again as she held the baby tightly and sobbed "We made it, kid!"

Soon Kathy was taken to the recovery area. Jackie personally made the transfer in a calm manner and cared for Kathy herself for the 2 hours she was in the postpartum room. Kathy fell into a relaxed sleep without medication. Her physical condition was normal. Jackie wrote down notes for the postpartum staff to alert them to Kathy's special needs and reactions.

Jackie arranged to visit Kathy the next day and together they relived the labor and delivery. Kathy remembered the events with some oversights of the most stressful moments. Kathy laughed and said, "It was no big deal at all, was it?" Jackie concluded that Kathy could recall most of what had happened and had come through the experience feeling confident and proud of herself. She would never know how Kathy might have reacted to the experience had not specific interventions been used to help control Kathy's anxiety but she believed that her intervention had helped a frightened and unprepared woman cope with a major stressful situation.

## SUMMARY

Anxiety is a familiar and common response to various types of threats. Anxiety is manifested in energy and each person develops unique control behaviors to cope with the energy of anxiety. Most useful are believed to be control behaviors which lead to the analysis of anxiety and behaviors which rid the individual of the excess energy in a healthful way. Anxiety is normally present to some degree in everyone. It can occur at several intensities. Learning and problem solving are believed to be most efficient at mild levels of anxiety. Anxiety is believed to be a learned response to adversity and exists throughout the life cycle after approximately six months of age.

Anxiety in patients and families is not to be avoided at all costs. Rather the nurse must be able to assess the individual's level of anxiety and its usefulness to him. She may be able to raise, maintain, or reduce an individual's anxiety level with therapeutic interventions.

The nurse will no doubt experience anxiety throughout her personal and professional life and can learn to recognize and cope with her own anxiety.

## REFERENCES

1. "Anxiety: Recognition and intervention." Am. J. Nurs. 65:131, 1965.
2. Benson, H.: "Your innate asset for combating stress." Harvard Bus. Rev. 52:49, 1974.
3. Boland, M., et al.: "Application of adaptation theory to nursing," in Murray, R., et al.: *Nursing Concepts for Health Promotion.* Prentice-Hall, Inc., Englewood Cliffs, N.J., 1975.
4. Brody, S., and Axelrad, S.: *Anxiety and Ego Formation in Infancy.* International Universities Press, New York, 1970.
5. Brownsberger, C. N., et al.: "Common psychiatric symptoms," in Solomon, P., and Patch, V. (ed.): *Handbook of Psychiatry.* Lange Medical Publications, Los Altos, Calif., 1971.

6. Brunner, L. S., and Suddarth, D. S.: *Textbook of Medical-Surgical Nursing.* J. B. Lippincott, Philadelphia, 1975.
7. Burkhardt, M.: "Responses to anxiety." Am. J. Nurs. 69:2153, 1969.
8. Burnside, I. M.: "Developmental reactions in old age," in Kalkman, M. E., and Davis, A. J. (ed.): *New Dimensions in Mental Health-Psychiatric Nursing.* McGraw-Hill, New York, 1974.
9. Burnside, I. M.: "Gerontion: A case study." Perspect. Psychiat. Care. 9:103, 1971.
10. Busse, E. W., and Pfeiffer, E.: "Functional disorders in old age," in Busse, E. W., and Pfeiffer, E. (ed.): *Behavior and Adaptation in Late Life.* Little, Brown and Company, Boston, 1969.
11. Chapman, A. H.: *Management of Emotional Problems of Children and Adolescents.* J. B. Lippincott, Philadelphia, 1974.
12. Cleland, V.: "Effects of stress on thinking." Am. J. Nurs. 67:108, 1967.
13. Drage, E. M.: "Recall of panic episodes." Am. J. Nurs. 68:1254, 1968.
14. DuGas, B.: *Introduction to Patient Care.* W. B. Saunders, Philadelphia, 1972.
15. Dylag, H.: "How difficult the 'I': The adolescent maturation of critical identity," in Hall, J. E., and Weaver, B. R. (ed.): *Nursing of Families in Crisis.* J. B. Lippincott, Philadelphia, 1974.
16. Ebersole, P.: "Geriatric crisis intervention in the family context," in Hall, J. E., and Weaver, B. R. (ed.): *Nursing of Families in Crisis.* J. B. Lippincott, Philadelphia, 1974.
17. Francis, G. M., and Munjas, B.: *Promoting Psychological Comfort.* Wm. C. Brown, Dubuque, 1975.
18. Haas, A.: "How youngsters survive trauma." Indianapolis Star Magazine, May 30, 1976.
19. Hitchcock, Janice E.: "Social and psychological crisis," in Kalkman, M. E. and Davis, A. J. (ed.): *New Dimensions in Mental Health-Psychiatric Nursing.* McGraw-Hill, New York, 1974.
20. Janis, I. L.: *Psychological Stress: Psychoanalytic and Behavioral Studies of Surgical Patients.* John Wiley and Sons, New York, 1958.
21. Kagan, J., and Moss, H. A.: *Birth to Maturity: A Study in Psychological Development.* John Wiley and Sons, New York, 1972.
22. Kalkman, M. E.: "Psychoneuroses," in Kalkman, M. E., and Davis, A. J. (ed.): *New Dimensions in Mental Health-Psychiatric Nursing.* McGraw-Hill, New York, 1974.
23. Manaser, J. C., and Werner, A. M.: *Instruments for Study of Nurse-Patient Interaction.* Macmillan, New York, 1964.
24. Michaels, D. R.: "Too much in need of support to give any." Am. J. Nurs. 71:1932, 1971.
25. Morrissey, J. R.: "Death anxiety in children with a fatal illness," in Parad, H. J. (ed.).: *Crisis Intervention: Selected Readings.* Family Service Association of America, New York, 1965.
26. Neylan, M.: "Anxiety." Am. J. Nurs. 62:110, 1962.
27. Parley, K.: "How to balance your tensions." Am. J. Nurs. 67:2099, 1967.
28. Peplau, H. E.: "A working definition of anxiety," in Burd, S., and Marshall, M. (ed.): *Some Clinical Approaches to Psychiatric Nursing.* Macmillan, New York, 1970.
29. Peplau, H. E.: "Anxiety," in Clark, A. L., and Affonso, D. D.: *Childbearing: A Nursing Perspective.* F. A. Davis, Philadelphia, 1976.
30. Peplau, H. E.: "Mid-life crises." Am. J. Nurs. 75:1761, 1975.
31. Pothier, P. C.: "Developmental reactions in infancy and childhood," in Kalkman, M. E., and Davis, A. J. (ed.): *New Dimensions in Mental Health-Psychiatric Nursing.* McGraw-Hill, New York, 1974.
32. Pothier, P. C.: *Mental Health Counseling With Children.* Little, Brown and Company, Boston, 1976.
33. Perls, F.: *Gestalt Therapy Verbatim.* Real People Press, Lafayette, Calif., 1969.
34. Reichle, M. J.: "Psychological aspects of the acutely stressed in an intensive care unit," in Bushnell, S. S.: *Respiratory Intensive Care Nursing.* Little, Brown and Company, Boston, 1973.
35. Saxton, D., and Hyland, P.: *Planning and Implementing Nursing Intervention.* C. V. Mosby, St. Louis, 1975.
36. Scipien, G., et al.: *Comprehensive Pediatric Nursing.* McGraw-Hill, New York, 1975.
37. Selye, H.: *The Stress of Life.* McGraw-Hill, New York, 1956.
38. Storr, A.: "The case of the unpleasant boss." Realities 278:30, 1974.
39. Verwoerdt, A., and Eisdorfer, C.: "Geropsychiatry: The psychiatry of senescence." Geriatrics 22:139, 1967.
40. Waechter, E. H., and Blake, F. G.: *Nursing Care of Children.* J. B. Lippincott, Philadelphia, 1976.
41. Walkup, L. L.: "The concept of crisis," in Hall, J. E., and Weaver, B. R. (ed.): *Nursing of Families in Crisis.* J. B. Lippincott, Philadelphia, 1974.
42. Wicks, R. J.: *Counseling Strategies and Intervention Techniques for the Human Services.* J. B. Lippincott, Philadelphia, 1977.

# BIBLIOGRAPHY

Holsclaw, P. R.: "Nursing in high emotional risk areas." Nurs. Forum 4:36, 1965.

Kennedy, M. J.: "Coping with emotional stress in the patient awaiting heart surgery." Nurs. Clin. North Am. 1:3, 1966.

Meares, A.: *The Management of the Anxious Patient.* W. B. Saunders, Philadelphia, 1963.

Nehren, J., and Gilliam, N.: "Separation anxiety." Am. J. Nurs. 65:109, 1965.

Powers, M. E., and Storlie, F.: "The apprehensive patient." Am. J. Nurs. 67:58, 1967.

Selye, H.: "The stress syndrome." Am. J. Nurs. 65:97, 1965.

# CHAPTER 7

# DENIAL

There is hardly any unexpected event which occurs to man that is not reacted to first by denial to some degree. This reaction can range from the complete denial expressed in, "Oh no! It can't be true!" to partial denial expressed as, "It's hard to believe." The nurse, regardless of the setting she works in, will see many patients and families who initially react to a stressful event or situation with disbelief. She will be involved with a lesser number of patients who persistently use denial to cope with anxiety. For these reasons, the nurse needs to be able to recognize denial, understand why denial occurs among patients and families, and be able to intervene appropriately with patients and families who are denying. The nurse, herself, may use denial both in her personal and professional life and this area will be explored with suggestions for recognizing when one is using denial and ideas on what to do to reduce one's use of denial.

This chapter will focus on normal and common forms of denial and not on pathologic denial.

## REVIEW OF THEORY

Denial can be defined as a mental mechanism of self-deception which affords protection to an individual, in whole or in part, from a given reality. The process is unconscious and not deliberate on the individual's part.[20] Denial is believed to be one of the first protective mental mechanisms which an individual develops, occurring first in infancy. Denial, or "shock and disbelief," is often described as the universal initial reaction of most individuals to an anxiety producing event.[6,11,15]

### The Anatomy of Denial

A further understanding of denial can be gained by considering in a simplified version how denial may occur.

1. A situation exists which is threatening in some manner to an individual.
2. The individual responds unconsciously with anxiety.
3. The anxiety is decreased by unconsciously and automatically rejecting or ignoring wholly or partially the reality of the situation.
4. Functioning of the individual is maintained.[7,13,25]

Denial serves then to protect the individual from a reality which he cannot face. Typically, after a period of time, denial gives way to a slowly developing awareness of the reality.[6] Denial is a basic and automatic protective defense but it requires considerable psychic energy to be maintained. As a defense, denial does not lead to problem resolution since one cannot analyze a threatening situation when he refuses to recognize the situation itself.

For these reasons, denial is often seen as an unhealthy, unhelpful, or destructive defense. It would seem more judicious not to rate denial as helpful or unhelpful in connection with its occurence but rather to consider it helpful or unhelpful according to the purposes it serves at the time. Denial which occurs immediately after a major threat is then judged differently than prolonged denial of an obvious reality. For example, denial may be helpful in the first days or weeks after a parent has been told his child has a life threatening but curable malignancy, but may not be helpful if it is still occurring several months later so that therapy has not been instituted. However, even prolonged denial may be advantageous in some situations as will be discussed later.

## Threat as a Cause of Denial

Denial may develop when an individual is faced with a major stressor or threat. The types of threats which are most likely to produce denial are those related to one's self-concept. Some particular threats to self-concept which seem likely to produce denial have been described in the literature.

The birth of a defective child seems particularly threatening to parents.[24,26,27,30] Denial is frequent and may persist throughout the child's lifetime although the parents may partially accept that the child is imperfect but deny the extent of the imperfection: "He's just a slow child. He'll catch up some day."

Another threat to self-concept involves illness. Illness requires that the individual accept that he is in some respects different than he was.[13] If the difference to be accepted involves a major change in self-concept which results in anxiety, denial may occur to protect the individual. The severity of the threat from the individual's perception will influence how profound the denial is.

Certain types of illnesses seem most likely to lead to use of denial:

1. Illnesses which are hard to disguise and therefore very obvious to others are likely to be denied. Examples include handicapping illnesses which will lead to the use of a wheelchair or special prosthesis, neuromuscular disorders, and disfiguring illnesses.

2. Illnesses which are seen as life threatening or usually fatal produce a major threat and are likely to be denied, such as cancer, myocardial infarct, and strokes.

3. Illnesses which may be seen as shameful or disgraceful may be readily denied.

Ten-year-old Bobby attempted to hang himself after his parents were divorced and his mother began dating again. Bobby's mother protested vehemently to any suggestion that Bobby had meant to kill himself and argued that the whole thing was an accident while Bobby was climbing in a tree. She insisted that Bobby was a happy, well adjusted boy who adored the man she was dating.

4. Addiction to chemical substances is frequently denied.

John was a junior in college when he began to drink alcoholic beverages heavily on the weekends. Now married and out of college for 4 years, he and his wife spend progressively more time drinking. John has lost two jobs because of excessive absences. John's mother has suggested that he needs treatment for alcoholism. John and his wife both deny that he is an alcoholic. They insist that his mother is prudish and old fashioned. After all, they say, all their friends drink as much as John does.

5. An individual may deny an illness when to admit it might involve others. A mother may deny symptoms of rheumatoid arthritis because she is unconsciously afraid that to admit them might make her a less effective mother to her children. A busy man may deny symptoms of an ulcer because his family is dependent on his income.

It should be noted that any one illness can represent several of these categories. For example:

Ms. Walker was admitted to the hospital with a diagnosis of chronic bronchitis. After preliminary tests she was told that she likely had lung cancer. She faced a life threatening illness, one which she interpreted as disgraceful because she had been advised many times to quit smoking, one related to addiction to cigarettes, and an illness which would involve others—her husband was dependent on her. She initially used complete denial of the condition.

It is important to remember that what may be a serious threat to one individual may not be to another. How the person involved reacts to the threat is of more importance than the objective truth related to the threat from the nurse's perception.

Denial is common when an individual is faced with potentially anxiety producing aspects of life apart from illness. For example:

Mrs. Weaver had a particularly long period of pronounced symptoms during the menopause. At the same time her son dropped out of college unexpectedly to join the Peace Corps and her daughter married unexpectedly against her wishes. Mrs. Weaver became convinced that her lack of energy and other symptoms were due to the fact that she had a number of nutritional deficiencies. She found relief from her symptoms and a rejuvenation of energy from taking high doses of expensive natural vitamins and through the use of a variety of organically grown health food substances. Through her health food faddism, Mrs. Weaver was able to divert her attention from the problems with her children and a changing self-concept that she could not face.

## Dimensions of Denial

Denial can occur in several forms. The most extreme form of denial is *complete denial.* This may be seen most often in the period immediately following exposure to a major threat.

Ms. Lee was told by the obstetric resident that her newborn son had Down's syndrome. She laughed at the physician. She explained that all of her babies had looked the same right after birth and that the new son looked just like his father who had almond-shaped eyes.

Mr. and Mrs. Saxon were called by the juvenile authorities after their 15-year-old son was arrested for molesting a 7-year-old girl in their neighborhood. They both insisted that a mistake had been made. Their son was probably helping the young girl undress for bed.

If temporary, complete denial is seen as normal and not serious. It is not considered normal for a person to evidence complete denial later than the initial period of shock.[13] One who does should be referred to an appropriate mental health source.

Mr. Ridpath's wife died after a prolonged illness. Mr. Ridpath was taken to the funeral and the burial. Four months later he still refused to part with any of his wife's personal belongings and insisted that she was still in the hospital.

While prolonged complete denial is uncommon and considered unhealthy in patients or parents, it is considered more normal in family and friends who are more removed from the immediate situation than the patient or parents. It is frequently evidenced as disbelief of a diagnosis.

Heather was diagnosed as having leukemia when she was 4 years old. After beginning chemotherapy, she returned to leading a normal life for 18 months. During this period, Heather's maternal grandmother refused to believe that there was anything wrong with her. She told Heather's parents that they were being "taken" by some physicians who wanted to make money. When Heather's symptoms returned, the grandmother believed it was caused by not getting enough fresh air and exercise.

The denial of others surrounding the patient or parents can be very difficult for the patient and those who are not using denial. They may be placed in the position of believing that they must continually prove the diagnosis. In addition, the denial of significant others increases the patient's and family's own inclination to cope through the use of denial.

Mrs. Larson was 19 when she abruptly began having grand mal seizures. Mr. Larson felt that the seizures were fainting spells caused by her "nerves" and worrying too much. He persuaded her not to see a physician and convinced her that she could control the "spells" if she tried hard enough. Mrs. Larson complied and did not see a physician. When her seizures increased in frequency and duration she did eventually seek medical help and was placed on medications. Mr. Larson continued to refer to the physician's diagnosis and treatment as a "bunch of nonsense" and encouraged Mrs. Larson to not take her medications.

Another form of denial is *partial denial.* Partial denial is very common and frequently seen in health care settings.

Partial denial is evidenced when an individual with an illness accepts some aspects of the illness but denies others.

Mr. Shaw was diagnosed as a juvenile-onset diabetic in his teens. Now at the age of 40, he recognizes that he has diabetes and routinely performs his related care activities. Despite the fact that he has repeatedly injured himself because he did not see hazards, he refuses to acknowledge that his vision is becoming seriously impaired.

Similarly, a parent may recognize a disability in a child but ignore parts of the manifestations.

Partial denial may present as accepting a diagnosis but denying its significance.[13] For example, one elderly lady knew that she had an abnormal growth in her breast but did not seek help because she was "too tough for anything to get her."

Partial denial can be seen as both helpful and unhelpful.[13] The individual who must live with a chronic disability or illness may need to partially deny aspects of his disability in order to maintain enough courage and hope to live. Similarly, the parents of a retarded child may use denial to partially blunt the impact of certain aspects of having such a child so that they are not completely overwhelmed by the burdens involved. On the other hand, partial denial is unhelpful when it interferes with possible correction or resolution of the threat being denied as in the example of Mr. Shaw.

Lastly, denial may occur as a *distortion of reality.* This represents some acceptance of the threatening situation but with distortion of the threat or situation so as to reduce its impact. The classic example of this involves the patient who recognizes symptoms of a myocardial infarction but insists that the symptoms are "gas pains" or "indigestion." Another example is the teenage girl who is not asked on dates who sincerely believes that it is because she is too good and refuses to engage in the "immoral" activities of all the popular girls.

Distortions of reality are frequently seen in health care settings. They present a challenge in that they are difficult to assess and resistant to reduction.

## Manifestations of Denial

While complete denial is usually obvious with careful assessment, partial denial is more difficult to pinpoint.

Some behaviors of the patient who is using partial denial may be very frustrating to health care professionals. The patient may flagrantly violate medical orders, fail to take prescribed medicines, miss return appointments, ignore his special diet, continually misunderstand what he has been told, and go from one health care facility to another.[13] Attempts at self-medication with megavitamins and illegal or "wonder" drugs may indicate that the patient denies the true cause or basis of the threat.

Denial may appear subtly as the avoidance of discussion of a specific topic. Or the patient may dwell on the past and exaggerate what his life was like in the past.[10] He is likely to avoid discussing the future.

The lack of the normal expected emotional reaction by an adult or child to a serious threat may indicate denial.[5] For example, the patient may appear inappropriately cheerful, or exaggeratedly optimistic in the face of a serious situation.[13,19] Another response may involve focusing on details of intellectualizing about a condition without any show of emotion. Failure to ask logical questions, seek specific information, or the avoidance of anyone's attempts at instruction are likely to indicate denial.[10] Joking about a condition or the inappropriate use of humor may indicate denial.[13] Even the failure to experience a phantom limb syndrome after an amputation is suspect.[7]

Subtle behaviors which show the denial of a restricting condition involve plunging into overactivity and unrealistic future planning.[10,13] Also of concern would be the patient who eats and sleeps well when he should not.[12] The patient may make an obvious pretense of vigor when he feels very ill. This might be seen as an overly robust and exaggerated handshake.[17]

Other attempts at denial may revolve around denial of symptoms or the minimizing of symptoms. Some patients may cope with symptoms through explaining them away.[10] Renaming a condition may indicate denial. Thus, obesity becomes "glandular problems" and the mentally retarded child becomes an "exceptional child." Even patients who talk about a specific illness may be denying the extent of the illness. "I had a slight stroke."[13] Another clue to denial occurs when the patient attributes confirmation of the illness to someone else: "The doctor said I had a stroke."[13] Other patients may seem to accept the condition but refuse to ever name the condition. What one is denying may be replaced by a contrary fantasy: "My husband loves me more than ever." Or a patient may say he is very unconcerned but appear tense and alert.[1]

Families who deny an illness of a family member may engage in the same behaviors described. In addition, they may attempt to hide or seclude the patient so that, since others cannot see the situation, maybe it does not really exist.[16] Families may be tempted to insist that the patient himself is not aware of the situation.[13] This in essence says, "It must not be very serious." Some families may be caught in limbo between proving to others that something is wrong and simultaneously trying to deny that there is any problem.[16]

The symptoms described here are common and may seem easy to diagnose but patients and families may express their denial in very subtle ways. It is essential to be alert for signs of denial because they may easily be overlooked. A common mistake in assessing denial is to assume that a patient or family who has lived with a threat for a number of years cannot still be denying the reality of the threat. Denial can last a lifetime—especially partial denial and distortions of reality.

Denial operates so swiftly and effectively in many situations that analysis is difficult. The best clue to the existence of denial is probably the absence of some emotion in a situation where it would seem to be logical for it to occur.

Tammy and Jack's first highly desired pregnancy ended in a stillbirth. Tammy's family and friends were amazed at how well she coped. She never cried and was never depressed or angry.

## Denial and Hope

Although hope and denial may not at first seem related, in reality hope may be thought of as a form of denial. The patient with a terminal disease who still hopes for a miraculous cure is in essence evidencing some denial that his condition is really terminal. The parents of a severely retarded child who hope for a normal life for their child are in part denying the seriousness of their child's condition and society's attitudes towards retardation. Hope is then in essence a form of helpful denial which occurs after reality has been faced and which softens reality enough to permit more comfortable confrontation. In some situations, denial may appear to be hope but in actuality be denial which is preventing one from ever facing reality. Contrast these two examples which may both superficially appear to represent hope.

Mr. Jenkins was told that he had an inoperable lung carcinoma. He reacted by reading his Bible and praying much of the time that he was awake. He stated that he had no fear of death but was ready to meet his God and receive His blessings. As his death became more inevitable, however, Mr. Jenkins found it more difficult to deny his fears of death and became severely anxious.

Kathy was diagnosed with lupus erythematosus at the age of 35. She slowly gained awareness of the implications of her disease and experienced depression and anger. She had always attended church and found her faith to be a major sustaining force as she faced her death. Shortly before she died, she planned her funeral, but still expressed hope that she might be cured.

The crucial distinction lies in the fact that hope only occurs after reality has been faced to some degree.

## DENIAL AND THE LIFE CYCLE

### Infants

Denial is believed to be used in infancy to handle anxiety automatically.[13] It is presumed that the child denies by closing his eyes to shut out reality or by withdrawing from unpleasant situations.

## Toddlers

The toddler uses verbal denial as if saying he did not do something can make it so.[7] The toddler's use of denial to cope with separation anxiety has been extensively described. It is felt that the toddler reacts to separation from a significant other through stages of protest, despair, and finally detachment.[3] In the stage of detachment he denies his need for the relationship as a way of protecting himself from further hurt. It is as if he were saying, "If I don't need my mother, then I can't be hurt because she is not here."

Symptoms of relationship denial in the toddler include apparent indifference to previously significant individuals and a resistance to forming attachments to others.[28]

## Preschoolers

The preschooler experiences many sources of anxiety which can potentially be handled through denial. He is supposedly anxious about the potential loss of the love of significant others, controlling aggressive and sexual impulses, and fearful over potential bodily harm.[22] Preschool children would seem to have more available means to deny reality and therefore control anxiety. For one, they can withdraw into a world of fantasy. Thus they may fantasize destroying a younger sibling who seems to be replacing them in their parents' eyes.[13] They can also project onto others unacceptable actions and thoughts. "Mother, B. J. was teasing the kitty. I wasn't." Withdrawal can also be used at this stage to help deny the external world.[18]

## School-aged Children

School-aged children may use denial to cope with anxiety over school success, physical competence, establishing peer relationships, and meeting parental and peer standards.[22] The school-aged child is notorious for his attempts to use false bravery to deny fears and concerns in the face of personal threats.[28] Denial can take the form of fantasy. For example, the young school-aged boy may fantasize that he has a twin brother who will always be his best friend.

When faced with a threatening situation in the future, school-aged children have been found to use an attitude of disinterest which is thinly veiled denial. Thus if they claim they know nothing about an impending event, such as surgery, and wish to know nothing, maybe it will not occur.[21]

## Adolescents

Teenagers may use denial when they are anxious over peer relationships, control of bodily impulses, developing independence from parents, death, and physical appearance deviations.

Denial behavior is often noticeable among teenagers in attempts to conquer death anxiety. This appears as risk taking behaviors such as excessive speeding in automobiles, chemical abuse, and so forth. The behavior is in essence an attempt by the individual to deny his vulnerability to death.

> Three young high school boys were killed in a car wreck when their car slipped off a rain-slick pavement into a tree at 90 mph. The local police officials expected that, at least for a few weeks, most teenagers in the same community would react by driving more sensibly. To their amazement, it seemed that speeding was worse than usual. What they didn't understand was that some of the teenagers were reacting to a very real anxiety producing situation with increased denial by striving to prove their own immunity to death.

A particularly interesting form of denial prevalent in teenagers involves the use of high idealism as a way of denying "unfit" thoughts and feelings.[28] Thus religious idealism may be used as a defense against sexual thoughts. Some religious groups have unwittingly capitalized on this period of reactive idealism by using this stage of life as a time to induct teenagers into commitment to a religious life.

Other forms of denial used by teenagers are similar to those used by adults.

## Adults

Denial may be used during adulthood to deal with anxiety of any proportion. Adults and teenagers use a still wider variety of denial methods than children. In addition to frank denial, many attempts at partial denial are prevalent. One interesting pattern of denial is to treat a threat as a joke.[5] Thus a man with prostatic hypertrophy may laugh and make embarrassing jokes to deny the significance of the illness.

Another denial behavior is using absorption in details to divert attention from a threat. Mrs. Weaver used this behavior to avoid facing her anxiety over the menopause and her children's behavior.

A common method of denial may involve philosophical rationalization.

> Betty had a very explosive and violent temper. She had occasionally injured her children in moments of anger. She explained to her friends that she had learned her behavior from her mother who had an uncontrollable temper. She rationalized that her temper wasn't nearly as bad as her mother's. How could she be blamed for her behavior?

## Older Adults

Denial may become a prominent way to cope with anxiety in elderly individuals. When resources diminish, complete denial, partial denial, or distortions of reality may be more comfortable to live with than facing unpleasant reality alone. In addition, society expects the elderly to deny many sources of anxiety. For example, the elderly are expected to deny fears of death.[1] As a result, others may assume that older adults are coping well with adjustments in their lives such as aging, relocation, and losses because they are not allowed to do otherwise. Because of this, they may not receive the intervention they need.

## NURSING INTERVENTION IN DENIAL

### Primary Prevention

Primary prevention of denial involves helping the patient or family to avoid using denial in situations where it is not appropriate. Health care professionals often unwittingly encourage patients to deny. Each nurse should analyze her area of practice to determine in which instances she might be tempted to encourage denial. This is the first step in reducing this practice. Secondly, the nurse can work to prevent this problem by analyzing what reaction she would expect the patient or family to have other than denial and permitting or encouraging the patient when he behaves as expected. This will be discussed in more detail later. The following illustrates how one nurse allowed a patient to react with expected emotions.

> Mrs. Nesson was injured in a car accident and suffered lacerations to her face and scalp and broken facial bones. The nurse expected her to react to her change in body image with anxiety, depression and anger. When Mrs. Nesson began to express any of these emotions, the nurse helped her clarify her feelings and communicated that her reaction was acceptable and expected. She provided opportunities for Mrs. Nesson to express herself. Mrs. Nesson never experienced any appreciable denial.

The nurse will find it more difficult to deal with anger, depression, and guilt than with denial which is much more comfortable for both the nurse and patient.

Another aspect of the prevention of denial involves reducing the strength of any threats which may produce anxiety and therefore result in denial.[13] If high levels of anxiety are lessened or prevented, the need for the use of denial will be much less. Specific guidelines for reducing high levels of anxiety are given in the chapter on anxiety.

Children may be likely to use denial when they are unable to understand what is occurring. Therefore, careful explanations and preparation at an appropriate level are vital.

Another important way to prevent denial involves using careful timing when presenting new information to a patient or family. The family and patient who are overloaded with information may use denial to handle their anxieties. The nurse who wishes to prevent denial must constantly monitor the patient's readiness for new information and plan her actions accordingly.

> Paul was 4 when he was discovered to have diabetes mellitus. His mother was a nurse so she had some information about diabetes but she was very anxious over learning to care for Paul. The nurse teaching Paul's mother very wisely avoided overwhelming her with responsibilities and instruction. She proceeded very slowly and allowed Paul's mother to determine the pace. The nurse unobtrusively took care of the other aspects of Paul's care until the mother was ready to partially and then fully assume them.

In addition to situations where a new condition is diagnosed, other situations exist in which patients and families might easily be overloaded with information. This well might happen when a patient is put into a special unit in the hospital such as a coronary care unit, an intensive care unit, or a special care nursery. Usually it is prudent to let the questions of patients and family members guide the presentation of information.

Another common practice which may encourage denial is vagueness when giving information or answering patient's questions. Concrete, specific statements or answers leave less room for intentional misinterpretation.

This material is summarized in Table 7-1.

**Table 7-1.** Possible nursing actions to prevent denial in patients and families

1. Avoid behaviors which might encourage denial.
2. Help patient to express and understand other responses to anxiety.
3. Reduce threats which may lead to denial.
4. Present threatening information slowly.
5. Avoid vague, nonspecific statements.

## *Secondary Prevention*

Secondary prevention involves planning and carrying out the appropriate intervention for the patient or family who is already using denial.

Initially the nurse must make a careful assessment of the situation in which denial is occurring. Primarily she needs to determine if the denial is mostly harmful or mostly beneficial in this particular situation. This judgment is based on several factors. Situations in which denial is likely to be mostly harmful include:

1. When the denial is very complete.
2. When the denial has persisted for a long period of time.
3. When the denial is adversely affecting the wellness of the adult, child, or family (i.e., interfering with treatment, limiting options, harming the development of others).
4. When the patient or family are consuming large amounts of psychic energy to maintain the denial.
5. When the need to maintain denial dictates adverse alterations in life style.

The following example illustrates one type of harmful denial.

> Becky was the second child of Dr. and Mrs. Holt. Mrs. Holt soon noticed that Becky was more difficult to feed and care for than her first child. She mentioned some of her observations to her family physician during checkups but he dismissed her concerns. By the time Becky was a year old, she evidenced uncoordinated spastic movements, difficulty chewing and swallowing food, and failure to crawl. At this time the parents were told by the physician that Becky was going to be a slow child but that if they worked with her, she would someday catch up. When Becky was 2, the physician suggested enrolling her in a special day care program associated with a community mental health center. Becky was first thoroughly tested and found to be moderately retarded but the test results were not explained to the parents. After Becky had attended the school for 5 weeks, the parents became convinced that Becky was regressing in behavior, and removed her from the school. They believed that she was learning several "bad habits" from some of the children at the center. The social worker from the center visited the Holt family and tried to encourage the parents to continue Becky's enrollment in the center. At one point the social worker stated, "Because Becky is retarded, she needs to begin some experiences earlier than a normal child." Both parents became quite upset and explained to the social worker that Becky was not retarded—only a slow child.
>
> Shortly after this experience, the Holts had new neighbors who had a 1-year-old baby. At first the two women visited frequently during the mornings. The 1-year-old was more proficient at locomotion, eating, vocalizations, motor skills, and socialization than Becky. Mrs. Holt soon stopped visiting the neighbor and returned to work leaving Becky with a housekeeper. Becky is now 4½. The Holts have become more and more withdrawn from their church and neighborhood activities. Becky is seldom taken out in public. Becky's older sister who is 7½ is a bright but lonely second grader. Both parents pour themselves into their professional activities and devote large amounts of time to writing, travel, and research. The mother expects to enroll Becky in a private kindergarten for the next fall although Becky walks only by holding onto objects, must be fed, is not toilet trained, does not make recognizable vocalizations, and spends most of her time in repetitive self-stimulating activities.

Situations in which denial is likely to be beneficial include:

1. Immediately after a major potentially anxiety producing event.
2. When the denial appears to be temporary.
3. When the aspects of the situation being denied are minimal.
4. When the denial is not resulting in lowered wellness.
5. When the denial allows the individuals involved to function more optimally because some unpleasant reality which probably cannot be changed can be ignored.
6. When there are not any other means available at the time for the individuals involved to cope with the anxiety.

While it may be tempting to think of harmful denial as chronic and beneficial denial as temporary, this is not always the crucial difference. The following case history represents a situation in which beneficial denial has lasted for several years.

> John and Anita had been married 5 years when they faced the fact that Anita hadn't become pregnant despite the discontinuance of birth control measures. They both were from large families and desired to have several children. After 2 months of indecision they decided to contact adoption agencies about adoption. After all, they said, there really were a lot of children who needed good homes. Their brothers and sisters had all had too many biological children anyway. They said they were very unconcerned about not having biological children and agreed that they probably could have conceived if they had wanted to go through with the expensive testing and treatment. Eighteen months after applying for adoption, a beautiful 4-day-old boy was placed in their home. They attended discussion groups at the adoption agency and read suggested materials on rearing adopted children. Two years later they received a daughter and they are now awaiting a third child. The parents and the children are thriving although the parents have never admitted that they are infertile.

It should be pointed out that differentiating harmful from beneficial denial is not always easily done. It may be useful to ascertain the opinions of several individuals who have assessed the patient or family if one is unsure. There are many situations in which the denial which is present has some beneficial and some harmful aspects. One must then weigh which aspects are more important.

If the nurse decides that the patient or family's denial is beneficial, she can allow the denial to continue but she should not participate in the denial or encourage denials.[5] The nurse would be participating in the denial if she engaged in denial behavior initiated by the patient and family. An example of this would be saying to a patient, "You must be right. The physician has made a mistake in your diagnosis" or "I agree with you. Your son must be innocent." The nurse would be encouraging denial if she initiates attempts at denial for the patient such as, "Why don't you go home and forget all about this. Maybe it's a big mistake" or "If I were you I wouldn't pay any attention to that." Another way to encourage denial is to cover up information or distort it so that reality is hidden from the patient or family. She might do this by hiding signs of deterioration of the patient's condition, for example. Other actions which might encourage denial include excessively promoting diversional activities.[5] Or the nurse might give false reassurance such as, "You'll get over this in no time."

Encouraging or participating in the patient's denial has several disadvantages. First, the patient or family member might be moving towards facing reality and the nurse's behavior might retard his progress. Secondly, when the patient is beginning to become aware of his denial, he may turn away from the nurse because he senses that she cannot help him.

In addition to avoiding participating in or encouraging denial, the nurse working with the patient whose denial is beneficial refrains from pointing out reality.[5] This would reduce the effectiveness of his denial as a way of coping with anxiety. She allows him to develop awareness at his own pace.

What can the nurse do to accept the patient's use of denial without furthering it? She can listen to and reflect the patient's thoughts and feelings accurately without adding to them: "You feel that your husband will come back to you." "You hope that the physician is wrong."

## HELPING PATIENTS AND FAMILIES FACE REALITY

For the patient or family whose denial is not beneficial, the nurse will want to help the patient face reality. This must be done slowly and only after the nurse understands the purpose the patient's behavior is serving. One of the primary methods the nurse uses is her presence. The fact that she is involved with the patient indicates that he has a need for help which she recognizes. Thus, she represents reality to the patient.[13] She never loses sight of the reality which the patient is not ready to accept.[5] The patient or family intuitively knows that she can be trusted to handle those aspects of the situation which they are ignoring. The nurse represents reality in addition because she does not participate in or encourage further the patient's use of denial.

> Mr. and Mrs. Johnson were told by their family physician that their 3-year-old son seemed to have a marked hearing loss. They were told that they should have his hearing evaluated more thoroughly and take any necessary steps to begin special education for him. The parents reacted with disbelief. They were sure that he could hear well but just didn't pay attention. They thought that he had a cold which interfered with his hearing test. The office nurse began weekly home visits to the Johnson family. She planned her visits to serve as gentle reminders of reality. She obtained information about sources of further speech and hearing evaluation and provided the information to the parents after a period of time. They eventually were able to follow through with the testing.

With the patient or family whose denial is more harmful, she may wish to do more than be present and reflect their feelings. She may make carefully chosen statements which represent reality.[13] These could be called "reality reminders" because they remind the patient or family of reality which they should already know but are trying to overlook. They do not present any new information which the patient or family are unaware of. Thus, she refrains from direct attacks on the denial.[13] Reality reminders are illustrated in these examples.

> Ms. Joyce:  Mother seems so much better today. She squeezed my hand.
> Nurse:      (Aware that the patient is getting worse) Your mother is very ill.
>
> Mr. Roberts: The police are driving us crazy. They seem to think we are covering up for our son. Why do they pick on him so?.
> Nurse:      Your son has been implicated in a serious crime.
>
> Mr. Davis:  My daughter will take care of me now. She won't let anything happen to her old dad.
> Nurse:      Your daughter has considerable responsibilities of her own.

Reality reminders must be used carefully and only when appropriate because an attempt at forcing awareness of reality may make the patient or family retreat into stronger efforts at denial. An appropriate reality reminder accepts the patient's denial, does not encourage or participate in the denial, and reminds the patient of a known reality.

As the patient and family begin to develop more awareness of the reality of the situation, it will be manifested very slowly. A reality that is faced on one day may be denied on the next. This may be perplexing to the nurse. She should focus on any association with reality when it occurs.[13] She must accept that the patient may return to denial later, however. As the patient begins to reduce his use of denial, he will experience more anxiety which may present as anger, depression, frustration, shame, guilt, and disappointment.[5,30] Although these emotions are challenging, the nurse should recognize these as signs of progress and encourage and facilitate them. This means communicating to the patient that his emotions are acceptable and understandable.[16] She should help him clarify them through her use of appropriate nondirective communication skills.[5] To stifle the expression of these emotions might encourage more denial. The nurse must remember that awareness is not synonymous with acceptance. If acceptance occurs, it will be much later.

In children, the stage of developing awareness is likely to be particularly tumultuous. The child may be demanding, irritable, emotionally labile, insultive, and generally obnoxious. The parents may be puzzled and attempt to control the child's angry outbursts through punishment. The nurse should explain the child's behavior to them as a sign of growing awareness. Play therapy may help the child express his anger and frustration at this time.[18]

Helping the patient to develop awareness carefully will reduce his use of denial. The nurse in many cases can time the presentation of more reality to the patient. The patient who finally has the courage to look at his new colostomy stoma is probably facing enough reality at that time. He will not be ready to learn about performing his irrigations until later. He will learn about alterations in his life style which may be necessary still later. To present him with all this at the first might be overwhelming and force more denial. The sensitive nurse lets the patient's questions guide her in presenting new elements of reality. This means that she must create an environment where the patient feels free to ask questions. She may have to tolerate the fact that the patient may reach the wrong conclusions initially before he asks for the truth.[10]

Many patients with physical conditions may be developing beginning awareness of a situation at a time when they are experiencing considerable pain or discomfort. Increasing awareness may occur because an increase in painful symptoms may make it more difficult to continue denying a situation. Proper nursing care measures and possibly the administration of analgesic medications may control pain and discomfort and help the patient develop awareness. Too little or inappropriately administered medication may aggravate the patient's problems as he copes with his pain and with his painful awareness of his situation simultaneously. Too much medication may retard the patient's development of awareness if he is excessively sedated.

During this time, the nurse should attempt to reduce the strength of the anxiety producing threat if possible. Reducing the patient's anxiety level will reduce his need to cope through denial and facilitate awareness.

> Mr. Bennett was experiencing frequent bouts of respiratory difficulties. His family physician told him he was developing emphysema and that he should stop smoking cigarettes. Mr. Bennett scoffed at the idea and claimed to know many people who had lived to be very old who smoked heavily and a like number of individuals who never smoked and who died young. Mr. Bennett's wife, who was always pushing him to quit smoking, increased her efforts. She used a scare tactic primarily. Mr. Bennett began smoking heavily at work. The industrial nurse persuaded Mrs. Bennett to reduce her scare campaign and Mr. Bennett's smoking reached a lower level. Mr. Bennett later joined the industrial nurse's group at work formed to help smokers quit although he requested that his wife not know.

It should be pointed out that the patient may require less intervention by the nurse than does the family.[13] By being removed from the situation, the family's awareness of the situation is often slower at developing. Parents especially are prone to use denial in coping with illnesses of their children because they are so very threatened and feel such guilt when their children are ill. The persistent denial of family members is usually very harmful to the patient. The nurse can plan specific contacts with parents and family members to help them develop awareness as she facilitates their expression of feelings.

Possible nursing actions to use with patients or families who are denying are summarized in Table 7-2.

## Tertiary Prevention

There are some patients and families whose use of denial is interfering with most important aspects of their lives and has become persistent. In these situations some direct attack on

**Table 7-2.** Possible nursing actions when patients or families are using denial

1. Assess to determine if denial is helpful or unhelpful.
2. If helpful:
   a. Allow denial to continue but do not encourage or participate in denial.
   b. Allow individual to approach reality on his own.
3. If unhelpful:
   a. Represent reality with presence.
   b. Use reality reminders.
   c. Be prepared to deal with responses as awareness increases.
   d. Present reality as individual asks for it.
   e. Control pain or discomfort.
   f. Reduce threats leading to anxiety and denial.
   g. Remember that the family may need intervention.

the denial may be warranted. Tertiary prevention of prolonged disruptive denial is not to be undertaken lightly but only when the situation is serious.

A technique to deal with massive denial has been identified.[14] The patient may be using evasive techniques to avoid facing reality. He may change the subject, withdraw, or generalize when the sensitive area is being approached. The nurse does not solve the patient's massive denial by giving him her version of the truth and exposing his denial. This approach is probably fruitless. Instead, she uses a communication pattern which demands specifics and she returns to subjects which were side-stepped by the patient or family. This focusing is reduced whenever the patient's anxiety level begins to interfere. In this approach, the nurse reminds the patient of conclusions he reached earlier to avoid his possible tendency to forget what he wants to later deny. For more information and an example of this process, the interested nurse should consult the article on denial by King.[14]

## A TOOL FOR ASSESSMENT AND EVALUATION

The tool in Table 7-3 can be used to assess a patient or family member's use of denial. Those whose behaviors predominantly appear to be "less optimal" should be considered at high risk.

The tool can also be used to evaluate the effectiveness of the nurse's interventions. The patient or family member should move from less optimal behaviors to predominantly more optimal behaviors.

## THE NURSE AND DENIAL

Nurses can use denial as a way of coping with unpleasant situations as readily as patients and families. One frequent pattern involves intellectualization. This may enable her to handle the anxiety caused by exposure to illness and suffering.

Nancy was a community health nurse. She could have identified very closely with one family she visited. The wife was a nurse about her age with young children the same ages as Nancy's own children. The husband in the family was an excellent accountant but also an alcoholic. Several attempts to stop the husband's drinking had failed. The wife was quite worried and the harmful effects on the family were becoming more obvious. Nancy told a coworker that she didn't really feel sorry at all for the wife because she had read that the wife of an alcoholic usually promoted her husband's drinking.

**Table 7-3.** Assessment and evaluation of denial

| Behavior | Less optimal | More optimal |
|---|---|---|
| Recognition of illness | Minimizes illness. Displaces concern to others "My wife thinks . . ." | Accurate assessment of illness—cause, nature, type |
| Focus of conversation | Avoids discussing denied areas, uses generalities, vagueness | Can discuss specifics |
| Degree of denial | Frank denial of long duration | Temporary partial denial |
| Reaction to unexpected threat | Unconcerned, unemotional | Appropriate to background and experience |
| Focus of attention | Dwells on the past, avoids future | Anticipates the future |
| Responses to care | Misses appointments, misunderstands, no questions, dismisses medical orders, etc. | Seeks information, follows medical orders, questions |
| Realism | Attributes serious symptoms to minor problems | Seeks to understand symptoms and condition |
| Relations with others | May withdraw | Unchanged |
| Mood | Inappropriate to circumstances, exaggerated cheerfulness or unemotional and analytical | Appropriate |
| Acceptance of limitations | Compulsive overactivity, denies limits | Realistic acceptance |
| Reaction to offers of help | Avoids offers of help | Uses assistance[8,10,13,19,23] |

Thus denial can be a way to avoid one's feelings of helplessness and frustration.[13] Questions the nurse can ask herself to possibly discover her use of denial with patients and families are:

1. How would I personally feel if I were the patient or family in this situation?
2. Can I allow myself to feel within safe limits the anxiety the patient might feel?
3. Have I blamed the patient or family for their problem so that I need not feel any concern for them?

In addition, health care workers may encourage patients and families in the use of denial as previously mentioned. If the patient and family avoid reality, the nurse will not have to face their anxiety with them. There are numerous accounts in the literature of common practices which encourage denial. Pregnant unwed teenage girls may be encouraged to disguise their pregnancies as much as possible, seek anonymity, give up the babies, and return to life as if nothing had happened.[2] With the birth of a stillborn infant the mother is likely to be put to sleep so she will not see the birth, the baby's body is secreted away, and the mother is placed away from other maternity patients so she will be spared from the sounds of baby cries. Recent attention is focusing on the need for the mother to see the baby and to be aware of her loss so that denial does not occur.[29] The mother who gives birth to a deformed baby may find her baby isolated from others and out of direct sight in the nursery. The staff may take her baby out last and return it first. In fact, the staff tends to withhold the baby from the mother.[27] Patients and families facing death are often surrounded by staff who may maintain a pretense of normalcy.[9]

Although only a few examples have been mentioned, the encouragement for patients and families in the use of denial by health care professionals is believed to be common. The use of denial is understandable in that it spares the nurse from facing the reality of the situation with the patient and family. But denial can also unfortunately encourage the patient and family to persist in denial behavior and limit drastically the supportive value of the nurse to the patient and family when they are ready to face reality. In fact, the patient and family may be placed in a situation where they feel they must maintain the charade to protect the nurse who cannot face the situation. The nurse might reflect on the following questions:

1. Am I avoiding reality under the pretense of sparing the patient or family?
2. Am I stifling the patient's expression of expected emotions?
3. Am I rewarding the patient or family for denial and refusing to let them face reality?

On the other hand, there are situations in which the use of denial by a patient or family is very frustrating to the nurse. She may believe she should force them to face reality. The harder she pushes for facing reality, the stronger becomes the denial of the family and patient.[14]

Connie was a 9-year-old girl with hyperactivity. Although she was on medications, her behavior at school was almost uncontrollable. Her parents set few limits at home and rejected her subtly. The school nurse was asked to work with the parents. The parents denied that Connie was ever a problem at home. Actually, they ignored her behavior at home. They felt that her school problems related to the fact that she was intellectually ahead of her class and generally bored with school. The school nurse tried to force the parents to realize that their daughter had numerous problems but the more she reported on Connie's behavior, the more the parents denied the seriousness of the behavior and defended her behavior as caused by others. The school nurse became increasingly frustrated and perplexed.

The nurse who works with patients or families who use denial is sometimes annoyed and may feel antagonism.[14] The following questions are suggested to help the nurse evaluate her tolerance of denial.

1. Do I see the patient's or family's denial as a way to cope with a situation they cannot yet face?
2. Am I presenting reality to the family gradually to avoid increasing their denial?
3. Am I planning my intervention to meet their needs or mine?

Health care professionals are likely to use denial in their personal lives in response to threats to their self-concepts. This often takes the form of intellectualization.

Angie, a nursing instructor, was diagnosed as having advanced renal disease. She expressed little emotion about her condition but studied diligently the medical aspects of renal disease and transplantation. When someone asked her how she was feeling, she replied with information on her BUN and creatinine.

It is very difficult to evaluate when one is using denial related to one's own responses to anxiety but the following questions may help the nurse to determine if she is using denial to cope with a personal threat.

1. Have I allowed myself to experience my true feelings about this situation?
2. What would be the worst possible reality related to this situation? Have I admitted to myself that this is possible?
3. If I were trying to avoid facing an unpleasant aspect of this situation, what would it be? Is it possible?

Another important way to protect against the use of denial is for the nurse to talk about stressful situations to others who listen well.[4] This enables the nurse to reduce her anxiety level and she may then gain awareness of situations she has been denying.

# AN EXAMPLE OF NURSING INTERVENTION IN DENIAL

The following example shows how a nurse helped a patient and his family lessen their use of denial and develop a more reality based perception of the situation.

A. J. Harris was eight years old when he was admitted to the hospital for corrective open heart surgery. A. J. had been hospitalized two times in the past for diagnostic procedures and palliative surgery. His last admission had been when he was five years old.

The nurse who was assigned as A. J.'s primary nurse had as a high priority assessing A. J.'s and his parents' needs for preparation for surgery and the postoperative period. In talking with the parents, she was amazed at their behavior. Most parents at this stage were anxious, full of questions, and hyperactive. A. J.'s parents were expecting this experience to be essentially the same as the other hospitalizations. They seemed to feel that there was little reason for concern and the mother kept repeating, "There's nothing to worry about." They did not ask any questions at any time during the initial interview. Later, the nurse realized that they never talked specifically about the surgery.

A. J. seemed disinterested in discussing his surgery at all. He denied any knowledge of what specifically was wrong with his heart or how it was to be fixed. He also asked no questions and busied himself with the TV. When the nurse mentioned that she was going to start talking with him about surgery that afternoon, he looked up alertly but then said he probably would be gone to x-ray or somewhere else.

The nurse felt that Mr. and Mrs. Harris were using some degree of denial to cope with the threat of their son's surgery. She believed A. J. to be trying hard to pretend nothing unusual was going on either. This was behavior she had seen occasionally in young school-aged children who thought they must be brave and who tended to deny interest in their care in the hopes that if they pretended nothing was happening, maybe nothing would. The nurse came to the following conclusions:

1. A. J.'s previous experiences at younger than 5 years of age do not guarantee that he is prepared for this experience.
2. A. J.'s surgical experience would probably be less traumatic if he understood what was happening, why, and how he could help.
3. Mr. and Mrs. Harris and A. J. are not asking questions about the approaching surgery which makes teaching more difficult.
4. It is unlikely that the parents are adequately prepared for what is ahead..
5. A. J.'s surgery is two days away. Mr. and Mrs. Harris are from out of town but staying near the hospital and planning to spend most of their time with A. J.
6. A. J. would be expected to look to his parents for support during the trying times ahead and Mr. and Mrs. Harris are unlikely to be supportive of A. J. if their present denial continues.

After considering this assessment of the situation, the nurse decided that an attempt should be made to increase the Harris' and A. J.'s grasp of reality because their use of partial denial was likely to become an ineffective way to handle anxiety as the time of surgery drew near. After considerable reflection and evaluating alternatives, the nurse decided on the following approach: She would proceed with a teaching plan for A. J. and his parents. She would modify her approach because of the denial present.

Normally, the nurse would have taught the parents and the child together but she believed that in this situation, she might be more effective if she worked with the parents and A.J. separately. She believed that the parents might be evidencing some pretense of normalcy out of the erroneous assumption that this would help A.J. If she talked with them separately, they might feel more free to express their own anxieties without fear of upsetting A.J. Similarly, she thought that A.J. may have sensed that his parents could not deal with the upcoming surgical experience and adopted their approach. If the nurse talked with him separately, he might feel more free to reveal his own anxieties without the need to pretend to be their brave son.

Second, the nurse decided to present her usual teaching plan backwards. She would therefore be talking about home care after discharge first, the postoperative period on the pediatric unit second, the stay in the intensive care unit third and so forth. She believed that this reverse order would allow her to begin teaching about an area where there would possibly be the least anxiety and therefore the least need for denial. Then she could talk about progressively more threatening areas while assessing the parents' and A.J.'s readiness carefully. If she were to teach in her usual order, she might not be able to get very far before the parents and A.J. became overwhelmed. The reverse order might allow the parents and A.J. to ask questions and focus on details with less anxiety associated. In essence, then, she was working from an area where there was little denial—A.J.'s homecoming—to areas where there was more denial.

Third, the nurse tried to increasingly use reality reminders as much as possible without unduly increasing everyone's anxiety. A.J. and his parents realized there was to be surgery but they were trying to ignore the fact as much as possible. She planned to gently remind them with references such as "After A.J.'s surgery is over and he goes home . . ." and "As you rest after your surgery . . ."

Fourth, the nurse planned to organize her teaching to provide as many opportunities for A.J. and his parents to concurrently release anxiety as possible. For example, she carried out her first session with A.J. while playing with him. Her first session with the parents was held during a walk she took with them during A.J.'s afternoon quiet time. She made her plan as informal as possible because they might be made more anxious by a formalized plan of instruction. Therefore, she used no notes, and rather discussed information with them much as in a friendly conversation.

Last, the nurse anticipated that A.J. and his parents might react somewhat differently from other parents and patients. She expected that they would ask fewer questions, seem less interested, and change the subject more often. From her experience with children A.J.'s age, she expected that he would listen intently while appearing not to. This knowledge plus the method of presentation during activities would mean that she would have less time than usual and would have to use the time available to the utmost. She selected content to teach which was important, general, and concise. She eliminated details and specifics usually taught. She realized that she would need to carry out her teaching with less feedback and less direction from the Harrises than she was accustomed to.

The nurse proceeded as she had planned. As she carried out her informal teaching sessions, Mrs. Harris became quite anxious but she was able to ask questions and focus on the situation ahead. The nurse found out that Mrs. Harris coped with anxiety by talking to others and the nurse not only spent extra time with her but arranged for other nurses to listen to her during the other shifts. Mr. Harris continued to dismiss any concerns about the surgery. He did listen closely to the nurse, however. Since Mrs. Harris would probably be able to support A.J., she elected to allow Mr. Harris to continue his avoidance of reality. When the nurse talked with A.J. he listened and could ask occasional questions but could not tolerate hearing any specific information about the surgery as related to his body. The nurse had to be very general and vague about that particular part.

After surgery, Mrs. Harris was obviously very relieved and much less anxious. She worked well with A.J. and was especially helpful when treatments which were uncomfortable had to be done. Mr. Harris remained distant and at times was very impatient with A.J.'s behavior which was entirely normal regressive behavior after such an immense threat.

The nurse concluded that she had been successful in reducing the use of denial by Mrs. Harris and partially so with A.J. but her approach had not worked with Mr. Harris. Given the time limitations she had worked in, she felt that she had enabled A.J. and his mother to function more optimally in a high risk situation than if she had not intervened to reduce their anxiety and lessen their use of denial.

## SUMMARY

Denial is an expected and common response to a major threat which occurs throughout the life cycle. It is a form of self-deception. Although denial is initially protective to the individual, it may become harmful if it interferes with optimal functioning. Denial can be complete, partial, or represented as distortions of reality. It is assessed primarily by noting the absence of an expected response to a threat. The nurse can intervene to prevent or reduce denial and aid developing awareness. The nurse, like all individuals, uses denial in her personal and professional life and she may be able to recognize and reduce her denial behavior.

## REFERENCES

1. Aguilera, D. C., and Messick, J. M.: *Crisis Intervention: Theory and Methodology*. C. V. Mosby, St. Louis, 1978.
2. Bernstein, R.: "Are we still sterotyping the unmarried mother?" in Parad, H. J. (ed.): *Crisis Intervention: Selected Readings*. Family Service Association of America, New York, 1965.
3. Bowlby, J.: "Childhood mourning and its implications for psychiatry." Am. J. Psychiat. 118:481, 1961.
4. Brunner, L. S., and Suddarth, D. S.: *Textbook of Medical-Surgical Nursing*. J. B. Lippincott, Philadelphia, 1975.
5. Crate, M. A.: "Nursing functions in adaptation to chronic illness." Am. J. Nurs. 65:72, 1965.
6. Engel, G. L.: "Grief and grieving." Am. J. Nurs. 64:93, 1964.
7. Francis, G. M., and Munjas, B.: *Promoting Psychological Comfort*. Wm. C Brown, Dubuque, 1975.
8. Freedman, A. M., Kaplan, H. I., and Sadock, B. J.: *Modern Synopsis of Comprehensive Textbook of Psychiatry/II*. Williams and Wilkins, Baltimore, 1976.
9. Glaser, B. G., and Strauss, A. L.: *Awareness of Dying*. Aldine, Chicago, 1965.
10. Hershberger, R. W.: "Nick; A sixteen-year-old new paraplegic," in Kalafatich, A. J. (ed.): *Approaches to the Care of Adolescents*. Appleton-Century-Crofts, New York, 1975.
11. Kalkman, M. E., and Davis, A. J. (eds.): *New Dimensions in Mental Health-Psychiatric Nursing*. McGraw-Hill, New York, 1974.
12. Kaplan, D. M., and Mason, E. A.: "Maternal reaction to premature birth viewed as an emotional disorder," in Parad, H. J. (ed.): *Crisis Intervention: Selected Readings*. Family Service Association of America, New York, 1965.
13. Kiening, Sr. M. M.: "Denial of illness," in Carlson, C. E., and Blackwell, B. (eds.): *Behavioral Concepts and Nursing Intervention*. J. B. Lippincott, Philadelphia, 1978.
14. King, J. M.: "Denial." Am. J. Nurs. 66:1010, 1966.
15. Kubler-Ross, E.: *On Death and Dying*. Macmillan, New York, 1969.
16. Lepler, M.: "Having a handicapped child." Matern. Child Nurs. J. 3:32, 1978.
17. Morgan, W. L., and Engel, G. L.: *The Clinical Approach to the Patient*. W. B. Saunders, Philadelphia, 1969.

18. Nahigian, E. G.: "Effects of illness on the preschooler," in Scipien, G. M., et al.: *Comprehensive Pediatric Nursing.* McGraw-Hill, New York, 1975.
19. Neu, C.: "Coping with newly diagnosed blindness." Am. J. Nurs. 75:2161, 1975.
20. Peterson, M. H.: "Understanding defense mechanisms—a programmed instruction unit." Am. J. Nurs. 72:1651, 1972.
21. Petrillo, M.: "Preventing hospital trauma in pediatric patients." Am. J. Nurs. 68:1469, 1968.
22. Pothier, P. C.: *Mental Health Counseling With Children.* Little, Brown and Company, Boston, 1976.
23. Redman, B. K.: *The Process of Patient Teaching in Nursing.* C. V. Mosby, St. Louis, 1976.
24. Schroeder, E.: "The birth of a defective child; A cause for grieving," in Hall, J. E., and Weaver, B. R. (eds.): *Nursing of Families in Crisis.* J. B. Lippincott, Philadelphia, 1974.
25. Schwartz, L. A., and Soloman, P.: "Psychoanalysis," in Soloman, P., and Patch, V. D. (eds.): *Handbook of Psychiatry.* Lange Medical Publications, Los Altos, Calif., 1971.
26. Tudor, M. J.: "Family habilitation: A child with a birth defect," in Hymovich, D. P., and Barnard, M. U. (eds.): *Family Health Care.* McGraw-Hill, New York, 1973.
27. VonSchilling, K. C.: "The birth of a defective child." Nurs. Forum 7:424, 1968.
28. Waechter, E. H., and Blake, F. G.: *Nursing Care of Children.* J. B. Lippincott, Philadelphia, 1976.
29. Zahourek, R., and Jensen, J. S.: "Grieving and the loss of the newborn." Am. J. Nurs. 73:836, 1973.
30. Zelle, R. S.: "The family with a mentally retarded child," in Hymovich, D. P., and Barnard, M. U. (eds.): *Family Health Care.* McGraw-Hill, New York, 1973.

## BIBLIOGRAPHY

Bascom, L.: "Women who refuse to believe: Persistent denial of pregnancy." Matern. Child Nurs. J. 2:174, 1977.
Gruber, K. A., and Schniewind, H. E.: "Letting anger work for you." Am. J. Nurs. 76:1450, 1976.
Weinstein, E. A., and Kahn, R. L.: *Denial of Illness.* Charles C Thomas, Springfield, Ill., 1955.

# CHAPTER 8

# ANGER

Anger is usually not considered a pleasant subject. Expressions of anger are, in most situations, considered distasteful or inappropriate. At the same time, it is assumed that anger is a natural, expected, and very common reaction to many situations which may confront a patient or his family in relation to health care and changes in health status. The stage is set for a difficult situation. Should the patient and family members express their anger, they may alienate others and embarrass themselves. Should they repress or internalize their anger, other equally troublesome problems may ensue. The nurse who understands the concept of anger, why it occurs, how it is expressed, and what to do about it can be of significant help to patients and families who are angry.

Nurses, too, get angry in their personal and professional lives whether or not they recognize it. The nurse needs to recognize anger she is feeling, learn ways to use it constructively, and learn to cope with anger projected towards her.

## REVIEW OF THEORY

Anger can be defined as a physical and emotional state in which an individual experiences a sense of power which compensates for an underlying sense of anxiety. There are other terms used to define states similar to anxiety such as aggression, rage, hostility, hate, and resentment. Numerous opinions exist on how to define anger and these related concepts and many pages could be devoted to definitively differentiating them. For the purposes of this discussion, they will be all considered as variations of anger. In simplified terms, *hostility* is usually considered to involve a desire to harm oneself or others.[17] *Aggression* is often used to describe actions which express anger or its related emotions. *Resentment* carries the implication that the person towards whom it is felt should experience guilt.[6,14,17] *Hate* can be thought of as prolonged anger, and *rage* as intense but short lived anger.

### The Anatomy of Anger

The following operational definition is offered to illustrate how anger may occur. It is a simplified version of several definitions found in the literature.

1. A situation exists in which one experiences a threat to security, self-respect, or a failure to reach a desired goal.
2. Helplessness is perceived which leads to unconscious anxiety.
3. Anxiety is converted unconsciously into a feeling of power.
4. Relief from anxiety is felt.[6,11,14,17]

Anger is believed to be one of several ways an individual can cope with the experience of anxiety. For many people, anger is a more comfortable emotional state than the state of anxiety.[6] It may also be more tolerable than feeling helpless and depressed.

One's ability to express anger is somewhat dependent on how one was taught to react as a child. Consider the two following incidents which illustrate how parents commonly respond to the expression of joy versus the expression of anger by a young child.

> Two-year-old Bobby is playing with a new toy his father has brought home. He giggles and beams with joy. His parents feel pleased, smile, and provide comments and attention which indicate their pleasure in his reaction.

> Two-year-old Jimmy is playing with a new toy his father has brought home. He is unable to make the toy perform as he desires. He bangs it on the floor, kicks his feet, and loudly cries in disappointment. His parents look disapproving and annoyed. They attempt to subdue his behavior by taking the toy away, withdrawing from him, and verbally admonishing him.

Some parents may attempt to deny or punish almost all expressions of anger. Others may allow anger in certain situations but not others. For example, a child may be permitted to express anger against people outside the family but required to suppress anger against any family member. It is likely that boys are permitted a wider degree of expression than girls. Many women will testify that their brothers were allowed to slam doors, kick the dog, and yell at playmates while they were not. This acceptance of anger more readily in males than females remains true for adult men and women.[1] In general, most individuals grow up repressing to some degree expressions of anger and feeling some degree of guilt if they do have angry thoughts or engage in aggressive actions. This leads many individuals to use considerable psychic energy to hide from themselves and others any trace of anger and results in a wide range of behaviors through which anger is expressed.

Because of the ways anger is expressed, it is often recognized as being one of the prime motivators of human behavior. In other words, much of what one does in the course of a normal day may be determined by the unconscious expression of anger.

> Ms. Lilly was angry with her husband because of a fight over money they had the previous evening. Although she was unaware of her intentions, she overslept, burnt the toast, and boiled the coffee as a form of retaliation. At work, she became very upset over not being able to locate a missing document a secretary had misfiled. She scolded her severely and then felt guilty. She skipped her lunch because she was too upset to eat. By midafternoon she was hungry and snacked on candy bars and a soft drink in spite of a low calorie diet she was trying to follow.
>
> As she drove home from work, she realized that she had forgotten to remove any meat for dinner from her freezer before leaving home in the morning so she stopped at a grocery store to pick up some hamburger and milk. She ran into an acquaintance in the grocery store who asked her to serve on a neighborhood committee related to establishing an art center. She really wasn't interested in the project but since she was tired, hungry, in a hurry, and still feeling traces of guilt about her day, she agreed just to get away.
>
> When she arrived home, she found her daughter waiting. She was supposed to be at a soccer game in 15 minutes but had forgotten to tell her previously. They jumped in the car and drove to the game with Ms. Lilly lecturing her daughter on her character flaws all the way. She watched the game in stoney silence not enjoying it at all. She was very hungry having had only the candy bars and soft drink since breakfast.
>
> After the game, partially due to her guilt over yelling at her daughter, she stopped at her daughter's favorite fast food restaurant and bought hamburgers and french fries to take home for supper although she knew they didn't need the calories or the cholesterol.

When she arrived home her husband innocently asked why she had left her milk and hamburger sitting on the counter top instead of putting it in the refrigerator. She angrily yelled at him and another fight ensued.

## The Manifestations of Anger

It is hypothesized that anger can be handled by the individual in a wide variety of ways. Some ways of expressing anger are outward, inward, through escape or withdrawal, and through learning.

## OUTWARD EXPRESSIONS

### Direct Outward Expression

Some outward expressions of anger may be directly aimed at the object causing the threat or blocking one's goal.[28] This is referred to as direct expression and may be physical, verbal, or nonverbal. Young children often quite naturally engage in physical attack when angry. Adults may engage in physical attack against certain objects but not against persons with whom they are more likely to use verbal attack. For example, it would not be unusual to see a secretary kick the door on a storage cabinet which will not open but less likely to see him kick his boss when she returns a letter to be retyped.

Verbal attack is highly influenced by culturally defined norms. A mother may verbally scold her child who spills a drop of his beverage on her new carpet but she may go out of her way to be comforting to her neighbor who spills a whole cup of coffee on the same carpet. The angry individual often appears flushed, anxious, tensed, and alert. He may appear physically ready to attack although he does not.

Direct nonverbal expressions of anger include glares, piercing stares, and "hateful" looks. Children (and less often adults) may stick out their tongues and thumb their noses.

Direct expression of anger in general is probably less frequent among adults than the forms which follow.

### Displaced Outward Expression

Outward anger may be expressed in a manner which is displaced. An object resembling the actual object of anger may be chosen for physical or verbal attack. The man who is angry at his physician may yell at the nurse who represents the physician. Often the object chosen for displacement of anger does not closely resemble the actual object but is instead a "safe" object on which to displace anger. Thus the man who cannot talk back to his boss may come home and displace his anger on his wife. The wife who cannot talk back to her husband may then scream at her son. The son who is afraid to express his anger to his mother may go hit his younger sister, and so on.

It should be pointed out that the individual involved in outwardly expressing displaced anger is most likely not aware that he is angry or of how he is displacing his anger.

Women and especially children are often "safe" objects on which to express anger because they usually do not have much authority or show much capacity to retaliate against the one who is angry. Inanimate objects are also safe objects on which to vent anger. Physical indirect expression of anger may involve slamming doors, kicking objects, throwing things, walking, or taking out one's frustrations on tennis balls or on the piano. Many individuals engage in these kinds of indirect physical expression of anger with partial awareness of their usefulness. It is not uncommon to hear someone say, "When I get mad I clean the house from top to bottom and I feel better." Children who are hyperactive or who engage in aggressive physical play activities may be expressing anger in this manner.[26]

## Indirect Outward Expression

Outwardly expressed anger may be shown in a manner that is indirect. In this mode of expression, the person involved does not directly attack an object but expresses anger by other less obvious behavior. For example, a child who is angry at his mother may continually wet his bed at night. A nurse who is angry at a physician may neglect to inform him of a change in his patient's health status or she might misplace his patient's chart. A patient who is angry at a physician may forget to take his medications, come late, or miss appointments.

Forms of verbal expression of indirect anger include gossiping, fault finding, and sarcasm. One who expresses anger in these forms may be thought of as quite witty by his friends. One who can poke fun at, laugh at, or expose faults in others feels some psychological power over them. There is a strong undercurrent of bitterness and jealousy in such remarks.

Again, indirect expressions of anger are almost always beneath the awareness of the individual involved. Indirect expressions of anger can be identified by the fact that they are designed to make the object of the anger irritated or annoyed. They often involve an element of obstruction.[5] They are often very subtle and difficult to pinpoint.

## INWARD EXPRESSIONS

Inward expressions of anger involve several methods. One common method is *depression* which is often defined as anger turned against the self. To be depressed is probably more accepted by society than being outwardly angry. Parents may strengthen the child's tendency to favor depression by shaming the child who displays angry actions and intentions. His guilt and shame may lead to depression which his parents more readily accept. Thus in the future, the presence of unconscious angry feelings automatically may result in depression. An extreme amount of anger against the self can culminate in suicidal behavior. Another chapter in this section focuses on depression.

Another way to control anger inwardly may involve *somatization*. A number of disease conditions have been reported as being related to anger such as rheumatoid arthritis, asthma, angina pectoris, peptic ulcer disease, migraine headache, chronic backache, and hypertension. The factual basis for this is nebulous at best but interesting to speculate about. Does anger lead to these conditions or does having one of these conditions tend to make one angry?

Another form of inward expression is *disowning*. In this phenomenon, the individual does not recognize that he is angry but instead behaves almost exactly the opposite of what one might expect. He may be overly polite, exceptionally kind, and engage in conversation which is "sugar coated." [11,14,17]

> The children in the family next door to Ms. Martin teased her dog, tore up her yard, messed up her garage, tromped on her flowers, and left toys strewn all over. Ms. Martin reacted by smiling sweetly at them. When their mother asked Ms. Martin if the children were ever a nuisance she talked at length using exaggerated terms about how wonderful it was to see them play and how much they reminded her of her own sweet children now grown and far away.

Patients may disown anger and unendingly and gratefully praise those who care for them. The nurse may "kill with kindness" demanding and obstinate patients. [11,14] This reaction probably occurs when the individual involved is very fearful of expressing anger. The key to identifying this response lies in recognizing the individual who is "turning the other cheek" when he has every right to be angry. [14] Again parents often unwittingly teach disowning.

> Julie and Jane were sisters. Jane worked carefully and consistently on her summer 4-H dress. Julie procrastinated until shortly before the judging contest. Mother finally helped Julie finish most of her dress in the nick of time. When Julie won a blue ribbon and Jane only a red, Jane was very angry with her sister and mother. Mother was shocked at Jane's anger and said, "You should be pleased and proud of your sister. Now tell her how glad you are that she won."

## ESCAPE AND WITHDRAWAL

Escape and withdrawal are used to solve anger by unconscious avoidance. This may take several forms. The individual may use fantasy to escape from the reality of the situation. He may project his anger onto another so that he visualizes that he was attacked by the other when actually he was the attacker. The abuse of chemical substances may provide a reliable withdrawal from a situation. An angry teenager may run away. Eating can be an escape. [3] Silence also is a form of withdrawal. Withdrawal is not always obvious.

> Mr. and Ms. Mattingly were not getting along well. When Mr. Mattingly was home there were frequent fights and disagreements. At about this time Mr. Mattingly began working later and later at his office. He frequently expressed how he hated being gone such long hours and not seeing his family as much. In reality he was creating busy work so he could avoid getting home until his wife was asleep.

## LEARNING

Last of all, anger may be expressed through learning behavior. [18] This occurs when the individual involved recognizes his anger and tries to determine why it is occurring, thus promoting increased self-awareness, and finally uses this knowledge to plan future action.

> Mark was having trouble concentrating on his homework. He found himself frequently pacing the floor of his room. He finally put his books aside and went out to practice basketball but he still was preoccupied with the day's events. He sought out his older sister to talk. Soon he was telling her about his day at school. As he talked about a committee meeting he had attended, his sister pointed out to him that he seemed upset. He realized that he was. He had been upset when his idea to revise the size and format of the school paper had been dismissed quickly. He explained that he really felt the idea was sound and had been enraged when it was casually ignored. After more discussion he commented to his sister, "I really have trouble accepting the fact that everyone else isn't in love with my ideas sometimes. I get angry and I attack them defensively for the rest

of the meeting. I still feel upset afterwards and hostile. I guess I have to learn to not take rejection of my ideas as rejection of me as a person. Next time I'll try to remind myself of that."

This method of expressing anger has obvious advantages. The anger is not used in counterproductive behavior which can lead to further problems as might occur if other methods were employed such as indirect attacks, somatization, or depression for example. Also, the individual learns more about himself, his anger, and how to cope with it. As the nurse works with angry patients and as she recognizes her own anger, it is hoped that this method of expressing anger can be used. More will be said about this when intervention in anger is discussed.

It should be noted that individuals are likely to have a consistent pattern of expressing anger. This pattern is based on early childhood experiences, later learning situations, and possibly on biologic factors. The particular source of anger influences how anger is expressed. For example, one may directly express anger at one source, but indirectly express anger at another source. This might be illustrated in the employee who directly vents his anger when aroused by a worker who is under his authority but who indirectly expresses his anger at his boss by procrastination and lateness to meetings.

It is likely that a particular individual cannot always give a reliable account of what makes him angry and how he expresses his anger although he may feel that he is very much in touch with his feelings. One's feelings of anger and the methods of its expression are often hidden from conscious awareness as noted previously. Usually one is aware only of circumstances surrounding direct expression of anger although one may not even be aware of this. This lack of objectivity about one's anger is also true of the nurse. Striving to become aware of one's less obvious sources of anger and methods of expressing anger is, therefore, a useful exercise.

As can be seen, anger is often more difficult to assess than other response behaviors.

## The Range of Expression of Anger

Expression of anger exists on a continuum from mild anger to extreme anger.[17] All forms previously described may be mild to extreme. For example, a direct expression of anger might be just a quick disgusted glance or it might be an extensive shouting tirade lasting nearly an hour. Similarly, indirect anger might be expressed as a nearly harmless sarcastic quip or in a wife's life long pattern of obstructionism toward her husband.

Mild expressions of anger are common and often fail to be identified as what they really are in normal day-to-day living. Stronger expressions of anger tend to be more noticeable and to make uninvolved observers uncomfortable.

Variability exists also in each individual's predilection to become angry. Circumstances which make one individual "fighting mad" may not perturb another at all. Some individuals may "fly off the handle" at what seems like the slightest provocation while others seem never to get angry. Some persons may be violently angry only to experience immediate calm while others seethe with anger or remain depressed for weeks. This variability in expression makes anger even more difficult to evaluate and assess.

## Chronic Anger

Certain individuals are believed to be especially prone to prolonged anger and may be said to have a "passive-aggressive" or a "hostile" personality.[2,5,17,21] It is believed that individuals with an unusual amount of dependency needs may become chronically angry. Because of their excessive needs, they are likely to be disappointed almost continually because others can seldom provide the great amount of security they need. They may feel helpless and secondarily angry. Usually the chronically angry person does not express anger directly because he is unconsciously afraid of driving away the very individuals on whom he is dependent. Instead his anger leaks out in other dimensions of his behavior. He may view the world from a very distorted perspective. He lacks trust in others and perceives hostile intentions in the behavior of others which in reality do not exist. He may become involved in life patterns which are designed to be secure and protective. The individual in this situation may find it extremely difficult to acknowledge his anger.

Examples of a chronically angry individual would be a wife who is never angry at her husband and a teenage son who is never angry at his parents and yet subjectively both seethe with signs of diffuse anger. The chronically angry individual is not the main subject of this chapter. For the most part, the nurse will be dealing with individuals with normal personalities and normal anger.

## The Patient, His Family, and Their Reasons for Anger

There are multiple reasons why individuals and their families may become angry when they enter the health care system.[17,29] First of all, the patient may be angry as a normal reaction to some illnesses. As described by Engel, he is likely to first experience denial. Later as symptoms intensify, denial may break down and awareness may increase, leading to anger among other reactions.[9] The individual moves from, "It isn't possible" to "Why me?" Anger is such a common part of an individual's reaction to illness that the nurse is often advised to be especially alert to the patient who does not experience anger. For example, the patient recovering from a stroke who does not express anger but instead remains apathetic is believed to have a poor prognosis.[29]

As the patient and his family contact and participate in the health care setting, threats which can lead to anger may occur. In almost all settings there is experienced some loss of self-esteem, increased dependency on others, impersonalization, uncertainty, exclusion from important discussions, unfamiliarity with the environment, and restrictions. For others there will be invasion and exposure of their bodies, pain, immobility, isolation, oral deprivation, embarrassment, disturbed normal patterns, inquiry into personal matters, loss of autonomy, imposition of authority, and confiscation of personal possessions.[29] The child in the health care setting is prone to experience even more anger than an adult who can usually comprehend the rationale for more of what is happening. The child may perceive evil intent and malice in much of what happens to him, depending on his age. He may also wonder why his parents are participating or at least fraternizing with his attackers. Anger towards his parents may put him in a psychological bind since anger towards parents is not very comfortable. His already prevalent feelings of being weak and powerless may be easily confirmed if he is ignored and restrained. It is amazing, not that patients and families become angry, but that they do not become more angry than they do![22]

Not only are sources of anxiety which may lead to anger prevalent when one has an illness or seeks health care, but methods for coping with anger may be restricted. An active teenage girl who defuses her anger through sports activities may be forced to limit her activities or even discontinue them. The man who copes with anger towards his wife by entertaining his fellow workers with satirical stories about her may be isolated from his friends and forced into close proximity to the greatest source of his anger. A young man who copes with anger through escape and withdrawal may find confinement to a hospital intolerable because he cannot pull his usual disappearing act. It is likely that all of these individuals react to the increased anxiety factors described and the unavailability of usual methods of expressing anger by venting anger through some other method. Frequently their anger may be directed towards the members of the health care team.

Another way to visualize the situation of the patient and his family is in terms of transactional analysis. In general, the patient and family may be treated in such a manner by those in authority that they may be encouraged to respond out of their "child" state. Their response is likely to be with the anger of the child state as expressed in, "I don't like you anymore," and "You're mean." The adult state, in which the patient and family and the health care personnel are able to think logically and factually about the situation and assert themselves positively without aggression or hostility, would be greatly preferable. This is the situation which this chapter will focus on achieving.

## Unhelpful Expression of Anger

The expression of anger an individual uses is considered unhelpful when the method interferes with his interactions with others and makes it harder for him to meet his personal needs. One form of expression cannot be considered always helpful and another form always unhelpful. The person who uses indirect means of expressing anger may create more work for himself, drive others away, and experience depression more than if he directly expressed his anger at its source. On the other hand, the individual who directly blasts anyone and everyone who makes him anxious might have more friends if some of his angry impulses were diffused in other ways.

## The Positive Benefits of Anger

Although anger is often seen as something to be avoided if at all possible, several benefits can occur from expressing feelings of anger.[7] As previously mentioned, anger may lead to learning. There are other possible benefits as well.

1. The expression of anger successfully in channels sanctioned by society may increase self-esteem.

   Tommy was the aggressive oldest son of very aggressive parents. He was frequently in trouble at home and at school and criticized and belittled by his parents. When Tommy joined the junior high football team, he played with daring and intensity. He received recognition from his peers, spectators, and coaches. As his aggressive football behavior continued, he was less trouble at home and at school.

2. Anger may lead to constructive and useful activity.

   Susan had always received high grades effortlessly in high school. When she started college in the summer on a preadmission program she drifted through her classes without expending much effort. At the end of the summer she was informed by the college that she would not be admitted in the fall due to her low grades in the summer. Susan was shocked and angry. She sought admission to another college and graduated three years later *magna cum laude.*

3. Anger may be substituted for other more devastating reactions.

> Marian's oldest child was found soon after birth to have moderate cerebral dysfunction. Although no one could be sure of the cause of the dysfunction, Marian was sure that it was due to inappropriate handling of the birth by her physician. She had a long list of criticisms which she expressed angrily. Her anger over the situation led her to devote considerable energy to therapeutic measures for her child and kept her from facing the possibility that she had conceived a defective child.

Thus anger has the potential for being both a constructive or destructive force.[1] And, any one expression of anger may simultaneously contain constructive and destructive elements. In judging the usefulness of anger, these need to be analyzed.

## ANGER AND THE LIFE CYCLE

### Infants

It is speculated that very young infants are capable of anger. Infants seem to make rudimentary movements suggestive of attack at an offensive object.[17] Anyone who has ever watched a circumcision on a newborn male infant might well conclude that he appears capable of rage! It is likely that for the infant, a total body response is evoked for distress of any form which interferes with his pleasure.[6] As he matures, his responses can be more differentiated. The older infant may express anger by spitting, vomiting, or biting.[27] The "failure to thrive" syndrome may represent the withdrawal and escape behavior of an angry infant.

### Toddlers

The toddler has several more developed methods of expressing his anger. He often projects angry intentions to others.[17] He may even project his anger onto objects.[6] He is often forced to use withdrawal and escape because he may not be openly permitted by his parents to express anger.[17] He is felt to be afraid of the anger he feels within himself and fears loss of control. If this is true, he probably appreciates limits which help him prevent loss of control.[24] He spends considerable time exploring what his limits are. This may be to reassure himself that he is safe. The notorious resistiveness and negativism of the toddler may represent a safe way of expressing anger at his parents. After all, he feels angry with them yet he is dependent on them to meet his needs.[6] If the toddler is provoked to anger yet not allowed to express it directly, he may resort to indirect expressions such as withholding feces or inappropriately releasing urine and feces. Temper tantrums may provide a legitimate release of anger when other channels are blocked.[4] The toddler is likely learning how to respond to his anger by assimilating his parents' behaviors.[14]

### Preschoolers

While the preschooler copes with an increasing number of anxieties which may provoke anger such as relations with peers, changing expectations by his parents, the presence of younger siblings, and supposedly jealousy towards the parent of the opposite sex, he is now less supervised and has a larger environment. These factors, along with his increased verbal and physical skills, give him more opportunities to dissipate his anger.

The preschool child is gaining more refined methods of expressing anger directly. He is becoming capable of more effective verbal expression of anger.[23] He may use name-calling, swearing, tattling, sassing, insulting, and shouting. His methods of physical expression may include punching, biting, shoving, hair pulling, kicking, pinching, and scratching. He is probably learning that the latter are seldom sanctioned and often lead to punishment.

It is speculated that if his strivings for independence are thwarted now, his repressed anger may predispose him to becoming an angry personality chronically.

The toddler who is ill may be more restricted, more supervised, and limited in physical and verbal expression and might be expected to accumulate more angry feelings.

## School-aged Children

The school-aged child has increased sources of anxiety such as concern over living up to parental expectations, peer group acceptance, and school performance. School-aged children show a wide and varied expression of anger. Extreme expressions are behaviors such as bullying, destructiveness, lying, stealing, school truancy, and underachievement. Milder more common expressions of anger are distracting, quarreling, fighting, disrupting, and uncooperativeness.[4,25,27] At this stage, parents now expect a greater degree of control of emotional expression by the child and probably disapprove of overt displays of anger. Fortunately, the school-aged child is often helped by the peer group and by neighborhood and school activities to express his anger constructively in competitive activities.[6] Handicaps and illness may inhibit peer group membership and interfere with competitive activities. The school-aged child who does not find his place in the peer group may be hampered in expressing anger.

## Adolescents

The teenager, trying to declare his independence from his parents, is often angry at his parents who he sees as forcing his continued dependency. He often overreacts in an attempt to show his independence and then compensates for the fear produced by again becoming dependent. Soon, however, he will become angry again and try again to assert himself.[6,7] This cycle will continue over and over until he can be independent without becoming fearful.

If the school-aged child's extreme expression of anger was not channeled into constructive action, the adverse behaviors associated with the outward expression of anger overlooked then are likely to become very obvious and very problematic when the child becomes a teenager. The parents are likely to seek help now while earlier they ignored or denied the behaviors. Examples of acting out behaviors seen in the angry teenager include stealing, lying, violence, sexual promiscuity, running away, truancy, and chemical abuse.[4] On the other hand, the adolescent who expresses his anger inwardly through somatization, disowning, or depression or through escape or withdrawal may not receive such notice.

## Adults

Adults are capable of all the behaviors described under the review of theory. The possible sources of anxiety and resulting anger adults experience are almost unlimited and change with the progression from young to middle to later adulthood.

Adults often get involved in a cyclic pattern related to anger which needs amplification. By adulthood, one is expected to be rational, mature, and in control of his feelings. Anger, jealousy, envy, and hate are emotions which one is expected not to feel. Only "positive" emotions such as love, joy, compassion, and hope are to occur. In reality, one functions in this world with a complete set of emotions, those considered by society both negatively and positively. Many individuals are able to do a good job of pretending to themselves and others to have only the positive ones, but the negative ones are still there repressed in the background. The result of this expectation is that one often feels depressed and guilty when one experiences an emotion such as anger which is defined by our culture as unacceptable. This results in a feeling of lowered self-esteem, depression, and eventually, more anger. McBride has referred to this cycle as the "anger-depression-guilt go-round" and writes about how it affects mothers when they feel angry with their children.[20] It can be applied to most of adult behavior, however. For example:

> Al and Janice had been married for only a few months. Al's parents had a habit of dropping in to visit them unexpectedly and staying for a meal. Janice was a busy student, the apartment was often untidy and the choices for a meal were often limited. Janice would usually experience considerable depression after Al's parents left because she felt she wasn't being a good wife if she couldn't adequately manage her home. She was becoming more angry and secondarily depressed all the time. As she talked with Al one night after one of his parents' unexpected visits during finals week, she realized that she actually was very angry with his parents, and also with him for not only allowing the situation to continue but actually promoting it. She also was angry with Al for not helping her with the housework and shopping. After the sources of her anger were recognized, they were both able to plan some changes. Janice's periods of depression became less frequent as a result.

When intervention in anger is discussed, suggestions will be given for breaking the anger-guilt-anger cycle common in adulthood.

## Older Adults

The elderly often have many reasons to be angry. They are often faced with rapid and significant losses which can create anxiety which may be expressed as anger. It is believed that the elderly often express their anger inwardly as withdrawal or depression. These behaviors may not be recognized for what they are and instead be assumed to represent senile changes. Thus, intervention which might help improve the quality of life for the elderly person who is angry might not be undertaken.

## NURSING INTERVENTION IN ANGER

## Primary Prevention

Primary prevention of anger concerns preventing anger from occurring through appropriate nursing action.

First of all, since anger may develop when an individual is faced with a situation which leads to anxiety and feelings of helplessness, the nurse can direct her actions toward promoting an environment as low in anxiety producing stimuli as possible. This would include measures which help the patient and family understand what is occurring, provide for their exercise of control appropriately, individualize the care to reflect the unique needs of those involved, and guarantee prompt, safe, and courteous care.

A similar focus for preventing anger might be on helping the patient and family to cope with anxiety as it occurs without allowing severe levels of anxiety to occur. The nurse does this by being alert to symptoms of anxiety and intervening to reduce anxiety as appropriate. More information on preventing and reducing anxiety levels is found in the chapter on anxiety.

Last of all, since anger by one person can easily provoke a similar response in another, the nurse needs to look carefully at how her behavior might be interpreted as hostile or aggressive. This is especially important when working with young children who are not able to understand the therapeutic intent behind nursing actions. One way to avoid provoking an angry response is to relate to the other individual with "adult" responses and not with "parent" responses. A nurse who says in an accusing tone, "Why haven't you been keeping your appointments at the clinic?" is more likely to evoke an angry response from a patient than a nurse who uses an "adult" factual statement such as, "I notice that you haven't gone to the clinic this month." It should be remembered that there are situations in which anger serves useful purposes and the nurse would be wise to assess for this possibility.

Primary prevention actions are presented in Table 8-1.

**Table 8-1.** Possible nursing actions to prevent anger

1. Reduce sources of undue anxiety and high levels of anxiety.
2. Use "adult" behavior which is less likely to be interpreted as hostile and responded to with anger.

## Secondary Prevention

Secondary prevention involves nursing actions designed to help an adult, child, or family member who is already expressing anger in some manner.

When working with the patient or family member whom the nurse believes to be angry, the goal the nurse is working towards is helping the individual to learn through his anger. Not only does this approach help to eliminate present problems but also may help the patient or family member to more effectively handle anger in the future.

The first step when intervening with a person who is angry is to validate that the individual is angry. This serves the purpose of verifying if the nurse is correct in her assessment and may be helpful to the patient in becoming aware of what he is feeling. She may wish to point out what manifestations she sees. The angry person is usually not totally aware of his anger. Since "angry" and "mad" have commonly been seen as unacceptable states, it may be wise to use less stigmatized terms. The nurse might say, "You seem to be upset by this" or "I imagine that you feel irritated, am I right?" It may be preferable to acknowledge the individual's anger and provide acceptance at the same time. She might say, "I would feel very disturbed if that happened to me." It is important that she use these statements only when she is confident that the patient is angry to avoid putting words in his mouth. If the patient agrees that he is angry, she can offer acceptance with statements such as, "I can understand how you must feel." The individual may at first or consistently deny any anger. In fact, the questions of the nurse may initially make him angrier because she has exposed within him an emotion he cannot admit to himself.[10] A child may confirm his anger through a story or a drawing but not verbally.

It is important that the nurse not try to persuade the patient that he is angry or use an accusatory tone.[28]

After the patient or family member acknowledges his anger, the nurse can help him to clarify the dimensions of his anger. If possible the person should explore how he feels, what may have caused his anger, and what the significance of the threat he perceived is to him.[28]

It may appear to the nurse that what the patient feels he is angry about is not really the true cause but she should refrain from enlightening the patient with her interpretation. The patient will need time to narrow down the source of his anger and he may never truly reveal it to himself. He often needs to learn if he can trust the nurse to tell her about his anger and this takes time.[17] Again children will often express themselves only indirectly. Not everyone will be able to explore these topics.

Learning about one's anger is not always accomplished quickly. The person may require considerable time for reflection. The nurse should try to achieve an understanding of the situation from the viewpoint of the individual involved.[28] Often, if the nurse has contact with the individual over a period of time, she or the patient may be able to see a pattern to the situations which led to his anger.

A community health nurse visited Ms. Nelson, the mother of three children, for health supervision. On several occasions, Ms. Nelson was angry and secondarily depressed. Each time the nurse helped Ms. Nelson explore her anger. On one visit, Ms. Nelson noticed that her anger was usually caused by a situation which illustrated that she was very tied down by her children and the expectations of her husband and this was basic to much of her anger and subsequent depression. The nurse and Ms. Nelson could then focus on this situation.

Later, the nurse and the person involved can explore possible solutions to the anxiety producing situation which is generating anger.[28] The adult or child may have many ideas of approaches which might work and, of course, the nurse encourages him to solve his problems in his own way. Part of the solution to the problem may involve exploring alternative ways of relieving angry feelings. Again, the person involved knows what is likely to work best for him. An optimal release of angry feelings combines as many of these elements as possible:

1. The activity used does not harm the individual who is angry.
2. The activity does not harm others.
3. The activity promotes insight into the individual's feelings.
4. The activity used provides some relief.
5. The activity is convenient and likely to be used.

Using these criteria will help in choosing an appropriate activity and in evaluating why one possibly did not work. Possible activities include crafts, physical exercise, housework, dancing, cooking, carpentry, and conversation.

The adult or child needs to know that changing his behavior will not occur rapidly. He needs to be encouraged by small steps he is able to take. For example, just learning to recognize and admit when one is angry is a large accomplishment. He also needs reassurance that he may frequently fail to respond as he wishes but should keep trying.

Ted was noted for having a violent temper. Several times in his sophomore year in high school he had gotten himself in trouble because of angry outbursts. He talked with the school nurse and tried to learn ways to control his temper. Often, however, he was unable to and reverted to angry outbursts. The nurse, rather than focusing on his failures, had him keep a list in the office of times when he was able to recognize his anger and avoid an outburst. As the list grew longer, he became more encouraged. Now, he still has days when he loses control but he can see past them towards greater improvement overall.

As solutions are tried, the nurse helps the patient to evaluate his progress and plan new steps as necessary. She can explain to the patient what they are doing so that as new problems arise in the future, the patient can use a problem solving approach on his own to learn from his anger.

Next, the individual may need to learn how he can identify when he is angry in the future. The nurse helps the patient to explore what makes him angry, how he feels when he is angry, nwhy he has difficulty admitting his anger, and what he can do when he is angry. She may need to again reassure the patient that everyone gets angry and that becoming angry is not a sign of poor mental functioning. Rather the important factor is what one does when one becomes angry.[20] This attitude may help to break the anger-guilt-anger cycle because anger can be recognized and accepted without the individual becoming secondarily depressed about his anger and then angrier still.

With children, intervention may involve helping their parents to realize that anger in children, as well as in adults, is normal.[3] The parents may need to talk about why they stifle expressions of anger by their children. Often, parents may force their children to rdpress their anger because the parents themselves are very afraid of their own anger. Discussing this area may not only be helpful but essential. Religious teachings are not uncommonly influential in leading to the repression or displacement of anger.[6] Parents may want to explore allowing their children to have angry feelings and how they can teach them to express such feelings constructively.

While there are varied opinions, the consensus is that young children should be permitted to express their anger openly as long as they do not harm themselves, others, or property. Nor should they be shamed or made to feel guilty afterwards. It has always been popular to consider "redirecting" as an optimal method of handling anger in children. "You cannot hit your sister but you can hit the pegs in this toy work bench." It is believed that this can help the child learn that he is angry, that it is all right to be angry, and how to express anger appropriately. Many children respond to this well. For some, considerable help is needed in learning ways to express their feelings which do not harm others or destroy property.[6,23,25] Often used are play activities such as punching a punching bag, tossing games, hammering, making up stories, physical activities, art projects, and playing "hospital."[24,27] The child may need to be encouraged and reassured, "It's okay to give the doll a shot. It doesn't really hurt anybody."

There is the possibility, however, that encouraging children to behave aggressively in any manner can lead to an escalation of aggressive behavior. Children can often express anger in nonaggressive activities and through talking with another person. Parents who believe their children to be excessively aggressive might consider the possibility that their children are being influenced by actions seen on television. Although the effects of TV violence on children are not certain, there seems to be mounting evidence that watching televised aggressive behavior is associated with increased aggressive behavior by children.[19] Programs designed especially for children, such as cartoon features, are often among the most aggressive.

Unfortunately, the nurse will encounter situations in which parents cannot tolerate any expressions of anger by their children. The nurse may be able to work with the school nurse or school counselor in designing situations where the child can play out or express his anger. If the child is hospitalized, she or the child life worker may be able to allow the child appropriate play opportunities. She should realize that parents often feel they are being judged personally by the behavior of their child in school, in the hospital, or in other health care settings, and they may feel a strong need to overcontrol and subdue their child.[24]

The child can learn through play activities to recognize and admit when he is angry and choose what to do about it. If the nurse must reprove the child for some behavior, she must be sure that she communicates that she likes the child even though she does not approve of his behavior.[6]

## INTERVENTION IN ANGRY EPISODES

Occasionally, the nurse is faced with an acute episode of directly expressed anger. The timing of her intervention becomes important.[28] It is likely that the angry person needs some time to cool off and gain control before talking with another.[29] He may benefit immediately from some physical activity that the nurse suggests. He may spontaneously seek a person to talk to afterwards.[1] Later, a problem solving approach can be pursued when the nurse senses that the time is right for intervention.[29] It is advisable to communicate to the patient that the nurse understands and can accept his anger.[14] It is crucial to focus on the person and not the behavior because the behavior may be reinforced by a lot of attention. This is especially likely with children.

> Neil had been burned over a large part of his body including his hands and face. As his condition became more serious, he was placed in isolation. The nurses and physicians began to spend less time with him. Shortly thereafter, Neil began venting his anger by destructive efforts aimed at the equipment and supplies in his room and by verbal insults. While the nurses disapproved of his behavior and told him so in explicit terms, they did move him closer to the station and checked on him more frequently. They noticed that his destructive behavior increased despite their warnings.

It is essential for the nurse not to react with anger of her own to the angry patient. Suggestions for accomplishing this difficult task are given later.

If the patient is violently angry and may possibly harm himself or others, help should be sought immediately and the situation considered a psychiatric emergency.[17] Table 8-2 summarizes secondary prevention.

**Table 8-2.** Possible nursing actions to reduce anger

1. Validate the presence of anger if possible.
2. Encourage acceptance of anger as normal to break anger-guilt-anger cycle.
3. Help individual explore present anger using a problem solving approach.
4. Help individual learn about how and when he uses anger in general.
5. Help parents deal with their children's anger.
6. In angry outbursts, allow individual time to calm down, provide physical activity, and focus on discussing anger and not behaviors used to express anger.

## Tertiary Prevention

Tertiary prevention deals with helping the patient, whose nearly constant anger has become unhelpful, experience less anxiety and, therefore, less anger. It is believed that patients who are continuously angry may be very dependent and feel continually disappointed in the attempts of others to meet their needs. Patients or family members who are continuously angry are often labeled as hostile or demanding. Any time a patient is classified as demanding, it should alert the nurse to the fact that the demanding behavior is a signal that anxiety is increasing and help is needed. The nursing intervention should be focused on increasing the person's feelings of security.

A vital way to increase the security the continually angry individual needs is by building his self-esteem through a helping relationship. Of greatest importance to such individuals is the establishment of a sense of belongingness and security within personal relationships.[1] This can be done when the nurse uses helping skills to relate to the patient as a unique individual in whom she is interested. More information on helping skills is found in the chapter on the helping process.

Termination with the demanding patient must be mentioned and planned for from the beginning of contact and done slowly to avoid increasing his feelings of dependency which may reactivate his anger.[1]

Another way to increase security is to decrease all perceived threats. Often, in health care settings, the largest threat a person experiences relates to fears about the unknown. The nurse can work to reduce this by providing the person with the information he needs to feel more secure in his situation. The nurse must, of course, be knowledgeable in the area of concern.

> Mindy, a teenager, was scheduled for a valve replacement. She gave the impression of being angry at the world. She was bossy, rude, and arrogant towards her parents, the nurse, and all who approached. The nurse astutely concluded that Mindy might be anxious over her surgery and life with an artificial valve. She overlooked much of Mindy's behavior and developed a teaching plan for Mindy with built-in opportunities for expression of feelings. As the teaching progressed, Mindy was able to begin to acknowledge her fears and her rudeness decreased somewhat.

Measures which allow the person to feel more in control reduce anxiety and increase security. This situation is one in which the nurse may not plan to allow the patient to face great amounts of decision making. Choices which lead to frustration may increase his anger.[1] Small measures to increase security can do much to decrease the individual's feelings of anger. With both adults and children, compliance to usual rituals and routines can be helpful.[24] The presence of family members and familiar surroundings can be comforting.

Another intervention to increase security for the angry patient and reduce his anxiety involves providing limits.[8,16,17] It is hypothesized that the presence of firm, concrete limits which are enforced consistently contribute to a feeling of being more protected—even from oneself. Most nurses have little difficulty setting limits with children but feel more hesitant to do so with adults. The following are examples of statements made by nurses to adults with demanding behavior which state limits and, therefore, provide protection to the person involved.

"I can only make a home visit to you once a week. You may choose what afternoon is best for you."

"I will be able to come to your room no more often than every 30 minutes. I will come then to check on you whether your light is on or not."

"This clinic is only for following healthy babies. I know you must be concerned because your baby is sick again and I know we let the doctor see her when she was ill last month, but we cannot do that any more. You will have to take her to the pediatric clinic at General Hospital or to a physician in the community."

To be effective, limits must be given without any hint of punishment or retaliation. They must be held firm even in the face of an angry outburst from the other person. The limits must be legitimate ones that the nurse has a right to impose.

One very difficult task for the nurse working with a person who is demanding or continually angry is to consistently focus on his underlying anger and not his behavior. It is very easy to get trapped into a battle with the person involved over the manifestations of his anger such as the demands he makes. Focusing on the forms of expression of anger can be reinforcing to the individual because of the attention he receives as a result.[1] The nurse should instead focus on his anger and on helping the person to learn from his anger. She does this by helping him learn through problem solving that he is angry, why he is angry, how he is expressing his anger, and what other possible solutions there are to his anger. This does not mean that she totally ignores the behavior and the demands the person makes. Often the complaints and demands are not truly the basis of the individual's anger but they may be evidence of displaced anger. The nurse who deals quickly and effectively with what may seem to her as trivial complaints will be showing the person her concern and he may eventually be able to more directly comprehend and express his anger as a result. She must take care of his complaints and demands without dwelling on them or making them the center of attention. Then she refocuses on helping the patient to learn from his anger. If the demanding individual does not seem able to learn from his anger, he may benefit from the application of behavioral modification learning techniques.

Possible nursing actions related to the tertiary prevention of anger are summarized in Table 8-3.

**Table 8-3.** Possible nursing actions to provide security for continually angry and demanding individuals

1. Use helping skills.
2. Reduce possible sources of anxiety.
3. Provide and enforce legitimate limits
4. Focus on underlying anger rather than on evidences of anger
5. Help patient to learn from anger through problem solving approach.
6. Use behavioral modification if necessary to extinguish anger.

## THE NURSE AND ANGER

The nurse is not unlikely to develop feelings of anger in her professional and personal life. The situation she works in, the patients she works with, and their reactions to her can contribute to anger.

The situation in which a nurse works can easily contribute to anger. She is often expected to effectively perform many diverse roles. She often works in a complex environment surrounded by technical equipment and populated by armies of individuals with varying backgrounds and focuses. Or she may work in cultural islands in the population where values, resources, and problems are totally different from hers. She is sometimes frustrated by shortages of personnel, supplies, and time. Reaction to this situation varies, of course, but it is not surprising that many nurses experience anger. While each individual expresses anger in a unique way, it is probable that most nurses are likely to avoid direct physical or verbal expression and instead use less obvious forms. Another possibility is that the nurse disowns anger for a while, and then gets really upset and creates a scene. Because many of the individuals who evoke the nurse's anger may have higher authority and the ability to retaliate, the nurse may express her anger indirectly through obstructive efforts. She may displace her anger onto others who have less authority over her and represent less threat—including patients and their families.

The nurse may react with anger towards the patients and families she cares for. Her anger may be caused by a lack of progress she sees in patients who ignore their health needs or by those who reject her efforts to improve their level of wellness.

Lastly, the nurse's anger may be defensive when she reacts in like manner to the patient who is angry with her. Patients may displace anger at the health care system in general onto the nurse in particular due to her visibility and availability. They may unconsciously consider the nurse a safer target for expressing anger than the physician. Children may find it more psychologically comfortable to displace anger at their parents onto the nurse. Similarly patients may become angry when they perceive the nurse as a threat or as an authority figure who is attempting to control them. She may be seen as one who violates the privacy of their bodies, performs painful procedures, forces movement even under painful circumstances, sends away visitors, disturbs their sleep, and limits diets, activities, and medications.[29] Children in particular are likely to see the nurse's actions as purely malicious. The overt and covert expressions of anger with which the adult or child responds are likely to promote an angry response from the nurse in return.

How the nurse deals with anger which occurs in her personal life or because of the situation she works in, and because of her relations with patients and families, has great significance for her practice. The nurse who is unaware of her own anger, unable to control her expression of anger, or who reacts in turn with anger when another does, deprives those she cares for of her full nursing capabilities.[28]

First, then, the nurse needs to learn more about her own anger. She can reflect on the following questions:

1. Do I see anger in myself as a normal and likely emotional response?
2. How can I tell when I am angry?
3. What anxieties lead to my anger?
4. How do I express anger?
5. Are there certain people to whom I am afraid to express anger?
6. When am I likely to displace or disown my anger?

The nurse will need to study herself repeatedly because learning about one's own anger is a life-long task. Practice will gradually lead to greater levels of awareness about anger. Talking with others who are qualified, such as supervisors, instructors, and counselors, can be beneficial.

## Facing Direct Anger

One of the most difficult challenges the nurse will face is working with individuals who directly express anger at her. It is logical for the nurse to feel upset and respond with defensiveness and anger of her own which limits her effectiveness. There are several ways for the nurse to learn to avoid responding with anger of her own to an angry individual. This is important because responding with anger often increases the other person's anger and may begin a cyclic pattern in which anger increases progressively.

First of all, the nurse needs to assume responsibility for what she is feeling. It is common for one to state, "He really made me angry." In reality, she should realize that she *chose* to become angry.[15] Thus, the first step in learning to respond to angry individuals is to learn that one need not automatically become angry even though angrily approached by another. One could choose to feel otherwise.

Secondly, the nurse can use the framework of transactional analysis.[13] The anger of the patient or family often leads the nurse to respond out of her authoritarian "parent" state or frightened defensive "child" state. The nurse can attempt to avoid entering her "parent" or "child" state and instead function from her "adult" state. The following interactions indicate how a nurse might respond to others in either a child state or an adult state.

Patient: Where have you been? I've been waiting for 10 minutes for you to answer my light. Can't you be more prompt!
Nurse: You're not the only patient on this unit, you know. Can't you be more understanding! [child state]
Nurse: It must be difficult to wait. [adult state]

Mother: Can't anyone around here do something for Timmy's pain? Do I have to call the doctor myself or have you got the guts to do it?
Nurse: If you want to try finding him go right ahead. I've called his office, his home, his answering service . . . [child state]
Nurse: I'm sure Timmy's leg hurts. We're trying to find Dr. Hunt. It must be frustrating for you seeing him in pain like this. [adult state]

The adult response avoids defensiveness and counterattacks. It focuses on giving and getting facts. The aim of the adult response is to encourage the other person to also communicate from his adult state. Only when this has been achieved can learning and problem solving about the person's anger occur.

Unfortunately, it is easier to think about defusing anger than to actually do it. Reacting defensively and angrily to an angry individual is very understandable. The nurse should expect that learning to maintain an adult tone and content to her communications will take time. She may be pleased when she can first learn to recognize when she is feeling angry. Later she may learn to recognize when she is responding with anger and then attempt to switch to her adult state. Still later, she can strive to remain in her adult state consistently with angry individuals.

Of course, there are situations and times when the nurse will find that she needs help and consultation with others. Often through discussions with colleagues a perplexing situation can be seen more clearly.[17]

The following questions have been suggested which may help the nurse when working with angry individuals.[29]

1. What behaviors indicate that the individual is angry?
2. How do these behaviors affect me?
3. How do others react to the same individual?
4. Am I able to see the purpose his anger is serving?

If the nurse finds that she is frequently subjected to angry verbal attacks by patients and families, she must give some consideration to the possibility that she is, by her behavior, provoking patients' or families' anger without being aware of it. She should reflect on whether she has been inconsiderate, impolite, intrusive, inattentive, or has projected her own anger onto the patient.[21] Has she appeared opinionated? Does her conversation have a distinctly parent-to-child flavor?[30] The continual presence of anger in those she cares for may mean that the nurse should more closely evaluate her behavior.[12]

## A TOOL FOR ASSESSMENT AND EVALUTION

The tool presented in Table 8-4 can be used to diagnose the presence of and the prognosis of anger in the behavior of patients and others. Individuals whose behaviors are predominantly "less optimal" are at high risk. The tool can also be used to evaluate the effectiveness of nursing action with the angry individual. The person should move from less optimal to more optimal responses if nursing action is appropriate.

**Table 8-4.** Assessment and evaluation of anger

| Behavior | Less optimal | More optimal |
| --- | --- | --- |
| Posture | Offensive position, alert, rapid reflexes, tense, voice changes | Relaxed or normal |
| Physiologic symptoms | Flushed face, anorexia, diarrhea, dilated pupils | Absent |
| Perception of reality | Believes world and other people are dangerous | Accurate perceptions |
| Use of humor | At the expense of others | Does not contain elements of ridicule |
| Cooperativeness | Sabotages plans, obstructs | Facilitates others |
| Viewpoint | Cannot modify when given new information | Can adjust to accommodate new information |
| Social behavior | Rude, demanding, or sugar-coated politeness | Normal |
| Acceptance of responsibility for errors | Projects responsibility onto others | Accepts |
| Evaluative abilities | Excessively critical | Can assess good and bad |
| Response to criticism | Attacks in return | Searches for elements of truth |
| Mood | Depression, withdrawal, fantasizing | Normal |
| Awareness of angry feelings | Denies | Acknowledges |
| Learning capacity | Minimal | Normal |
| Security | Based on deficiencies of others | Based on personal attributes[6,8,11,15,17,27-29] |

## AN EXAMPLE OF NURSING INTERVENTION IN ANGER

The following example illustrates how a nurse with limited formal authority was able to help an individual who was continuously angry and demanding.

Ms. Arnett was to bring her son into the allergist's office every Thursday for a desensitization injection. A regular time slot had been agreed upon and 4:45 p.m. was set aside for the injection. However, Ms. Arnett was usually late and arrived just as the office staff was hurrying to finish the day's work at 5:15. Ms. Arnett would leave her two other children in the reception area to amuse themselves. She detained the physician as long as possible once he entered the examining room with demands that he listen to other problems and sometimes followed him down the hall still talking. She regularly roamed through the office and perused the supply room for samples of medications she took home for herself and her other children. She antagonized the office nurses with behaviors such as treating them as servants and criticized their promptness in seeing her. On other occasions, she and her son would not appear until late on Friday without notifying the office. She would walk into the nursing area marked "private" and insist that her son be seen right away. If they protested she would say, "It's just a shot. Why should we have to sit out there with all those people sick with heaven knows what?"

Norma, who was one of the office nurses, decided that the difficult and uncomfortable relationship she had with Ms. Arnett should be improved. She planned first to set a limit related to the appointment time. She phoned Ms. Arnett at home and asked if 4:45 on Thursdays was still a convenient time for her son to be seen. Ms. Arnett replied that it was. The nurse then explained that her son would be seen then and only then. If they could not be there by 5:00 her son would have to be seen on another day and she would have to call ahead to arrange an appointment. Ms. Arnett seemed unconcerned.

The next week Ms. Arnett came in at 5:10. Norma got out the appointment book and pleasantly inquired about when they could come on Friday. Ms. Arnett became very agitated when she realized that Norma was serious about the time restrictions. Some of the patients in the waiting room began to watch the nurse and Ms. Arnett. Ms. Arnett insisted that her son be seen that day. The nurse explained that he had missed his appointment and that there were other patients waiting for theirs. She responded with, "How petty!" and again demanded that since she was paying exorbitant prices for medical care, her son had a right to be seen right then and there. The nurse replied calmly, "I know this must make you angry but we see all patients by appointment only here as you know and I'm afraid I must ask you to obey the same policies and come back when we can schedule another time." Ms. Arnett then stated that she couldn't come back Friday and that she was afraid of what would happen to her son without his injection. The nurse, striving to maintain a calm and factual approach, again stated that she would have to make another appointment. Ms. Arnett then demanded to see the physician. The nurse replied that he would be with patients the rest of the afternoon but she could certainly talk to him about the situation during her son's next appointment. At that, Ms. Arnett turned, collected her children, and marched towards the door, remarking loudly, "We'll see how he feels about this when he finds out that you girls are driving all of his patients away!"

Ms. Arnett was not heard from again until the next Thursday when she and her children appeared at 4:40. She gave the appearance of being quite angry—her eyes were wide open and her jaw and fists were clenched. She did not speak to any of the nurses although they attempted to converse with her and her son.

She did, however, talk to the physician when he entered the examining room to see them. She loudly issued a series of complaints. The physician took care of the son, sent him to the waiting area, and then suggested that Ms. Arnett talk with Norma. Although Ms. Arnett was reluctant at first, she later agreed.

Norma came into the room, closed the door, and sat down near Ms. Arnett. She had prepared herself to listen carefully, use helping skills as best she could, and to try to keep the conversation on an adult-adult level. Ms. Arnett proceeded on her tirade of complaints and injustices. Norma listened carefully. Some of her complaints were justified. For example, Ms. Arnett pointed out that she was expected to always be on time and yet her son was never seen at 4:45 even if he was there because the office was almost always running 20 to 30 minutes late. Other complaints were based on misconceptions but Norma avoided her desire to correct them, allowing Ms. Arnett an opportunity to freely express herself. Norma encouraged expression by statements such as, "I can see how that would make you feel" and "Yes, I see what you mean." Ms. Arnett's tone eventually became less agitated as she continued. Norma struggled successfully to concentrate on Ms. Arnett's conversation and use empathy and concreteness. Ms. Arnett's conversation began to hint at her frustrations with life, her husband, and her children. She became quite dejected and very unlike the haughty, bossy woman Norma had known her to be.

After 30 minutes of conversation, Norma felt that she understood Ms. Arnett as never before and that she was, in many respects, a frightened and insecure person. Norma tried to focus on Ms. Arnett's anger and reasons for its occurrence. Ms. Arnett intimated that she sometimes behaved as she did towards others because she was afraid they would ignore her otherwise. For some of Ms. Arnett's specific objections related to the present situation, Norma and Ms. Arnett agreed on some solutions to try. When Norma and Ms. Arnett parted, Ms. Arnett seemed much less angry than initially.

The next few visits of Ms. Arnett and her son to the office proceeded smoothly. They always arrived before 5:00. Ms. Arnett began to talk to Norma more on each visit. Many of the things Ms. Arnett mentioned were concerned with her personal life and her insecurities. Because the need for weekly visits to the allergist was soon to be over, Norma suggested that Ms. Arnett might enjoy regularly talking with a counselor and when Ms. Arnett showed interest, she prepared a list of counseling services available in the community. Later Ms. Arnett told Norma that she had gone to see a counselor and was working on some of her problems with her. Gradually the demanding behavior of Ms. Arnett became more infrequent.

## SUMMARY

Anger is a common though often denied human emotional response to overcome feelings of anxiety and helplessness. Anger may be expressed in numerous ways, many of which are covert. Anger appears to be present throughout the life cycle in various forms. The nurse can help the angry person by acknowledging and accepting his anger, and by helping the individual to analyze and explore his anger. Continually angry individuals may be helped by measures which lead to the feeling of greater security. The nurse may herself experience anger in personal and professional situations. Although developing self-awareness is difficult, she can learn to use her anger to learn about herself. She may, in addition, learn to respond to angry patients without anger of her own.

## REFERENCES

1. Brooks, B. R.: "Aggression." Am. J. Nurs. 67:2519, 1967.
2. Brownsberger, C. N., et al.: "Common psychiatric symptoms," in Soloman, P., and Patch, V. D. (eds.): *Handbook of Psychiatry.* Lange Medical Publications, Los Altos, Calif., 1971.
3. Bry, A.: "How to make your anger work for you." Family Circle 89:55, 1976.
4. Chapman, A. H.: *Management of Emotional Problems of Children and Adolescents.* J. B. Lippincott, Philadelphia, 1974.

5. Clancy, J., et al.: "The hostile-dependent personality." Postgrad. Med. 55:109, 1974.
6. Coffman, J. A.: "Anger: Its significance for nurses who work with emotionally disturbed children." Perspect. Psychiat. Care 7:104, 1969.
7. Denyes, M. J., and Altshuler, A.: "Effects of illness on the adolescent," in Scipien, G. M., et al.: *Comprehensive Pediatric Nursing.* McGraw-Hill, New York, 1975.
8. Dixson, B. K.: "Dealing with passive-aggressive behavior." Nurs. Forum 8:276, 1969.
9. Engel, G. L.: "Grief and grieving." Am. J. Nurs. 64:93, 1964.
10. Francis, G. M., and Munjas, B.: *Promoting Psychological Comfort.* Wm. C. Brown, Dubuque, 1975.
11. Gahan, K.: "Everybody gets angry sometime." J. Psychiat. Nurs. Mental Health Serv. 12:27, 1974.
12. Gruber, K. A., and Schniewind, H. E.: "Letting anger work for you." Am. J. Nurs. 76:1450, 1976.
13. Harris, T. A.: *I'm OK—You're OK: A Practical Guide to Transactional Analysis.* Harper, New York, 1967.
14. Hays, D. R.: "Anger: A clinical problem," in Burd, S. F., and Marshall, M. (eds.): *Some Clinical Approaches to Psychiatric Nursing.* Macmillan, New York, 1970.
15. James, M., and Jongeward, D.: *Born to Win: Transactional Analysis With Gestalt Experiments.* Addison-Wesley, Reading, Mass., 1971.
16. Kalkman, M. E., and Davis, A. J. (eds.): *New Dimensions in Mental Health-Psychiatric Nursing.* McGraw-Hill, New York, 1974.
17. Kiening, Sr. M. M.: "Hostility," in Carlson, C. E., and Blackwell, B. (eds.): *Behavioral Concepts and Nursing Intervention.* J. B. Lippincott, Philadelphia, 1978.
18. Lego, S.: "Frustration and conflict," in Clark, A. L., and Affonso, D. D.: *Childbearing: A Nursing Perspective.* F. A. Davis, Philadelphia, 1976.
19. Liebert, R. M., and Baron, R. A.: "Some immediate effects of televised violence on children's behavior." Devel. Psychol. 6:469, 1972.
20. McBride, A. B.: "The anger-depression-guilt go-round," in *The Growth and Development of Mothers.* Harper and Row, New York, 1973.
21. Morgan, W. L., and Engel, G. L.: *The Clinical Approach to the Patient.* W. B. Saunders, Philadelphia, 1969.
22. Moritz, D. A.: "Understanding anger." Am. J. Nurs. 78:81, 1978.
23. Nahigian, E. G.: "Effects of illness on the preschooler," in Scipien, G. M., et al.: *Comprehensive Pediatric Nursing.* McGraw-Hill, New York, 1975.
24. Penalver, M.: "Helping the child handle his aggression." Am. J. Nurs. 73:1554, 1973.
25. Petrillo, M., and Sanger, S.: *Emotional Care of Hospitalized Children.* J. B. Lippincott, Philadelphia, 1972.
26. Pillitteri, A.: *Nursing Care of the Growing Family. A Child Health Text.* Little, Brown and Company, Boston, 1977.
27. Pothier, P. C.: *Mental Health Counseling With Children.* Little, Brown and Company, Boston, 1976.
28. Thomas, M. D., Baker, J. M., and Estes, N.: "Anger: A tool for developing self-awareness." Am. J. Nurs. 70:2586, 1970.
29. "Understanding hostility (Programmed instruction)." Am. J. Nurs. 67:2131, 1967.
30. Veninga, R.: "Defensive behavior: Causes, effects, and cures." J. Envir. Health 37:5, 1974.

# BIBLIOGRAPHY

Eng, M.: "Letter to a patient." Am. J. Nurs. 78:434, 1978.
Janis, I. L.: *Psychological Stress.* John Wiley and Sons, London, 1958.
Kleeman, S.: "Psychophysiologic disorders," in Soloman, P., and Patch, V. D. (eds.): *Handbook of Psychiatry.* Lange Medical Publications, Los Altos, Calif., 1971.
Peplau, H. E.: *Interpersonal Relations in Nursing.* G. P. Putnam's Sons, New York, 1952.
Schroeder, E.: "The birth of a defective child: A cause for grieving," in Hall, J. E., and Weaver, B. R. (eds.): *Nursing of Families in Crisis.* J. B. Lippincott, Philadelphia, 1974.
Travelbee, J.: *Intervention in Psychiatric Nursing: Process in the One-to-One Relationship.* F. A. Davis, Philadelphia, 1969.
Velazquez, J. M.: "Alienation." Am. J. Nurs. 69:301, 1969.
Wachter-Shikora, N.: "Scapegoating among professionals." Am. J. Nurs. 77:408, 1977.

# CHAPTER 9

# GRIEF

Almost every nurse will at some time have the difficult task of caring for an individual or family who is grieving after a loss. The nurse's ability to help grieving individuals is dependent on her understanding of the grieving process and how the process can be assessed and facilitated.

The nurse herself will experience losses during her lifetime. An understanding of the grieving process can help her understand her personal reactions. She must also seek to desensitize herself to death if she is to support others who have faced a death.

Although the grieving process can be initiated by any significant loss, this chapter will focus on the nurse's role in grieving caused by the death of another person. Information in this chapter can be applied to grieving caused by other losses as well. The chapter in this book on fatal illness contains additional information related to death and dying.

## REVIEW OF THEORY

All individuals in the process of development experience losses of various kinds: friends move away, items are lost or broken, capabilities diminish. The death of another person represents severe object loss which is irreversible and seems irreplaceable. A profound reaction ensues which eventually leads to adaptation to the loss. This is referred to as the grieving process.

### The Grieving Process

The grieving process provides a method through which an individual suffering a loss can become detached from the lost object, adjust to his world without the lost object, and become open to other objects of replacement.[7] The grieving process takes considerable time but the passage of time alone is not sufficient to assure that proper grieving has occurred.[3]

Engel has proposed a description of the grieving process which has been widely accepted. He suggests that there are three stages an individual passes through as he adjusts to the loss of a significant person in his life.[8]

## SHOCK AND DISBELIEF

This stage is described as stunned numbness. The individual does not appear to actually quite comprehend the meaning of the event. Some individuals may appear to be functioning cognitively and planning but may show little emotion. Emotional acceptance of the loss always lags behind intellectual acceptance. This latter stage usually does not last more than a few days and may last only for a few hours.

## DEVELOPING AWARENESS

Eventually the individual becomes more consciously aware of the significance and reality of the loss. This occurs on a continuum beginning with little awareness and lasts until the individual usually experiences complete awareness accompanied by intense anguish, pain, and a need to cry. Other emotions are periodically expressed during this stage, such as guilt, anger, hostility, sadness, anxiety, and helplessness. This stage can last several months or years and it is a very difficult stage for the one who is grieving.

## RESTITUTION

This stage lasts for at least several months and begins when the individual is fully aware of his loss. The individual involved then begins the slow and painful process of coping with the loss and rebuilding his psychic self without the lost object. This is referred to as grief work.[25] During this stage the individual initially becomes preoccupied with the lost object and reflects on the positive qualities so that the one who died may become idealized. The individual may attempt to incorporate some of the lost one's behaviors or attitudes as his own. Emotional pain and anguish as well as the other emotions described continue periodically throughout this stage while gradually becoming less intense. Eventually the individual emerges from this stage able to occupy himself with other events and with a realistic memory of the one who died.

Progression through these stages is not neat and orderly. Nor is it always possible to exactly pinpoint where in the process an individual may be at a given time.

The experiences, thoughts, and feelings described by individuals who have experienced a significant loss have been collected by Lindemann and help to explain what the individual involved in coping with a loss perceives.[25] Lindemann recognized three types of manifestations.

## SOMATIC MANIFESTATIONS

Individuals who were grieving described an overwhelming distress syndrome manifested by tightness in the throat, an empty feeling, a loss of appetite, muscle weakness, shortness of breath, sighing respirations, and crying. These sensations came in waves lasting up to an hour at a time and were precipitated by reminders of or thoughts of the one who had died. The individual attempted, therefore, to avoid any situation which would precipitate their return.

## PSYCHIC MANIFESTATIONS

Reported psychic feelings included mental pain, a sense of unreality, preoccupation with the lost person, irritability, anger, guilt, a dislike for the presence of others, a desire to be alone, and the imaginary presence of the lost person. These symptoms troubled individuals in that some felt they were becoming insane, particularly because of their hostility towards others and their fantasy of the deceased as an imaginary companion. These symptoms lead the individual to participate in social relationships in a very contrived manner without genuine emotions.

## PSYCHOMOTOR MANIFESTATIONS

Individuals often reported restlessness, aimlessness, overactivity, the search for something to do, nervous speech, and an inability to carry out formerly automatic activities. This resulted in an inability to initiate and carry out the usual routines of living and resulted in a feeling of helplessness.

Lindemann found that, over time, these manifestations progressively decreased.

## *Factors Influencing Loss*

While there is a general pattern related to how individuals adapt to a loss of a significant other, several factors can lead to variations in the grieving process. The *closeness and intensity of the relationship* between the survivor and the deceased is a good clue to estimating how severe the grief reaction will be. Even a strong adverse relationship can lead to severe grieving because of the intensity involved. For example, the death of a sibling may be more profound for the sibling who continuously fought with the deceased than for the sibling who got along with the deceased well.

The *significance of the lost individual* to the survivor is another consideration. One of the most significant losses which can occur is death of the mother of a young child once he has become attached to her. The potential for harmful effects on the child's development is believed to be grave.[3,5] Another significant loss which characteristically leads to prolonged and profuse grieving and extreme adaptation methods is the loss by parents of a child.[18] Parents rarely expect one of their children to die. They are supposed to protect and defend their dependent children from harm. The death represents loss of the parents' link with the future[31] and loss of their creation.[10] The presence of small nuclear families means that a replacement for a lost child is less available.[10] For these reasons, loss of a child usually leads to exquisite anguish, guilt, and difficulty grieving.

The *age* of the one who dies is sometimes significant. Generally, the younger the person who dies, the more pronounced is the grief reaction.

The *circumstances surrounding the death* are factors to be considered. For example, suicide is not a noble form of death and those who mourn may feel anger, embarrassment, and guilt.[4]

The *predictability of a loss* is also a factor to be considered. For example, the sudden unexpected death of a young healthy person is usually more traumatic than the gradual death of an elderly person in poor health.

*Previous losses* an individual has experienced can be influential in increasing the severity of grieving. For example, a mother who has previously lost a child will likely grieve more intensely over the death of an infant than a mother who has never lost a child before.

The *replaceability of the loss* to the individual is worthy of consideration. For example, the loss of an only child would theoretically be more traumatic than loss of a child with seven other siblings who remain as survivors.

Another factor to be considered relates to the *amount of change* in the survivor's life which will result from the death. For example, a wife who was very dependent on her husband emotionally and financially will likely suffer more grief than a wife who was less dependent.

The survivor's *stage in the life cycle* is also important. Losses occurring to an individual at a young age or when elderly seem more difficult to adjust to than losses occurring at other ages.

Of course, the *emotional strengths* of the individual suffering the loss are relevant to the grief reaction he will have. Emotional strengths include such capacities as defense and coping mechanisms and resources.

Grief reactions can be more pronounced when the survivor believes that he has *responsibility* for the death of another in some way. This again accounts for the severe distress felt by parents who most likely will feel responsible for the death of a child.

In addition, grief reactions conform to *cultural expectations*. It is very difficult to know how different families expect their members to grieve but these expectations can lead to compliance or to guilt if one does not comply.

Reviewing these factors may alert the nurse to the possibility that many of them can exist at once. It is not always possible for the one observing the grief reaction of another to be completely aware of the meaning of the loss. In addition, the grieving individual is the only one who really knows how much grief he feels. However, an awareness of these factors can help the nurse to anticipate to some degree the severity of the grief reaction which may occur.

## Chronic Sorrow

Prolonged grieving can occur in some situations when an individual suffers a partial loss which lasts over a period of time. The classic example of this concerns the birth of a defective child. In this situation it is proposed that the parents mourn the loss of the perfect child they did not produce and continue to feel sorrow until the defective child dies. Obviously, chronic sorrow can last for years. The parents in this example must not only cope with their sorrow over their loss but also must attempt to raise and relate to the child who continuously reminds them of their sorrow.[27] It is believed to be possible for the family to reach some degree of awareness or restitution which allows them to accept and relate normally to the child.[34] Unresolved and recurrent mourning can occur in other partial losses in addition.

## Pathologic Mourning

In some situations the grief process does not follow the favorable course, grieving is not complete, and the ties with the lost person are not severed.[25] Difficulties with the grieving process can arise at any stage. In a sense, the bereaved cannot then maintain a normal life because he has not freed himself from the deceased.[3]

Several symptoms of pathologic mourning have been described. First of all, an individual may persist in denying that the loss occurred.[8] Or, an individual may acknowledge the loss but deny the significance.[8] Another reaction is the development of symptoms of a disease which afflicted the one who died. Development of a psychosomatic disorder, such as asthma or ulcerative colitis, is another possibility. Some adverse reactions result in social isolation or activities which in reality serve to punish the griever and subconsciously reduce his guilt such as squandering his life savings. Persistent hostility towards someone who is felt to have harmed the deceased is another maladaptive response. Other neurotic and psychotic reactions are possible. Occasionally pathologic mourning takes the form of expecting another individual to take the place of the lost object. These reactions are the remnants of unsuccessful efforts to avoid grief expression.[28] Pathologic mourning is characterized predominantly by feelings of emptiness and numbness rather than pain and loneliness.[25,35]

Maladaptive grief is not synonymous with intense grief but rather represents normal symptoms manifested in excessive intensity. Thus, the line between normal intense mourning and pathologic mourning is indistinct.

Some suggestions have been made about who is likely to experience pathologic mourning. Isolated families without familial or community ties seem most prone.[32] It may be that maladaptation responses by the informal leaders of a family or a group predispose the members of the group to similar maladaptation.

## Delayed Mourning

In a few situations the grief reaction does not occur within the usual span of time but is delayed. This sometimes occurs when an individual busies himself supporting others and with details so that he represses his own grief. This repressed grief may be activated later when another loss occurs or may emerge spontaneously. Because individuals differ in regard to how much they will allow themselves to experience emotional states and openly grieve, the amount of attempt to repress grief will vary. It has been noted that males and the elderly frequently experience delayed mourning.

## GRIEVING AND THE LIFE CYCLE

Some generalizations about how an individual views death and grieves can be gained from looking at the typical characteristics of an individual at various points on the life cycle. Of course, in addition, one's attitudes about death are influenced by one's previous experiences, intelligence, personality, family relationships, religious training, and so forth.[15]

## Children Under Three

The child under three is very affected by the death of individuals who are significant to him and to whom he is attached. After an infant is attached to his mother, her death especially can have extreme consequences. His reaction to death is similar to his reaction to any separation which is how death appears to him.

The young child is very prone to develop pathologic mourning because he passes through the grieving process very quickly and detaches from the lost object prematurely without fully expressing his emotions and awareness of the loss. Especially, he may not fully express his anger at the lost object.[5]

## Preschoolers

Between three and five the child becomes more curious about death as he discovers dead animals or witnesses someone being "killed" on television. Immobility is associated with death so that in his play the one who is shot lies down and "plays dead" for a period of time and then resumes play. He may feel that there are many variations in being dead such as "sort of dead" and "really dead."[23] His views of what causes death are very egocentric and often magical.[22] Therefore, he may attribute death to "stepping on a toadstool." He feels that death is reversible like being asleep and then being awake.

> A 5-year-old boy watched his kitten being buried after it was hit by a car. His mother and father explained about the kitten's death in terms they thought he would understand. A few days later he asked his mother if they could dig up the kitty so he could play with her again.

Between three and five the child reacts to the death of a significant other as the loss of a love object. He may expect the object to return, or believes the dead person is at some other place such as at work.

The child of this age mourns in a fashion somewhat similar to that of adults. This reaction to separation was first noted in children separated from their mothers by hospitalization.[5] At first after a separation, the child engages in a period of *protest*. This is analogous to the stage of shock and disbelief. He fully expects the lost person to return and angrily demands the same. This is a stage of scolding the lost person. The child probably expects reunion more than the adult in this stage because his grip on the reality of the situation is less. Next the child enters a period of *despair* which is analogous to the stage of developing awareness. He is despondent and unresponsive as he mourns for the lost love object. Eventually the child experiences *detachment* which corresponds to restitution. He can think of the lost person with less pain although he may occasionally return to despair.

The child passes through these stages much more quickly than an adult and has difficulty in mourning for any length of time.[16] This may perplex the adults in his world who wonder why he is not as despondent as consistently as they are.

It is proposed that the preschooler may have death wishes towards others such as siblings or parents and his guilt may be unbearable if death does occur to one of these people because he may believe he caused the death.[4] The preschooler does mourn more effectively than the younger child so he recovers with less probability of pathologic mourning.

## School-aged Children

During his early school years the child learns that death is irreversible and the difference between things that are alive and things that are dead. He believes that violence is the most likely cause of death.[13] When pressed for a specific cause of death he will likely cite objects such as "guns," "dope," or "poison."[22] By 12 his answers will be more conceptual such as "illness," "accidents," or "old age."[22] The school-aged child will usually view death as synonymous with mutilation and injury.[4]

At the beginning of this period the child may believe that he is immune to death but by 8 or 9 years of age he comes to the gradual realization that he too can die. Death is frequently personified,[23] perhaps as a bogey man, and superstitions about cemeteries, caskets, funeral homes, and ghosts abound. As the child reaches the preteen years he begins to see death as not only irreversible but also as inevitable. He may express his fears of death in morbid stories and jokes which give him an impression of mastering death.[2] Superstitious behavior may be used to sublimate his intrigue with death.[15]

The school-aged child mourns more effectively than the younger child. He may be inhibited in expressing his emotions. He easily feels guilt over the death of a loved one. His natural curiosity about death may lead him to talk and behave inappropriately in the opinion of adults. In addition, he will recover more quickly than an adult due to his ability to more easily substitute love objects.

## Adolescents

The teenager has an almost mature conception of death. He is aware that death is inevitable and he is especially impressed that death is so unpredictable. The teenager may handle his fears of death by behaviors which deny death. Examples of this risk taking include driving at high speeds, drug abuse, taking dares, and smoking. The ability to laugh off his own mortality may help him to master his real fear that he too is mortal.[13]

The adolescent mourns much as an adult except that he reaches resolution more quickly.

## Adults

There is, of course, no accurate picture of how all adults feel about death. Many believe that basically adults in our culture are very afraid of death and that death is one of the greatest fears man has if not the greatest fear. How the adult views death is dependent on many variables.

Age is one consideration. The average person in his 20s or 30s is usually seldom touched by death. By his 40s, the death of one or both parents becomes more probable. The man in his 40s may be startled and frightened by the unexpected death of a friend his same age. The woman in her 40s may have a friend who has a malignancy. Death suddenly becomes more present and for many more fearful as they realize that it could happen to them.

As the individual passes through his 50s, both parents may have died as well as an older brother or sister. Death may be a more familiar experience and possibly less frightening.

Waning health and an aging body remind the individual that he is certainly not going to live forever. Planning for retirement is in a sense planning where and how to live the last of one's days. Death is still feared but it is less deniable. When retirement occurs and the 60s and 70s are reached and friends gradually die, one is continually reminded that he is old and near death.

In addition to age, one's previous experiences with death can be important. Previous experiences can contribute positively or negatively. Parents losing a child may benefit to the extent that they change some of their life priorities and learn to enjoy the fleeting time one is alive more fully. Other parents may have been left with bitterness and emptiness and a view of life as unjust and unfair. Thus, the previous experiences an individual has had need to be examined in terms of their influences on his perspective on death and his familiarity with death.

Death comes to be represented in different ways for adults. Some may see death as a curse, others as a fulfillment, still others as a punishment for misdeeds. How one views death is usually reflective of one's view of life.

## Older Adults

Older adults view death from varied perspectives. It is unjustified to believe that all older individuals are comfortable with death. It is possible that because of myths about how the elderly view death they are not expected or allowed to grieve appropriately over losses. It is probable that older adults will grieve more than a younger adult over a similar loss.

It has been suggested that the older adult is likely to experience delayed mourning so that he grieves later for a loss which he accepted stoically at the time. Those around him may not recognize his distress as grief.[6]

It may be that the elderly person is more likely to experience losses only partially and thus develop chronic grief responses.[14] If he appears angry and irritable, others may incorrectly assume that his behavior is evidence of senility and avoid helping him to grieve.

Lastly, the older adult may manifest his grief through somatic symptoms which may again be seen as something other than symptoms of grief.

For all these reasons, the older adult may need help in realizing his losses and support through a helping relationship to work through the grieving process.[6]

# NURSING INTERVENTION IN GRIEVING

## Primary Prevention

Because the grieving process is a healthy response to a loss, the nurse should not attempt to prevent grieving. Rather primary preventive efforts can focus on facilitating healthy attitudes about death and grieving among the individuals she works with and society in general.

First of all, the nurse should do what she can to produce attitudes conducive to acceptance of death as a natural and inevitable event in life in those she has contact with. A good place to start is with children. Parents may not ask about death education until a death has occurred in the family. The nurse may want to talk to families she works with about death education before a death occurs.

Initially, the nurse should encourage parents to explore their attitudes and beliefs about death. It is helpful to discuss with them how they learned about death. Understandably, many parents will have difficulty discussing death and may not wish to discuss the subject with their children. They should realize that avoidance of the subject can teach the child fear and leads to fantasies.[19] Some parents may be able to recognize that it is easiest to teach their child about death when it can be approached casually and in a nonemotionally threatening situation first. They may also see the merits in teaching their children about death themselves as opposed to letting them learn about death from television, snatches of adult conversation, or from older children.

If parents do want help the nurse might offer the following suggestions based on the advice of individuals in this field.[11,16,22] First, it seems advisable to reduce attempts to avoid the subject of death in normal living. For example, parents might be tempted to quickly remove a dead bird from the yard before a child can see it but this would deprive the parents and child of a natural and casual opportunity to discuss death. Similarly, parents may avoid stories or prayers which speak of death although these might logically serve to familiarize the child with death in a natural way. Too, parents can refrain from trying to soften the word death by use of terms such as "passed away." These terms can confuse the child and lead to misconceptions.

Next, the parents can use specific planned situations to explain about death such as plants dying of frost or a dead bug on the sidewalk. The child will probably want to know details little by little such as what is death, why do things die, what happens when things die, and will he ever die. Parents should answer these questions as matter-of-factly as possible, calmly, and without evasive statements.[16] Parents do not have to offer definitive answers but should admit their uncertainty about some things, suggesting, "No one really knows. What do you think?" Encouraging reflection and consideration of alternatives is necessary. Some questions the child asks may have a hidden meaning. When he asks, "Why do birds have to die" he may also wonder if he will have to die. General discussions about the differences between living and nonliving things can help too. And children can learn about the grieving process and write notes to people who have had a loss.[22]

Parents may need help in explaining death to children when a death has occurred. Some statements parents could make when someone dies can cause conflicts or confusion for the child and are best avoided even though the parents themselves heard them and they are commonly used. For example, telling the child that "Aunt Helen is sleeping" or has "gone to eternal rest" may lead the child to persist in denying the death or could possibly make the child afraid of going to sleep. Telling fairy tales or glamorizing death is sometimes tempting but the story will have to be later unlearned and the child may later feel the parent was dishonest. For example, one child was told, "Your little baby sister has been taken to heaven to be an angel. She can now fly around with golden wings." The child may feel jealous that he did not get to go too and he may literally believe the story which must later be rejected.

Another commonly used statement contains the philosophy, "Daddy was such a wonderful person that God wanted him to come live in heaven with Him." The child may wonder if he should try to be good any more because he does not want to die. Mother must not have been wonderful because she is still alive. He probably also wonders how his father got to heaven when he saw him buried in the ground.

Statements which stress the joy of death such as, "We are celebrating because your grandmother has gone to heaven and we are all glad that now she is in peace" communicate to the child double messages. He should be glad but he feels sad. And why are so many people crying if death is so joyous?

It is also unwise to tell a very young child that someone died because of illness. He may be afraid that he will die the next time he is ill. This approach also encourages the child to equate illness with punishment. In general, death should not be linked with sin and punishment. The older child will be able to understand the difference between being ill and being very ill. Other evasive statements which are in essence half truths are, "He has gone on a long journey" and "He has gone to do God's work."

What can parents say? It is best to stick to truths such as, "Grandfather has died. He will not be with us anymore. His body will be put in a special box and buried in the ground. Even though Grandfather is gone we can still remember him in our hearts." The parents may be guided by remembering to not tell their child anything they themselves would not accept and thus avoid trying to "pretty up" death for children.

Maybe the real problem with using well known cliches with the child is that they prevent a chance for honest discussions of the meaning of death. The cliches may become meaningless when the child matures. An honest discussion with the child will be more difficult so the parents may want to read more on the subject. There are books for children which the family can read together which discuss death. It has also been suggested that pets can be used effectively to teach the child about death and grief.

In addition to helping parents with death education, the nurse may be able to promote death education content in preschool, elementary, junior, and senior high schools and in adult groups. Such content could focus on historical, philosophical, and religious perspectives related to death and the grieving process. Sometimes older students wish to visit mortuaries and plan and conduct a mock funeral.

The nurse can make it a point to help families talk about death whenever the opportunity arises. All of these activities help to desensitize death so that the participants can think more clearly about life and death with less fear.

Another primary prevention activity is related to promoting healthy attitudes about grieving among adults and children. Our society seems prone to deny the necessity of grieving. Individuals who are grieving often feel great pressure to "cope" quickly, bear up in public at least, and return to living unaffected. These attitudes often cause difficulty for the one who is grieving because he finds it impossible to live up to these expectations. In addition, he feels isolated from and unsupported by others around him who act as if they cannot personally tolerate his continuing grief.

Primary prevention actions are summarized in Table 9-1.

**Table 9-1.** Possible nursing actions to promote healthy attitudes towards death and grieving

1. Teach parents how to help their children learn about death as a natural and inevitable part of life.
2. Promote death education discussion groups in schools and elsewhere.
3. Promote healthy attitudes about grieving and the grieving process.

## Secondary Prevention

Secondary prevention concerns working with the individual or family that is grieving.

There are many situations where the nurse has contact with an individual or family that is faced with an unexpected loss. In these situations the actions of the nurse can help the individuals involved to grieve in a healthy way. It is important to remember, especially when the death has been unexpected and unsettling, that the goal of nursing intervention is not to abort or subdue grieving but to foster an appropriate and healthy grieving process.[33]

If the nurse is present before the actual loss occurs, she can help the family to anticipate what the loss might mean.

> Jerry and Joyce had given birth to a very small premature baby whose condition was growing worse with every passing hour. The neonatologist had discussed the baby's situation with the parents at length and they knew he had no chance of survival. The nurse in the intensive care unit sat down with the parents and helped them to discuss their feelings about the premature birth and what the loss of this baby would mean to them. The baby died less than a day later.

When the family is in the stage of shock and disbelief the nurse may be tempted to request and administer sedatives. While this may give the illusion of calming family members, some feel that sedation at this time can produce a sense of unreality and possibly interfere with the grieving process.[30,35]

The family at this time needs privacy which the nurse can provide. They may need permission to express themselves. Many families desire to see the body of the one who has died and this is usually advisable. The nurse should prepare them for the appearance of the body and especially for the possibility of rigidity and coldness of the body. The body can be treated with respect by the nurse and prepared for the family as positively as possible. For example, a stillborn can be wrapped in a soft blanket. Viewing the body represents reality and helps dispel denial of the loss.[35]

Because the family is in a state of shock it is important to guide them through what needs to be done. It seems important for family members to be allowed to stay together at this time. If the family was not present when the individual died, they may appreciate being told how he died by someone who was with him. If realistic and truthful, they appreciate knowing that the deceased was calm and free from pain. The family should be asked if they would like to see a chaplain or have another person from a particular religious denomination contact them.

As the family gains awareness of the death, the nurse should provide for frequent contact. Even "close" families need an outside presence to express their thoughts to. Many people are helped by having the grieving process and the manifestations of grieving explained to them. It may help them to be told that what they are experiencing is normal, that it will someday end, and they will be able to return to an enjoyable life. They may especially appreciate knowing that it is natural to experience guilt and anger at the one who has died, feel hostile towards others, and experience a desire to be left alone. It may be helpful to prepare them for fantasies of being in the presence of the deceased. Not everyone in the family will reach the same stage at the same time.[21] Many individuals have commented that some of the symptoms of the grieving process have led them to believe that they were going insane.

Most important, the nurse can help with the individual's overwhelming and relentless feelings of guilt, anger, hostility, and depression by listening and accepting them as the individual does his difficult grief work. She should avoid platitudes and instead seek to develop empathy.[26] The nurse can help the family if she listens as they go over their memories of the deceased and the relationship and recount the losses they have suffered.[25] She should remember that the initial memories may be idealistic. Short but frequent visits may be best.

The circumstances surrounding the individual's death are important for the nurse to know as this information may help her to understand the grieving process.

Mrs. Jones was a 57-year-old widow whose son was shot and fatally injured by the police when he was apprehended during an armed robbery attempt at a liquor store. He had just returned from the Army two days before and it was later revealed that he was suspected of being chemically addicted and had planned the robbery to obtain money for drugs. Mrs. Jones' grief was mixed with anger at her dead son for bringing shame and publicity to her family, guilt related to her sense of failure in raising her son without a father, and generalized hostility that she had suffered so much in losing her husband and son. The nurse helped Mrs. Jones to express and cope with these emotions but she grieved for an unusually long time and remained frequently depressed afterwards.

Mrs. Smith was a 57-year-old widow whose son was killed while serving as a missionary in a remote part of Central America. Mrs. Smith felt proud of her son's life and death which received notice in the newspapers and among church leaders. She was honored and supported by the community in her grief. She grieved deeply but in a period of a few months was back to her normal life.

Obviously the role of the nurse in these two situations would be very different with different goals.

If the deceased individual died in the hospital, some individuals may like to return to visit after a few months. This visit can help them to work through painful memories and may provide reassurance that they are remembered.[17] Contrary to lay belief, bringing up the subject of death again is not opening up healed wounds and the nurse may find it often useful in helping the family reach a new level of resolution.

Most families find it important to know why the death occurred if the reason is not obvious to them. They may appreciate hearing the coroner's report or the autopsy reports. In some situations where this is not done the family may develop less satisfactory coping and they may become convinced of their own private rationale for the death.[17] Having a readily identifiable reason for the death can be as simple as, "His lungs were too immature to work properly and he finally wore out from the effort of breathing." Recently it has been suggested that the parents whose infant dies of crib death will cope better if they are given the diagnosis of Sudden Infant Death Syndrome as an identifiable concrete condition. This is easier for them to explain to themselves and others than "No one knows how the baby died."

Those who are mourning have an increased risk of death themselves especially in the first year after the death of a spouse.[29] The nurse should be alert to this possibility and take measures to help insure the survivor's health.

Many families will have to continue to relive over and over the patient's life and last days. They may dwell on condolences they received such as the unhelpful remark, "When God reads someone's name in His book there is nothing you can do." The nurse should recognize these instances of anger and hostility as expression of normal emotions in the grieving process and not take a defensive attitude.

Some individuals may become overprotective of those around them in an attempt to ward off future losses.[24] They need help realizing that this is occurring and that it can be self-defeating.

The individual who has spent considerable time caring for a fatally ill family member may need help reentering the family which has become functional without him.[24] Communication patterns which have broken down should be reestablished.[24] In addition, changes in family goals and relationships due to the absence of the one who died may need to be discussed.

The individual who is less able to express his emotions openly and fears loss of control will have more difficulty completing his grieving process.[4] This is often more true of men than women.

## WHEN A CHILD IS GRIEVING

Parents and others may need to be reminded that children grieve too and need some support when they have suffered a loss. The common assumption that "he'll get over it" may not be true. The child needs specific help with each stage. During shock and disbelief, the child should be gently faced with the reality of the situation to counteract his abilities to fantasize that the death has not occurred. Involvement in the planning stages and actual funeral and burial may be appropriate if the child desires. In addition, the parents should avoid forcing the child into denial of the loss that has occurred. He should not be told for example, "Don't cry, we'll get you another puppy." He should instead be allowed to accept the loss without a substitute until resolution has occurred.

During the stage of developing awareness, it is good to help the child with his grief work by encouraging him to recall the memories of the one who has died and assure him that these memories will always be with him. It is sometimes comforting for the child to realize that the ones who live thereby keep a little part of the one who has died. Parents should be alert to the possibility that the child will feel a need to attempt to fulfill the role of the one who has died and adopt his behaviors. The parents can gently discourage any excessive amounts of this behavior and assure the child that they want him to remain himself.

It is important to allow the child to express his feelings during this stage and to not be made ashamed of how he feels. "It's all right to feel sad and to cry when you think of grandmother. I miss her too." The child who sees his parents grieve is assured that what he is feeling is natural. Thus parents should avoid any attempt to hold back their grief "for the sake of the children." The sometimes used phase "We must be brave now and go on with life as Daddy would have wanted us to" stifles grief and denies loss.

Children often feel guilt for a death even though, to the adults, it seems ridiculous. A word of assurance that nothing one did or did not do caused the death is in order. When a sibling of the child has died he may feel guilty that he was not the one to die instead.[20] The parents can assure the child of their love and their joy that he is alive.

The child can be helped to realize that his anger and irritability at others including the deceased is acceptable and can be dealt with in ways that will not hurt others. He may need to know that he may feel the one who has died is present from time to time and to discuss this with his parents when it happens.

When the child is unprepared for death and poorly supported, serious difficulties can occur.

When Jane was 6 her parents explained to her that they were going to have a baby. Jane wasn't at all pleased with the news and openly stated that she didn't want a brother or sister. When her mother was in her sixth month she went into premature labor and the baby died at birth. Jane was staying with her aunt who explained to her that her baby brother had gone to heaven to be with Jesus and was growing in heaven as a beautiful flower. As other relatives gathered, they cried openly and hugged her so tightly she thought she couldn't breathe. Her parents were moody and depressed and paid little attention to her. Everyone talked incessantly about the baby and frequently she heard, "If only it hadn't been a boy." Jane was so angry that all this fuss was about some little brother who had upstaged her even in death. She decided she never would go to heaven because she certainly didn't want to be with her brother. On the afternoon of the burial, she ran through her mother's flower gardens and stomped every plant to the ground. Her behavior became almost uncontrollable after that. Her confused parents retaliated with more harsh punishment to no avail. It was over a year before the parents sought help and steps were taken to help Jane work through her anger.

If the parents are temporarily not capable of helping their child grieve, the nurse must provide extra support herself or through appropriate referrals.

As the family reaches the stage of restitution, they may need permission to again enjoy themselves without feeling disloyal to the deceased. Holidays and the deceased's birthday may lead to a reactivation of the pain and sorrow believed to be conquered previously.[24] The grieving person may feel dispair as he wonders how long his grief will last and if he will ever enjoy life again.

Some individuals may need the nurse's help in returning to an external focus after their months of self-absorption. They must eventually visualize a future life without the deceased. There are many groups with special purposes which may help. Parents who have lost a child may find a parent group useful.[1] Parents in these groups often state that they benefit by learning that others have lived through and survived what they have encountered. Widows or widowers may benefit from an appropriate group such as Parents Without Partners. Many individuals who have been through a loss report that one of the best ways to recover was by becoming involved in helping someone else who is going through what they just did.

This information on intervening to promote grieving responses is summarized in Table 9-2.

**Table 9-2.** Possible nursing actions to promote healthy and complete grieving

1. Help prepare individuals for loss if possible.
2. Avoid actions which subdue or abort expressions of grief.
3. Provide privacy.
4. Promote the expression of grief reactions.
5. Promote reality by allowing access to the deceased person's body.
6. Guide survivors through necessary business.
7. Keep family together.
8. Provide information about the deceased's last moments.
9. Provide for a continuing contact with another helping person.
10. Instill hope that grieving will eventually lead to an enjoyable life.
11. Explain grieving process and manifestations.
12. Listen and help individual do grief work.
13. Learn about circumstances surrounding death and how these affect the perceptions and grieving of the survivor.
14. Consider a visit to the hospital if appropriate for the one who is grieving.
15. Discuss the cause of death concretely.
16. Accept hostility and anger.
17. Caution against the development of overprotective tendencies.
18. Help families restructure goals and relationships and reintegrate family members.
19. Teach parents to help their children grieve or provide outside support.
20. Give family permission to enjoy life again without guilt.
21. Help development of outside interests.

## Tertiary Prevention

When the nurse encounters grief reactions which she feels are not progressing appropriately or reactions which appear chronic, delayed, or pathologic, she can assess thoroughly and collect careful details of her perceptions and refer the patient to an appropriate source. She may be able to continue to work with the family or individual with suggestions and support from others.

## THE NURSE AND GRIEF

Before the nurse will be able to greatly help grieving individuals, she should make a planned effort to get in touch with her feelings about death. At first she will find that it is difficult to think even for a few minutes about her own mortality without finding herself feeling anxious and thinking about something else. The following suggestions are designed to help in a systematic attempt to encourage reflection about death and thereby remove some of the fear associated with it.

First of all, the nurse might find it useful to reflect on what she was taught about death as a child and how this has affected her views. What things does she still believe to be true and what things does she now believe to be untrue?

Later the nurse should assess her beliefs about death. Why must individuals die? What causes death? What happens to people after they die?

Next, the nurse can recall if anyone close to her has died and remember the experience. How did she grieve? What reactions did she go through? What things happened which were helpful and what things were not?

Eventually, the nurse can consider how she would feel if specific people close to her were to die. She should reflect on how she would feel, how she would cope, and how realistic is it to pretend that those close to her will never die.

Finally, the nurse can reflect on her own death. How would she want to die? Would she want to know if she had a fatal illness? How would she choose to live the last day, week, month, or year?[12] What would she want others to feel? How would she want her body taken care of? How would the world be without her? What would she like others to say about her after she had died?

Discussion groups can sometimes be useful in examining one's view of death although anxiety in the group will often be initially high and the group may discuss safer topics such as ethical questions in the beginning. It may be useful to write down one's thoughts about death which can be reviewed from time to time so that one sees progress in facing the inevitability of death.

It has been suggested that individuals with a high degree of death anxiety may be attracted to the health care fields.[9] This may be because they subconsciously believe that as health care professionals they may become immune to death. The nurse can ponder her reasons for choosing to enter nursing and search for evidences of this attitude. While these exercises may seem morbid, it is believed that each time one reflects on one's own death, it becomes less frightening. What is desired is for the nurse to recognize death as a natural and inevitable part of life—even her life. She can stop hoping she will live forever because she will not. She can start learning to live with the knowledge of her own mortality so that her dying will be less cause for alarm and regret. It has been proposed that everyone would lead a much different life if they stopped to remember each day that they were dying.

Once the nurse has conquered some of her own death anxiety, she will be more effective at helping others who are grieving over the death of a loved one. She will then be less likely to avoid the grieving individual because the situation reminds her of her own mortality.

Not only must the nurse face her own mortality but she should learn how she grieves over losses. She can decide what losses she has faced and how she reacted to them. She may be able to learn in which situations her grieving responses have been facilitated or inhibited. She can learn how to seek help in fully grieving when she is faced with a loss.

Similarly, the nurse can analyze how she responds when those she works with are grieving. The nurse who works with the grieving individual or family may find her work with them to be very difficult. As the individual experiences each devastating emotion, the nurse may react with a similar emotion. She should be prepared for hostility which the individual may occasionally direct at her even though he needs her support. She may find herself discouraged about the individual's progress as he becomes repeatedly bogged down in his despair. She may be agitated because she views his situation as an outsider and sees opportunities and reasons for hope which he does not. She may find his bouts of self-pity mixed with idealization of the deceased unrealistic and futile.

To make matters worse, she cannot help but be exasperated by her own helplessness in the situation. She cannot offer magical words or heal the pain with medications or medical treatments. She must accept her role as one of striving to empathize completely with the one who is grieving and experience his world as if she were in it as she allows him to do his grief work. She must realize that only the one who grieves alone can remedy his situation. The time he needs is extensive and the anguish he will go through and communicate to the nurse may seem unrelenting. She can reflect on these questions.

Can she cope with her own helplessness?
Is she able to accept and tolerate another's grief.
Does she become overwhelmed herself?
Is she unable to relate to some grief reactions over certain types of losses?

Each nurse must learn ways to seek personal support when she works with individuals and families who are grieving because it is often a personally threatening and emotionally draining experience.

## A TOOL FOR ASSESSMENT AND EVALUATION

The information in Table 9-3 can be used to help the nurse assess the risk involved for individuals who are grieving. Those whose behaviors are predominantly less optimal are at high risk of unsuccessful grieving.

The nurse can also use this information to evaluate the response of the grieving individual to her nursing interventions. The individual should evidence more optimal behaviors predominantly with time if he is progressing normally in the grieving process.

## AN EXAMPLE OF NURSING INTERVENTION IN GRIEF

The following example illustrates how a nurse helped a family cope with an unexpected death as she coped with her own reactions.

Joan, a community health nurse, had been visiting the Martinez home for several years. Four-year-old Julie Martinez had cerebral dysfunction and the visits were to help the family provide the most optimal environment possible for Julie. Joan enjoyed her visits with the family. Julie was lovingly cared for although her care required considerable time from both parents. Julie's mother and father seemed accepting of her limitations and she was regularly taken to the clinic. Julie's older sister, Jody, was a bubbly and very intelligent first grader.

**Table 9-3.** Assessment and evaluation of grief

| Behavior | Less optimal | More optimal |
|---|---|---|
| Use of denial | Continued frequent denial of death or the significance of the loss | Initially high but diminishing with time |
| Crying | Unable to cry or express sadness | Frequent crying |
| Psychic manifestations | Emptiness or numbness | Pain and loneliness diminishing with time |
| Guilt | Persistent and extended | Initially high but diminishing with time |
| Hostility and anger | Focused on one or a few individuals and persistent | Sporadic, diffuse, and diminishing |
| Disengagement from usual activities | Extended apathy | Increases activities gradually |
| Possessions of the deceased | Kept intact | Gradually disposed of or reallocated |
| Development of other reactions | Appearance of insomnia, anorexia, depression, morbid preoccupations, or illness of the deceased | Minimal |
| Adoption of behaviors and ideals of the deceased | Total preoccupation and change in behavior | Minimal |
| Idealization of deceased | Unceasing | Diminishing with time |
| Feelings toward self | Negative self-concept | Returning to positive self-concept |

Mr. and Mrs. Martinez were proud of their family and, although money was not abundant for them, they provided for their daughters a pleasant and enriched environment filled with harmony and love. Mr. and Mrs. Martinez were especially pleased to discover that Mrs. Martinez was pregnant and thrilled when they soon discovered that they were to have twins. Mrs. Martinez was very receptive to Joan's prenatal teaching and the pregnancy progressed normally.

Joan was surprised one morning to find a note on her desk taken from Mr. Martinez who had called to inform her that Mrs. Martinez had gone into labor unexpectedly, lost the babies, and was at the University Hospital. Joan was able to stop at the hospital around noon. She found out at the nurses' station that Mrs. Martinez had delivered two very small male infants who had both died immediately.

Before going to Mrs. Martinez's room, Joan stopped to collect her thoughts. She felt very sorry for the Martinez family and she knew that seeing Mrs. Martinez would be very difficult for her. She realized that the main thing she could do for Mrs. Martinez was to listen if she wanted to talk about what had happened and to facilitate her grieving processes.

Joan was at first surprised at Mrs. Martinez's appearance. She had never seen her looking so haggard and unkempt. Her usually bright and shining eyes were red and swollen. Mrs. Martinez smiled thinly when Joan entered and asked her to sit down. Joan felt almost unable to speak as she became more aware of the meaning of the situation to Mrs. Martinez. She sat down and said nothing.

Mrs. Martinez asked if she had heard about the babies. Joan nodded. Mrs. Martinez began to cry softly and commented that she never knew anyone could cry for hours. Joan felt overwhelmed and helpless. She felt compelled to offer comforting words but she sat silently. Mrs. Martinez started talking about the events leading up to the delivery and Joan found it easier to ask questions and pursue that topic. Mrs. Martinez had thought the babies would be bigger than they were and expected that they would live. She was angry that no one told her that they would be too little to live. She had wanted to see them and touch them but no one responded to her request although she asked repeatedly. She wanted to be with her husband when he was told that they were dead but she was not. She expressed other complaints at the personnel and physicians.

After a while, she expressed bitterness and recounted all of life's slights she and her husband had received. Joan listened and tried to maintain eye contact. After what seemed to Joan like hours, Mrs. Martinez began to talk less and her tone grew less angry. Joan asked how Mr. Martinez and the girls were taking the news. Mrs. Martinez talked about how sorry she felt for him to lose two sons and she expressed guilt over not being able to give him a boy. She said the girls were both very sad and were being taken care of by her mother. Joan asked about plans for the burial and Mrs. Martinez explained what was to happen.

Joan tried to tell Mrs. Martinez how sorry she was about what had happened. Her words seemed trite and meaningless in the face of Mrs. Martinez's loss. She asked how she was recovering physically from the delivery which was apparently good. Joan asked if she would like her to pay a visit after she went home and Mrs. Martinez asked her to come soon with tears in her eyes. As Joan left she walked from Mrs. Martinez's room past the nursery and saw two proud mothers peeking in the windows of the nursery and laughing at their babies. In her car she sat overwhelmed with feelings of sadness. She knew that she needed to discuss how she was feeling with her supervisor before she could begin planning to help the Martinez family with their grieving.

The goals which she eventually established for the family were to: (1) give each family member opportunities to verbalize about the loss, (2) assess and support each member's grieving process, and (3) explain the grieving process to the family.

Joan next went to visit the family on the evening of the first day Mrs. Martinez had come home from the hospital. Jody and Julie were out for a walk with their grandmother. After talking with Mr. and Mrs. Martinez, she felt that they were grieving appropriately. Mrs. Martinez was still expressing considerable anger at the hospital staff for various actions although Joan noticed that Mrs. Martinez seemed less bitter when she talked than she had seemed in the hospital. Both were able to talk about the loss and how sad they felt. Mr. Martinez expressed surprise at how badly he felt about two babies he had never seen and added that many people did not understand the pain of losing a baby. Joan explored this and discovered that he was upset because his employer was allowing him to take off only the afternoon of the burial from work.

Joan explained the grieving process to them and they both nodded as she mentioned the bodily sensations and typical feelings. She prepared them for other troubling emotions such as the desire to be left alone and the possibility that Mrs. Martinez might imagine that she was still feeling fetal movements. She asked them to describe how Jody and Julie were reacting. From the report of the parents they were both openly expressing their sadness at times and being supported by their parents. Joan explained how children of their ages usually view death and cope with grief. Neither parent had thought that the girls might feel guilt over the deaths of the babies and they agreed to casually bring up the idea that no one had caused the babies to die just in case.

The burial was to be the next day and there would be a large family gathering. It appeared that Mr. and Mrs. Martinez were both receiving considerable help and support from their families which they accepted as a matter of course.

Just before Joan started to leave, the grandmother and Jody and Julie returned home. The grandmother was dressed in black and had taken over child and home management completely. Joan decided after talking to her that this was her way of coping with the situation. The girls seemed overly excitable and anxious. Joan felt that this was due to the tensions in their parents along with the presence of their grandmother. They both talked freely about their baby brothers who had died and how they were going to wear their best dresses tomorrow. Joan believed that this reaction of the children seemed appropriate for their ages.

After leaving, Joan called the school nurses at Jody's school and the rehabilitation center where Julie attended nursery school, and the industrial nurse where Mr. Martinez worked to alert them to the fact that there had been a death in the family.

Joan's next visit was a week later near time for school to be out so she could talk to Mrs. Martinez alone and then see the girls. Mrs. Martinez stated that she was very depressed. She had just received a bill for "extras"nassociated with the delivery and hospitalization that were not included in the clinic fee and was concerned about how they were going to ever pay it. Mr. Martinez earned just enough money to prevent them from receiving any extra aid for Julie's health care but barely enough to meet normal expenses. Mrs. Martinez stated that she was tired and discouraged over the future. She described Mr. Martinez as very irritable. His employer was complaining about his work and he was worried about losing his job. Joan suggested that Mrs. Martinez's discouragement and Mr. Martinez's irritability might still be related to their responses to loss of the babies. Mrs. Martinez seemed hopeful that this was indeed true. Mrs. Martinez also thought the bleak long winter was depressing too. She stated that she cried over any slight insult from her children or husband and was angry and demanding toward the girls for little reason. She was unable to keep up with the housework. Joan reassured her that she would slowly feel more energy and less anger towards others. Mrs. Martinez was considering getting a part time job until spring or summer because she was bored and lonesome and they needed the money. Joan used the problem solving process and they discussed the consequences and possible actions.

Joan asked if Mr. and Mrs. Martinez had discussed the possibility of a future pregnancy. Mrs. Martinez said that they had and that they were not sure how they felt although they both seemed to be hesitating about planning another pregnancy right away. Joan mentioned that it is often best to wait until one is completely over a loss before becoming pregnant again because it is difficult to thoroughly grieve over the past while preparing for another child. Mrs. Martinez seemed to comprehend the idea well and agreed that it made sense. Joan inquired about the availability of birth control measures and found out that they were available.

Mrs. Martinez said that the girls were still talking about their baby brothers who had died and sometimes they pretended that they were alive and were playing with them. She felt uncomfortable when they did so. Joan explained that both of them probably could not yet totally understand the absolute irreversibility of death and suggested that the parents try to talk with them about their brothers occasionally and maybe visit the cemetery again. Mrs. Martinez felt she couldn't go to the cemetery yet but maybe her husband could take them.

Jody came home from school and talked to Joan about her day at school. Joan decided that she was somewhat less enthusiastic than usual and was probably affected by her parents' lack of usual responsiveness. Julie was soon brought home by the van from the rehabilitation center. She looked tired and was very irritable. She was still receiving her exercises and Joan felt her physical care was probably being adequately carried out. Joan decided to watch the girls' behavior and reactions closely through frequent visits to make sure that the present situation was resolved.

Joan found the family gone one week later but at home two weeks later. She came in the evening so she could see the whole family. She found that they had all just cleaned the house from top to bottom and were rewarding themselves with popcorn. The conversation was lively and seemed the usual happy patter Joan associated with the Martinez family. The girls were put to bed after showing Joan the tiny tomato and pepper plants they were starting for their garden in the spring.

Mrs. Martinez had taken a job as a waitress in the mornings and enjoyed her job except that her feet hurt at night. Mr. Martinez teased her that it was because her feet were too big to begin with. Mrs. Martinez said that she now had more "good" days than "bad" days but that the bad days were very painful. Joan asked her what she did on the "bad" days and she stated that she cried a lot which helped. She asked Mr. Martinez how he felt about her frequent crying and he said that he realized she had to cry to get over the loss. He stated that he felt better about losing the babies and tried to keep busy now so he would not have to think about it. They said they still talked about losing the babies sometimes. They had decided to have another baby again but not now. Mrs. Martinez reported that the girls did not get on her nerves as much and that they all felt closer now than they had been although there were times when they both wanted the girls to leave them alone. Joan assured them that this was normal. Mr. Martinez was happier with his job but still didn't like his boss. The entire family had gone to the gravesite after all and Mrs. Martinez was glad that she had gone. The girls had made tissue paper flowers to put on the grave. They rarely pretended to play with their baby brothers now. Joan explained that their play had probably helped them to work through their feelings. Mrs. Martinez was still angry with the clinic and hospital and insisted that she would never go there again. She was not intensely hostile but Joan decided to follow this lest it become an overwhelming theme.

Joan continued to visit the Martinez family periodically and they did recover in about three months. Mrs. Martinez was angry about her hospital stay but she began to add comments of understanding after expressing her anger, such as "They have so many of us at one time I guess they can't do everything the way each of us wants." Joan advised Mr. and Mrs. Martinez to continue to periodically talk to the girls about the deaths because their questions and understanding of the situation would change as their maturation increased. She also told them that they all might expect to have periods of time when they were reminded of the deaths and felt sad all over again. The Martinezes became more active in the neighborhood as the weather was warmer. Joan next planned to talk with them about death education with Julie and Jody since the subject had been brought to the fore.

## SUMMARY

Nurses often have contact with persons who are grieving after the death of someone significant to their lives. The nurse must understand the process grieving individuals go through to separate themselves from the lost person and reestablish a life without him. She should be aware of how individuals in various phases of the life cycle view death, how they typically grieve, and what other factors can influence grieving.

The nurse can organize nursing actions to promote helpful attitudes about death and grief reactions and to help individuals grieve completely and appropriately. The nurse must be aware of her own attitudes about death and learn to become less fearful of death so that she can be of greater service to persons experiencing grief.

# REFERENCES

1. Anglim, M. A.: "Reintegration of the family after the death of a child," in Martinson, I. M. (ed.): *Home Care for the Dying Child*. Appleton-Century-Crofts, New York, 1976.
2. Arnstein, H.: *What to Tell Your Child*. Bobbs-Merrill, Indianapolis, 1960.
3. Benoliel, J. Q.: "Loss," in Clark, A. L., and Affonso, D. D.: *Childbearing: A Nursing Perspective*. F. A. Davis, Philadelphia, 1967.
4. Benoliel, J. Q.: "The terminally ill child," in Scipien, G. M., et al.: *Comprehensive Pediatric Nursing*. McGraw-Hill, New York, 1975.
5. Bowlby, J.: "Childhood mourning and its implications for psychiatry." Am. J. Psychiat. 118:481, 1961.
6. Burnside, I. M.: "Grief work in the aged patient." Nurs. Forum 8:416, 1969.
7. Carlson, C. E.: "Grief," in Carlson, C. E., and Blackwell, B. (eds.): *Behavioral Concepts and Nursing Intervention*. J. B. Lippincott, Philadelphia, 1978.
8. Engel, G. L.: *Psychological Development in Health and Disease*. W. B. Saunders, Philadelphia, 1962.
9. Folta, J. R.: "Perception of death." Nurs. Res. 14:234, 1965.
10. Fond, K. I.: "Dealing with death and dying through family centered care." Nurs. Clin. North Am. 7:53, 1972.
11. Frjiberg, S.: *The Magic Years*. Charles Scribner's Sons, New York, 1959.
12. Francis, G. M., and Munjas, B.: *Promoting Psychological Comfort*. Wm. C. Brown, Dubuque, 1975.
13. Fredlund, D.: "The remaining child," in Martinson, I. M. (ed.): *Home Care for the Dying Child*. Appleton-Century-Crofts, New York, 1976.
14. Gramlich, E.: "Recognition and management of grief in elderly patients." Geriat. 23:87, 1968.
15. Green, M.: "Care of the dying child." Ped. 40:492, 1967.
16. Grollman, E. A. (ed.): "Prologue," in *Expaining Death to Children*. Beacon, Boston, 1967.
17. Gyulay, J. E.: "The forgotten grievers." Am. J. Nurs. 75:1476, 1975.
18. Gyulay, J. E., and Miles, M. S.: "The family with a terminally ill child," in Hymovich, D. P., and Barnard, M. U. (eds.): *Family Health Care*. McGraw-Hill, New York, 1973.
19. Hardgrove, C., and Warrick, L. H.: "How shall we tell the children?" Am. J. Nurs. 74:448, 1974.
20. Kastenbaum, R.: "The kingdom where nobody dies." Sat. Rev. 56:36, 1972.
21. Klepser, M. J.: "How long does grief go on?" Am. J. Nurs. 78:420, 1978.
22. Koocher, G. P.: "Why isn't the gerbil moving anymore: Discussing death in the classroom—and at home." Child. Today 4:18, 1975.
23. Krause, D. M.: "Children's concepts of death," in Martinson, I. M. (ed.): *Home Care for the Dying Child*. Appleton-Century-Crofts, New York, 1976.
24. Levitt, C. J., et al.: "Parent support groups for the grieving parent," in Martinson, I. M. (ed.): *Home Care for the Dying Child*. Appleton-Century-Crofts, New York, 1976.
25. Lindemann, E.: "Symptomatology and management of acute grief." Am. J. Psychiat. 101:141, 1944.
26. McLaughlin, M. F.: "Who helps the living?" Am. J. Nurs. 78:422, 1978.
27. Olshansky, S.: "Chronic sorrow: A response to having a mentally defective child." Soc. Casework 43:190, 1962.
28. Parkes, C. M.: *Bereavement*. International Universities Press, New York, 1972.
29. Peretz, D.: "Reaction to loss," in Schoenberg, B., et al. (eds.): *Loss and Grief: Psychological Management in Medical Practice*. Columbia University Press, New York, 1970.
30. Petrillo, M., and Sanger, S.: *Emotional Care of Hospitalized Children*. J. B. Lippincott, Philadelphia, 1972.
31. Share, L.: "Family communication in the crisis of a childs' fatal illness. A literature review and analysis." Omega 3:187, 1972.
32. Vollman, R. R., et al.: "The reactions of family systems to sudden and unexpected death." Omega 2:101, 1971.
33. Weisman, A. D.: "Coping with untimely death." Psychiat. 36:374, 1973.
34. Young, R. K.: "Chronic sorrow: Parents response to the birth of a child with a defect." Matern.-Child Nurs. J. 2:38, 1977.
35. Zahourek, R., and Jensen, J. S.: "Grieving and the loss of the newborn." Am. J. Nurs. 73:836, 1973.

## BIBLIOGRAPHY

Ammann, A. J.: "Sudden, unexpected, and unexplained death in infancy," in Waechter, E. H., and Blake, F. G.: *Nursing Care of Children.* J. B. Lippincott, Philadelphia, 1976.

Aronson, M. J.: "Emotional aspects of nursing the cancer patient." Ment. Hyg. 42:267, 1958.

Burnside, I. M.: "You will cope, of course. . . ." Am. J. Nurs. 71:2354, 1971.

Crate, M.: "Nursing functions in adaptation to chronic illness." Am. J. Nurs. 65:72, 1965.

Davis, R.: "Psychological aspects of geriatric nursing." Am. J. Nurs. 68:802, 1968.

Geis, D. P.: "Mother's perceptions of care given their dying children." Am. J. Nurs. 65:105, 1965.

Jackson, E. N.: *Telling a Child About Death.* Hawthorn Books, New York, 1965.

Jackson, P. L.: "Chronic grief." Am. J. Nurs. 74:1288, 1974.

Jensen, G., and Wallace, J.: "Family mourning process." Family Process 6:56, 1967.

Kennell, J. H., et al.: "The mourning response of parents to the death of a newborn infant." New Engl. J. Med. 283:344, 1970.

Levin, S.: "Depression in the aged," in Berezin, M. A., and Cath, S. H. (eds.): *Geriatric Psychiatry: Grief, Loss, and Emotional Disorders in the Aging Process.* International Universities Press, New York, 1965.

Mandell, F.: "The tragedy of the sudden infant death syndrome." J. Assoc. Care Child. Hosp. 4:4, 1976.

Miles, H. S., and Hays, D. R.: "Widowhood." Am. J. Nurs. 75:280, 1975.

Mills, G. C.: "Books to help children understand death." Am. J. Nurs. 79:291, 1979.

Nakushian, J.: "Restoring parents equilibrium after sudden infant death." Am. J. Nurs. 76:1600, 1976.

Sheer, B. L.: "Help for parents in a difficult job—Broaching the subject of death." Matern.-Child Nurs. J. 2:320, 1977.

Ujhely, G. B.: "Grief and depression: Implications for prevention and therapeutic nursing care." Nurs. Forum 5:23, 1966.

# CHAPTER 10

# DEPRESSION

Depression probably affects all individuals to some degree at some time in their lives. It is estimated that 5 out of every 100 adults will have an episode of depression serious enough to adversely affect their functioning for a period of time during their lifetime. Nurses and the consumers of nursing care are no exceptions.

Nurses are prone to develop feelings of depression for reasons which will be explored later. Patients and families may develop states of depression because of the alterations in their life style or health status which frequently bring them in contact with the nurse. For these reasons, the nurse needs a working knowledge of the phenomena of depression, how to deal with it in her personal and professional life, and how to assist patients and families to prevent or cope with their feelings of depression. This chapter will focus on assessing and intervening only in the less prolonged and less severe states of depression that are frequently encountered in general health care settings.

## REVIEW OF THEORY

Depression is difficult to define because the term has been used to describe a feeling state, a symptom, a syndrome, a mood disturbance, and an emotional disorder. It is not known whether depression exists as the many manifestations of one basic process or whether it is many different processes. Whatever depression is, it is an uncomfortable emotional and physical experience of remorse, sadness, discouragement, and dejection. It is also very common. Depression often exists as a normal, short lived reaction to adverse situations after one has developed awareness of his situation. For this reason depression can be thought of as a preliminary sign of psychological recovery from a serious problem or a setback because it connotes realization and an attempt to cope.[14] Depression may provide the individual with time to worry and reconnoiter.[15]

Depression is not an easy entity to comprehend because of the many complex factors associated with it as will be explored. Depression can be precipitated by clear-cut events or by obscure ones. These events can vary from long desired achievement to shattering failure and from expected life events to unanticipated events. Depression can vary in the manner in which it manifests itself, presenting no symptoms at all, symptoms which mimic physical illness, or symptoms which denote mental illness. Depression may last from a momentary second to several years. Depression may vary in intensity from a slight feeling of sadness to an utterly devastating mood of hopelessness and helplessness which inactivates both mind and body. Depression can occur to anyone from infancy to old age.

## The Anatomy of Depression

Most of the commonly appearing theories on the dynamics of depression are elaborations on the speculations of Sigmund Freud. These theories and their variations propose that a series of events has occurred in the life of the infant:

1. The infant's needs are effectively met by a "love object" (usually the parents) on whom the infant develops dependence.
2. Alterations in this primary infant-love object relationship occur. These alterations may be, for example, death of a parent, a change in the expectations by the parent of the child, or a decrease in contact with a parent. The degree of alteration does not seem of significance.
3. The infant attempts unsuccessfully to reestablish the previous relationship with the love object and experiences frustration, anxiety, and feelings of ambivalence toward the love object.
4. The resulting anxiety and the anger at the love object are decreased by turning the anger upon the self, and feelings of self-blame or guilt over the loss are engendered.
5. Depression occurs for a period of time, leaving the infant sensitized to repeat the same sequence whenever an object loss occurs again.[2,17,18,21,29,31]

Of course, this proposed sequence of psychological events is speculative. Others accept the concept of object loss as a precipitating factor in depression, but feel that the loss can occur at any time during life and mus  not necessarily occur during infancy.

Individuals frequently do develop feelings of depression shortly after suffering a loss of some kind. Losses may be of a very real nature or may be symbolic, imaginary, past, present, or foreseen. Real losses which are very observable and may lead to depression include, for example, loss of a job, death of a friend, loss of an extremity by amputation, divorce, abortion, separation from family or friends, loss of a previous level of body functioning, or loss of a prized possession.

Most losses which lead to depression are not as obvious and have symbolic or intangible meaning to the individual. For example, depression may result from loss of status at work, loss of prestige after retirement, loss of self-esteem after an illicit love affair, loss of freedom after marriage, loss of reputation after being charged with a crime, loss of reproductive capability after a hysterectomy, or loss of control over life after institutionalization. These losses even though real to the individual, may be illogical. For example, depression may occur in a man who feels loss of sex appeal after a vasectomy.

Depression may occur after losses which occurred in the distant past. For example, a man may experience depression every year on the anniversary of the day that his wife died. Depression may occur over present events which may represent anticipated losses such as waning health, fading beauty, decreasing sexual ability, advancing age, declining productivity, aloneness, or financial insecurity. This is particularly pertinent with aging individuals but not exclusive to them. The depression occasionally experienced during pregnancy may be related to the loss of freedom anticipated once the baby arrives, or depression when reaching the 30th birthday may be related to a perceived future loss of youthfulness.

The following points must be considered in assessing losses which are associated with depression.

1. The individual experiencing depression may not be consciously aware of the loss or losses precipitating his depression even though others may be aware of his losses. It may be possible, however, to identify such losses upon reflection.
2. Depression is probably precipitated by many losses occurring together. Thus, a pregnant woman may experience loss of her ideal body image, loss of sexual desire, loss of control of certain bodily processes, anticipated loss of freedom, and loss of girlhood which she reacts to with the development of feelings of depression.
3. It is not always possible to predict how one will react to any particular loss or series of losses. As in the example above, the pregnant woman may develop depression as described, but most women do not. Other individuals may become depressed over what we consider to be a trivial loss. Therefore, the tendency to develop depression varies widely with all individuals and varies from one situation to another depending on one's previous life experiences and the interpretation one makes of his situation.
4. If an individual is able to pinpoint a specific event which he feels has led to his depression, he may or may not be accurate. For example, an individual may believe that his depressive feelings stem from his recent failure to receive a desired promotion when in reality the person's depression occurred much earlier and resulted in a gradually deteriorating work performance which negated the opportunity for the promotion.
5. It is believed that the individual experiencing depression after a loss frequently has experienced ambivalence about the lost object and anger which has not been expressed outwardly but instead turned in upon the self. Therefore, where depression exists, there is almost always ambivalence and hidden anger.
6. An individual's perception of the significance of his loss is more relevant than an outside observer's perception of the loss. Thus, a young married woman's depression after a cross word from her husband may seem disproportionate to an observer who is not aware that she may fear her marriage is failing because she has been married for six years and her parents were divorced after six years of marriage.

There are always exceptions to every rule, and depression occurs in situations where it is impossible to determine that a loss has occurred.

Some authorities attribute depression to a lack of social skills.[22] The individual who has suffered a loss or disappointment may develop depression when he is unable to search out or attract others for comfort because of his deficit of the necessary interpersonal skills. Another suggestion is that individuals with low self-esteem may develop unrealistically high expectations of themselves so that they will fail, thus living a "self-fulfilling prophecy" of failure leading to depression.[22]

Still another view on the causation of depression suggests that some individuals may develop "learned helplessness."[22] These individuals may have concluded that they cannot cope with certain situations and are reinforced for their helplessness by others around them. This would seem to help explain why women are more frequently afflicted with depression than men since women are expected to be the "weaker sex," and why youngest daughters seem prone to depression since they may be socialized as the helpless and protected "baby" by their families.

Researchers have uncovered physiologic changes in depressed individuals which might suggest a biochemical causation of depression.[20,29] Most plentiful have been studies which demonstrate changes in adrenocortical functioning and in amine metabolism. These changes are very complex and only rudimentary knowledge exists about them at present. Unfortunately, it is unknown whether these changes contribute to depression or merely reflect the presence of depression in the body.

Depression also seems to be easily communicated, as most emotions are, from one individual to another. It seems likely that this is not pure contagion but rather occurs when the depressive feelings of one individual strike a responsive chord in another individual.

It is suspected that genetic factors may play some role in depression.[13,20,33] Studies with identical twins have shown that if one twin develops depressive illness, the other twin is much more likely to develop the same condition than would be generally expected. The children of depressed mothers seem more likely to suffer depression during their lives. It must be emphasized that it is difficult to separate the effects of genetics from the effects of environmental conditioning, however.

Socioeconomic status has been shown to have a possible influence.[17,18] Depression is reportedly more frequent in the upper classes than the lower classes although this could easily reflect a diagnostic and treatment bias rather than a real difference.

Personality characteristics which predispose one to develop depression have been described by several authors.[3,9,20,22,29,31] Individuals who are prone to develop depression are seen to be "worriers" and dependent on others for support or praise to constantly affirm their self-worth and competence. They are more concerned with evaluation by others than self-evaluation so that they tend to order their lives in an attempt more to gain praise and avoid the criticism of others than to achieve personal goals. They are frequently from homes where the moral and religious standards were rigid and difficult to achieve. They are thought to be near perfectionists who lead lives of few interests and have few close friends outside of their families. Depression prone individuals may demonstrate an undue concern about doing what is proper and with promptness. They may be so concerned about fulfilling their obligations that they overextend themselves. They may become noticeably depressed when their schedule is interrupted by a cold or the flu. Those prone to depression have been described as having a narrow range of emotional expression. They are frequently respected for their reliability and perseverance. The usefulness of this personality description to predict depression is limited by the fact that it was presumably compiled by retrospective evaluation and is extremely subjective.

A similar personality description related to children who are prone to depression has been compiled.[3,17,18,21] These children have been described as being "little adults" who seem prematurely old. They are overly concerned with a fear of punishment for infractions and appear unusually serious or earnest. They demonstrate a strict and overwhelming conscience which restricts their ability to play with and relate appropriately to their peers. The middle child may be particularly susceptible since he has no "special" place in the family. This personality sketch is also limited by the same factors as the adult personality sketch.

It is important to note that women are much more likely to suffer depression throughout their lives than men. Some possible reasons can be given. First of all, even in our present culture, the female is still largely socialized to be dependent, other-oriented, and "helpless" in the presence of males. She is discouraged from displaying anger or strong negative emotions and taught that angry outbursts and cursing are not "ladylike." It is felt that men may discharge repressed anger by engaging in sports activities or active physical work. This option is not encouraged for women who usually perform more routine repetitive tasks which take more toll in boredom than physical exertion. For example, little girls help mother dust while little boys mow the yard.

Physical illness is frequently accompanied by depression. While this may be related to the concept of loss or biochemical change as discussed earlier, it seems possible that as yet unknown biochemical factors contribute to depression before, during, or after physical illness. A number of conditions are repeatedly mentioned as being associated with depression. These include:

Mutilative surgery: hysterectomy, mastectomy, colostomy, amputation.
Infectious diseases: common influenza, mononucleosis, bacterial infection.

Metabolic diseases: pituitary disorder, diabetes mellitus, thyroid disorders, drug intoxication.
Cardiovascular disorders: stroke, hypertension, arteriosclerosis, angina.
Nutritional deficiency states.
Malignancies: leukemia, brain tumor, lymphoma.
Immobilizing conditions: burns, fractures, myocardial infarctions.
Obesity.
Chronic handicapping conditions: hemophilia, arthritis, congenital defects, epilepsy.
Uremia.
Neurologic disorders: cerebral arteriosclerosis, tension headaches, migraine headaches.
Hepatitis.

It may be possible that depression adversely affects the body's defenses against illness.[28]

Depression may occur when severe, prolonged stress or crisis exhaust the individual's coping mechanisms so that depression eventually ensues as a protective mechanism. It is usually felt that stress occurring in one's personal life is more disturbing than stress occurring at work.

It has been hypothesized that depression can occur when the grief work for a previous loss was incomplete for some reason. At a later time, possibly because of a similar loss, the individual recommences the grief work with more difficulty and intensity. Some possible situations which could lead to a delayed grief reaction include those in which the individual was prevented from grieving appropriately or where the loss was not realistically appreciated.[29] Individuals experiencing this type of depression are believed to be consciously unaware of the etiology of their depression and, therefore, the grief may never fully abate but become chronic.

Depression is commonly seen as a side effect of a number of pharmacologic agents such as tranquilizers. In addition some sedatives, antihypertensives, diuretics, and steroids have been noted to cause depression.[13]

The prevalent religions in our Western culture may be interpreted as augmenting feelings of depression. Consider the level of perfection that one should strive to achieve. There may be emphasis placed on regularly facing oneself with how poorly one is meeting these standards.

A particularly puzzling form of depression is the feeling of sadness and remorse which frequently occurs after one has achieved a much desired and diligently pursued goal. For example, the graduate student who finally receives his Ph.D. or the Olympic gold medal winner may go from elation to depression within a few hours or a few days after their achievement. This depression may represent a symbolic loss of goals and may persist until new goals are found, or perhaps there is a special melancholia in having all things finished.[20]

It has been proposed that depression can occur when one has outgrown one's present life style.[12] This might occur when one retires, when one's children leave home, when an individual is divorced or separated, or when a spouse dies, for example. It is true that these are in fact times when depression is frequently seen. This rationale would also help explain the development of depression after success.

In conclusion, the speculations on the factors associated with the development of depressive feelings are varied and vague. Fortunately some basic ideas can be selectively and tentatively enumerated which can give the nurse a starting point from which to work. Depression appears to commonly relate to a loss of a real or symbolic nature. The significance of the loss is unique to each individual at any given time. The depressed individual may or may not be cognizant of the identity and nature of the loss. Other factors such as heredity, physical disease, biochemistry, and learning experiences seem also of relevance in unknown ways. Within the dynamics of depression, there probably exists ambivalence about the lost object or symbol, and anger which is hidden. Factors often leading to depression and hopelessness are extensive illness, loss of supportive resources, invasion of privacy, unrelenting pain, and fatigue.[16]

## Manifestations of Depression

Depression has been called the great masquerader because it can mimic other conditions. There is, however, a classic form of depression which is probably the most frequent and the easiest to recognize. This pattern is associated with disturbances in appearance and emotional, intellectual, and physical functioning. Although depression exists in less severe intensities as will be described later, the more extreme manifestations will be described in each area to show the direction in which depressive behavior may proceed.

### APPEARANCE

The very depressed individual looks sad and dejected. His body may be slumped and his head lowered. He sits quietly and seems to be almost asleep or he may prefer to lie down continually. His clothes may show a lack of attention. He may neglect personal hygiene such as combing his hair or brushing his teeth. If engaged in conversation his speech is hesitant and frequently focused on a few preoccupations. The depressed individual seldom begins a conversation himself and he may lose his train of thought in the middle of a sentence. At mealtime he picks at his food and eats very little. At night he may lie awake for hours before falling asleep or he may awaken several hours before he normally would and lie awake until morning. Every activity seems to require superhuman effort. He appears tired, unresponsive, and withdrawn. This "slowed down" behavior is referred to as psychomotor retardation. He may cry or appear ready to cry at any time. If he can still attend to work, he is likely to start his day's work later than usual and fail to complete as much as he previously did. Even his gait is slowed and lifeless and his posture appears rigid. He appears older than his stated age.

### EMOTIONAL FUNCTIONING

The very depressed adult reports that he feels great emotional discomfort. He sees no hope in the future and feels helpless to change his current situation. He may mention that he is unimportant and worthless. He may say that he does not like himself and feels he is being punished for some sin. He states that he never sleeps well, never feels rested, and hates the morning. His mood may improve somewhat as the day progresses. He may mention that he has lost interest in some of his previous projects and has no motivation to work on them or to begin anything new. He may have noticed that he no longer desires food, sex, activity, or sleep. The depressed person may conclude that the world would be a better place if he did not exist or that death is the only way to escape his present misery.

## INTELLECTUAL FUNCTIONING

An adult who is very depressed may fear that he is "losing his mind" because he can no longer remember things, seems unable to concentrate, and finds that his mind is filled with unrelenting thoughts about his miserable state—even at night when he tries to sleep. He states that he can hardly attend to what he is reading. He may be worried about his lack of interest in his job, his declining efficiency, and his loss of ambition.

## PHYSICAL FUNCTIONING

The very depressed adult may experience changes in several body processes due primarily to a decreased basal metabolism rate. He may experience a dry mouth, loss of appetite, poor digestion, constipation, and weight loss. He may feel vague "light" feelings in his chest. He does show a change in his sleep electroencephalogram with more light sleep and fewer periods of deep sleep. In the female, menstruation may cease and she may become nonorgasmic. The male may become impotent. A number of vague somatic complaints such as headache may develop. He may show a lack of muscle tone and increased fatigue. An increased secretion of adrenocortical hormones has been demonstrated as occurs in most instances of illness or stress. In depressed individuals the peak of adrenocortical hormone secretion occurs at 2:00 or 3:00 a.m. rather than at 6:00 a.m. which is normal. The reasons for this or the effects this may have upon the normal circadian rhythms of the body are unknown at this time.

Depression may manifest itself in ways other than the classic symptoms described. For example, some depressed individuals present only with physical complaints. These complaints are likely to be mild or vague headaches, pain in the chest, extremities, or abdomen, chronic constipation, dizziness, pervasive fatigue, nausea and vomiting, or loss of sexual drive. These are referred to as "depressive equivalents." Because these individuals do not clearly manifest the other symptoms previously described, they may never be suspected of being primarily depressed and the diagnosis of depression may easily be missed.[8] It may be that some individuals unconsciously mask their depression under physical complaints such as those above because physical illness is more acceptable than emotional disturbance both to society and to health care professionals. Therefore, any person who has physical symptoms which are found not to have any detectable organic basis or logical causation may actually be depressed.

## *Agitated Depression*

Occasionally the depressed adult exhibits his anxiety through agitation which accompanies his depression.[5,29] This is seen as a physical restlessness with activities such as hand wringing, pacing, and excessive verbalization. The depressed person who is agitated may state that he feels like he is about to "jump out of his skin" or "about to burst." The recognition of the person with agitated depression is crucial because he is at high risk for attempting suicide.[29] Agitated depression may at first glance resemble anxiety which is less likely to result in suicide. Table 10-1 represents some differences between agitated depression and neurotic anxiety which the nurse may assess.[5]

**Table 10-1.** Some differences in behavior in agitated depression and neurotic anxiety

| Behavior | Agitated depression | Neurotic anxiety |
| --- | --- | --- |
| Motor behavior | Paces in a given route Repetitious movements such as hand wringing | Random, unpredictable movements |
| Verbal behavior | Monotone voice | Variable verbal tones |
| Thought content | Persistent expression of a few worries | Wandering conversation, on many subjects |

## Manic-Depressive Illness

A small number of depressed individuals have episodes of extreme elation which may alternate with severe episodes of depression.[3] These episodes are referred to as periods of mania and the individual is referred to as having manic-depressive illness. During the manic phase, the individual exhibits almost the extreme opposite of depressed behavior. He is euphoric and rarely eats, rests, or sleeps. He has grandiose plans which he thinks are of extreme importance. He is the epitome of self-confidence. This chapter will not discuss nursing intervention with this individual. The interested nurse should consult textbooks of psychiatric medicine or nursing.

## Suicide

Because of the correlation between suicide and depression, the depressed individual may have suicidal thoughts, make suicidal threats, or actually attempt suicide. There are many ways to commit suicide such as drug ingestion, drowning, hanging, and self-inflicted wounds in addition to what appear to be obvious attempts.[12] It is possible that many high speed car accidents with stationary objects and private plane crashes are actually suicide attempts. Similarly, one may wish to commit suicide when one refuses to seek treatment for illnesses, refuses to participate in medical treatment plans, abuses toxic substances such as alcohol, drugs, or nicotine, overeats, and participates in crimes. Such subtle acts of self-destruction are in some instances more socially acceptable than suicide. Some feel that individuals who are accident prone are likely to be depressed and subtly indicating their desire for self-destruction.

The presence of the following factors in a depressed individual increases the risk of suicide:

1. A serious depressive state.
2. A recent death in the family.
3. A previous suicide in the family.
4. A suicide note by the individual.
5. A means to commit suicide readily available.
6. An individual who has made previous suicide threats or attempts.
7. An individual who has no close personal relationships.
8. Agitated behavior in the depressed person.
9. A setback in recovery from a condition.
10. A recent discharge from a hospital.
11. Signs of leave-taking (i.e., making a will, giving away belongings).[3,29,35]

Although there is an increased risk of suicide with a severe level of depression, the individual who attempts suicide usually does not make the attempt at the depths of his depression but when he is beginning to recover from his depression. Various reasons have been offered as explanations for the increased incidence of suicide following improvement in depression.[2] Some authorities feel it is due to a decrease in psychomotor retardation making the attempt more physically possible. It may be that the improvement helps the individual to see how difficult total recovery will be. Or it may be that the decision to destroy himself leads to a sense of peace which appears as improvement but is soon followed by the suicide attempt.

The nurse should assess whether the patient has thought about committing suicide. If he has, she can find out how preoccupied with suicide he is by asking him if he has thought how or when he will kill himself. Individuals who have definite plans are in need of immediate help. It is not true that people who talk about suicide never kill themselves.

## Differentiation of Depression from Other Similar States

It is possible to confuse depression with two other states in particular—neurotic anxiety and certain forms of schizophrenia. Neurotic anxiety is an extreme state of anxiety. Schizophrenia is a profound psychological disturbance which requires intensive psychiatric intervention. Some individuals with schizophrenia appear depressed. Anxiety and depression are parallel emotions in some respects. An anxious individual may become secondarily depressed over his anxiety. A depressed individual may become secondarily anxious over his depression.[5] Table 10-2 shows some general parameters to illustrate some of the differences.

The purpose of this chapter is to help the nurse to intervene in the more commonly seen mild or moderately severe states of depression. If the nurse determines that the individual's depression is severe, if there is agitation, thoughts of suicide, delusions, or if the individual is manifesting only depressive equivalents, she should seek validation and consultation with resources beyond this book.

**Table 10-2.** Some differences between certain behaviors in depression, anxiety, and schizophrenia

| Behavior | Depression | Anxiety | Schizophrenia |
|---|---|---|---|
| Speech | Focused on a few topics, pessimistic tone | Wandering, many subjects | Tangential, loose associations |
| Movements | Slowed | Hyperactive or normal | |
| Relation to time of day | Feels worse in the morning | Feels worse in the evening | |
| Mood | Consistent sadness | | Great variability |
| Affect | Appropriate | | Inappropriate or lacking |
| Willingness to discuss problems | Reluctant, does not immediately feel better | Eager, feels better after talking | |
| Internal thoughts | Feels sad | Feels anxious | Feels puzzled and empty |
| Bowel habits | Constipation | Diarrhea | |
| Appetite | Decreased | Eats well | |
| Value of sleep | Little value | Feels better | |

# DEPRESSION AND THE LIFE CYCLE

Depression is a conclusion that is inferred from observing the behavior of an individual. There is no one clear pattern of behavior which is always indicative of depression for all ages of people. In order to best reflect the complexity of the manifestation of depression, it is helpful to consider depression as it is seen during the different stages of the life cycle.

## Infancy

The first descriptions of depression in infants were derived from observations in institutions or hospitals of infants who had no mothers or mother substitutes available to them. The most classic studies were reported by John Bowlby and Rene Spitz.[1,30] The infants they studied were characterized as listless, poor eaters, underweight, highly susceptible to disease, underresponsive to stimuli, and apathetic. This behavior could be detected by six months of age and was described as anaclitic depression. The depression of these infants was reversible if they were provided with a mother substitute or series of mother substitutes who cared for and cuddled the babies regularly. If this was not provided, the babies frequently died.

It is hypothesized that infants manifest depression in their behavior so readily because they are unable to verbalize about their feelings and have almost nonexistent defense mechanisms so that mood states are easily seen in behavior.[6] Fortunately, depression is believed to be easily relieved in infants because they appear to have the ability to easily substitute love objects and because, like all children, they have a "push for growth" which tends to sustain hope and optimism in the face of obstacles.

## Children

The presence of depression in children has only recently been generally accepted as a real entity. Depression rarely exists in an easily observable state but is felt to exist in forms which are more difficult to detect. The period of time that the depression is evident is much shorter in children than with adults. A framework of the levels of childhood depression was formulated by Cytryn and McKnew[6] and demonstrates the elusive nature of childhood depression. They suggest that depression exists first in the child's fantasy, then in the child's verbal behavior, and lastly in mood and behavior. This outline will be used to describe the symptoms of childhood depression as reported by them and others.[3,8,17,18,25,29,33]

## LEVEL I

Level I is believed to be fairly common but normally unobserved in the child because the feelings of depression are detectable only in the child's fantasy life. These feelings might be expressed in the child's play activities and his dreams, and might be demonstrated through projection techniques such as having the child describe what he sees happening in a picture which is subject to many interpretations. The themes to listen for are those related to death, suicide, mistreatment, loss, abandonment, blame, personal injury, criticism, or thwarting.

## LEVEL II

Level II is believed to be less frequent than Level I and more easily observed in the verbal conversation of the child. The themes to listen for in his conversation are related to suicidal thoughts, helplessness, hopelessness, being unloved, being guilty, being worthless, or being undesirable.

## LEVEL III

Level III is less frequent, readily observable, and expressed in both mood and behavior. Depressed children may try to escape their feelings of depression by acting out through aggressive behavior, provocative behavior, angry outbursts, defiance of authority, inattention, or the development of phobias. They are sometimes sadistic and enjoy the misfortunes of others. Depressed children may mistakenly be diagnosed as hyperactive. Their rich fantasy life may lead them to tell exaggerated and complex stories. They may be excessively interested in death and relish "bloodthirsty" stories. Joking and clowning are used to gain attention in school. Frequently one or both parents also suffer from periodic depressive episodes and consciously or subconsciously reject the child. His home environment is frequently one of constant criticism or lack of attention to his needs. The child's parents may react to him with anger in return and he easily may become the family "scapegoat." He is likely to believe that he is a burden.

Another pattern of depression in childhood is more similar to the typical adult manifestations of depression and this also is infrequently seen. Severely depressed children look sad, dejected, and unhappy. They may demonstrate a poor self-concept, frustration, self-blame, and irritability when they are unsuccessful. Achievement may make the child uncomfortable. His mood tone may be one of pessimism. He is frequently a loner and slow to form friendship. He is described by his parents as mature, conscientious, and serious. He may be found crying when alone. He may be successful in school because of his fear of performing poorly and behaving improperly. He may demonstrate a vague feeling of guiltiness although he is not aware of why he feels guilty. His parents may feel he is ill or a weak child because he so often appears tired and lacking in the spontaneity and responsiveness of other children. Children who manifest these behaviors frequently have one or both parents who experience episodic bouts of depression.

Other symptoms of childhood depression may be self-destructive elements evidenced in the child's behavior. These might include playing in hazardous situations, continual accidental injuries, and behaviors which provoke aggression in others.[7]

Depression in children may be associated with an absence of behavioral symptoms and the presence of entirely somatic complaints such as headache, abdominal pain, insomnia, anorexia, dizziness, nausea, encopresis, and enuresis. The child is more likely to be brought for health care because of these symptoms than because of the previously mentioned behavioral ones and the possibility that depression exists is almost always overlooked according to some authors.

Although suicide (which is associated with depression) is rare in children under the age of 12, it does occur.[25] Children are usually not very adept at suicide because they have a limited knowledge of how to kill themselves and few means available. Suicide attempts commonly take the form of hanging, drowning, and poisoning—all of which may appear accidental and be taken by the parents and others as such.

Depression in childhood is probably seldom evident because a child is presumably better able to prevent or rid himself of the symptoms of his depression than are adults.[6] Children have a poorly developed superego and, therefore, feel less guilt. They also have a poorly developed ability to test reality and are left freer to use newly acquired defenses such as denial, magical thinking, or projection to distort reality when their psychic equilibrium is challenged. Children have an increased verbal ability which allows them to "discharge" some feelings. And, like the infant, they seem to be able to substitute love objects and maintain hope and optimism as a basic mood. Thus a child may manifest observable symptoms of depression only when these defenses fail. Before these observable changes occur, however, it may be possible to demonstrate elements of depression in the fantasy life or the verbal expressions of the child. Because this is seldom pursued, some feel that depression in childhood is grossly underdiagnosed.

## Adolescents

The presence of depression in adolescents is more commonly reported.[3,17,18,25,29] It is difficult to diagnose even though it is sometimes more like the adult response.

Adolescent behavior is notoriously erratic and mood swings are exaggerated and frequent. The depression seen in adolescents varies from mild to severe. Adolescent depression is commonly related to developmental tasks such as developing relationships with others, identity, authority, and dependence-independence. Therefore, adolescent depression is frequently precipitated by loss of friends, fights with parents, or rejection by others. Adolescent depression may present with apathy, withdrawal, and inactivity. Overeating and excessive sleeping are occasionally seen. The adolescent may appear tearful, overly sensitive, confused over his identity, unable to satisfy himself, and chronically in search of affection and approval at any cost. Sometimes depression is manifested by periodic "acting out" behavior such as drinking, delinquency, drug use, stealing, school truancy, and promiscuity. The acting out behavior is thought to represent attacks upon the outer world to help relieve the misery of the inner world. This behavior may be followed by intense guilt and lead to the symptoms first described. As can be seen, there can be a narrow border between "normal" adolescent behavior and preadult depressive states.

Suicide behavior is discouragingly prominent in adolescents and young adults and a high risk for those between the ages of 15 to 25 years, among whom it is presently the third leading cause of death in the United States.[3] The adolescent who resorts to suicide usually shows loss of interest in himself, a preoccupation with thoughts of death, an isolation from others, and a history of disturbed behavior.[25] Unfortunately, the depression of the adolescent may not have been recognized until a suicide attempt occurred. Suicide is felt to represent the ultimate form of self-punishment and atonement for guilt as well as an expression of anger.

Depression is thought to be more commonly seen in adolescents because they lack the defenses of the younger child: reality testing is more fully developed; love object substituting is more difficult; the superego is more mature, leading to the possibility of guilt; and fantasy is not as available as an escape.[6]

## *Adults*

Some periods occurring in adulthood are seen as vulnerable times for depression to appear. It is widely reported that many women experience some degree of depression shortly prior to the beginning of menstruation. This "premenstrual tension" is assumed to result from hormonal factors and reportedly leads to irritability, feeling "blue," crying, and emotional instability. Recently the presence or absence of premenstrual tension has become a controversial issue with some believing it is grossly exaggerated and others believing it is underinvestigated and devalued.

There also appears to be a tendency for some women to develop feelings of depression during the period following the birth of a child.[24] The mother reports feeling sad and unable to cope with the demands of her home and her infant. She may regret the pregnancy and birth although a few days earlier she was ecstatic. She may cry easily and not know why. This is sometimes referred to as the "baby blues" and presumed to be due to pain, tension, fatigue, and hormonal influences. It is interesting to note that adoptive mothers also report feelings of depression after the placement of children in their homes. Normally the depression associated with the postpartum period is mild and abates in a few days but the depressed state can be of varying intensity, even to the point of becoming a severe depression with delirium, agitation, confusion, and the possibility that the mother might attempt destructive actions toward herself and the baby. This behavior, referred to as postpartum psychosis, is felt to be due not so much to the birth of the child as to the combination of a previous marginal psychological equilibrium disturbed by the events of pregnancy, parturition, and biochemical factors.[4]

In men, particular proneness to depressive symptoms appears to occur near the 40th birthday. The individual may become disinterested in his work, unhappy with himself and his family, and in general discontent with his life. He may become particularly sensitive to comments about his thinning or greying hair and may desire to spend more time alone than previously. Most men recover after a few mild episodes of dejection and resume their usual lifestyle. Some may attempt to soothe their depression by exaggerated attempts to hide their age, forbidden sexual encounters—usually with younger women—and attempts in general to acquire what they feel are more youthful behaviors and habits.

In both men and women, involution can be a time of potential depression.[23] This is sometimes referred to as menopause in the female and andropause in the male. Involution occurs in the 40s and 50s for women but later in the male, and corresponds to atrophy of the ovaries in the female and testes in the male with resulting changes in hormone secretion and balance, and changes in the function and appearance of sexual organs. The individual may be facing retirement and this is frequently the time when children are leaving or have left home—the "empty nest syndrome." Both women and men may find themselves with role confusion. The depression in both men and women at this time seems to manifest itself with restlessness or agitation. Some feel that the individual with a compulsive-obsessive personality is particularly vulnerable to involutional depression.[9,20]

Depression in adulthood may be the cause of other conditions which may be treated without consideration for the possibility that underlying depression exists. For example, a depressed individual may find that alcohol will temporarily relieve his depression and he may eventually become a heavy drinker. Attempts to treat his alcoholism may be unsuccessful because his unrelieved depression will again lead him to seek the solace of alcohol.[20]

Depression may become chronic at any stage of the life cycle, but chronic depression is probably more widely recognized in adulthood. Chronic depression is usually of mild severity but can be of any degree of intensity. It is recognized as any depressive state which persists over a period of years.

Much too numerous to elaborate on are other developmental and situational events which are related to depressive states in adults. Some of these are popularly recognized as the "marriage blues," the "postcoital blues," and the college graduation letdown.

## Older Adults

The aging stage of the life cycle is frequently associated with depression. It is not difficult to imagine the totality of possible losses than can occur with a changing body image, changing functioning of the body, loss of friends, loss of familiar objects, and loss of identity to name only a few. The elderly individual who is depressed is likely to be quarrelsome, agitated, pessimistic, and complain of insomnia, constipation, headache, fatigue, loss of appetite, and other previously described symptoms of depression.[29] It is likely that depression is very prevalent in the older population and also likely that the symptoms are assumed to be normal or evidence of early senility. The distinction between depression and senile changes of aging is important because the depressive state can often be relieved with proper counseling and care.

# NURSING INTERVENTION IN DEPRESSION

The nurse is in an important position to prevent or detect depression. She is frequently the only health care practitioner who may be looking at the entire individual, both mind and body. She is in frequent contact with individuals who are at risk to develop depression. Because early intervention can often prevent serious depressive episodes, her actions are important.

## Primary Prevention

Much could be done to prevent depression before it starts. One obvious area is related to the grieving process. It has become desirable in our society for the grievers to "not break down" and to conceal or deny their grief. This can lead to incomplete grieving and depression. The nurse can help both children and adults who are grieving to do their grief work and to avoid denial of the loss. This means that the painful reality of a loss must be faced squarely.[8] This is discussed further in the chapter on grief and grieving.

Another area of primary prevention is helping the individual learn to express anger in ways that are appropriate for him so that his anger does not become the forebearer of depression. Having strong emotional feelings is not unhealthy. It is one indication that one is alive and responsive to his environment. Knowing how to deal with them is important.

The nurse can help others to get in touch with their feelings of anger by careful confrontations such as: "You really look fit to be tied" or "You're feeling really upset with your mother and father for bringing you here, aren't you?"

It is most commonly felt that emotions such as anger are best expressed outwardly in physical activity or in verbal activity leading to learning, and harmful if turned inward. Many individuals who have long conditioned away any expression of anger will have difficulty learning how to discharge anger without guilt. The nurse may help them by giving them permission to be angry. She may want to use terms which are easier for some to admit to at first. For example, the nurse may comment to a patient, "I would be upset if my husband left me with five children to raise by myself" or "I would be very indignant if my sister-in-law expected me to babysit all the time." Because anger may be dissipated in physical activity, some may be helped to learn to use activity when they are uncomfortable. Even activities such as needlework, piano playing, or solitaire with cards, even though not rigorous activity, are therapeutic to some. Working with houseplants also seems to be particularly therapeutic. Children often use physical activity instinctively but some may need help. Most importantly the nurse can help patients and family members learn from their anger. This is discussed in the chapter on anger.

For a number of adults, depression might be prevented if they could learn to lead lives with variable interests. Many depressive episodes seem to center around situations where individuals are leading lives of limited focuses and interests. When they are forced for reasons such as retirement, divorce, illness, or departing children to change their focus, they may be unable to cope.[9,12] Helping individuals to plan ahead through anticipatory guidance might help some situations. Otherwise, being there when the change occurs might help.

There are numerous other situations where depression is likely to occur for both adults and children which should alert the nurse to efforts at prevention. These might be events such as admission to a hospital, loss of some bodily functions, presence of a physical illness, pregnancy, impending surgery, accidental injury, chronic illness, acute disabling disease, changes (favorable or unfavorable) in life style, separation, criminal charges, loss of employment, birth or adoption of a child, school entry, moving, graduation from school, and loss of friendships. The nurse can intervene in these situations in the interests of primary prevention.

1. She can help the individual to verbalize about what losses he may experience. She encourages him to explore what the loss will mean to him.
2. She can help the individual to keep in touch with his emotional reactions to what is happening to him and facilitate his expression of them.
3. She can mobilize other resources to help compensate for the approaching loss. For example, if an individual is approaching the dissolution of his marriage, the nurse might help him to get involved in other sources of socialization.

This content is summarized in Table 10-3.

**Table 10-3.** Possible nursing actions to prevent depression

1. Help individuals grieve completely.
2. Teach patients and families to express anger appropriately.
3. Help individuals diversify their lives.
4. Provide support when life style changes occur.

## Secondary Prevention

Secondary prevention involves intervening to reduce mild or moderate depression. Probably the most important function of the nurse in intervening in depression is to provide ego support to the depressed individual through use of the helping process.[34] The nurse demonstrates interest and concern by her attitude, and communicates that she values the individual who is depressed by her attention. This is accomplished by visiting the child or adult frequently, listening to him actively, and focusing intently on his problems and concerns. She is subtly communicating hope which he can draw upon to replace the hopelessness he feels.[32] She is by her actions saying, "I refuse to give up on you. You are a person of worth."

The nurse should seek validation that the individual feels he is depressed.[16] Some individuals may not have been able to come to grips with their unhappy state and may feel better when they are able to verbalize that they are depressed. Emotional feelings are easier to discuss when labeled.[31] They can then be coped with more easily since the mind "thinks with language." If the individual was already aware of his depression, acknowledging his depression to someone else may make him feel less alone and as though he has someone to share his burden with.

The nurse can carefully assure the individual that he will eventually feel better since most instances of depression are short lived and he may be glad to know that depression occurs to almost everyone sometimes.[3,10,20] This assurance may help to reestablish hope in the future. The nurse can point out improvements she notices. This should be done in a concrete and objective manner.[2] "You have washed your hair today. You look like you feel better." If she tries to give broad reassurance or compliments, the patient may feel he must deny them or they may make him feel more unworthy.

The nurse must guard against any impulse to be overly cheerful. This makes it more difficult for the individual who is depressed to relate to her.[10,26] The nurse should strive for a calm attitude and minimal verbal activity. She should keep the environment at an appropriate level of low stimulation.[10,26,31]

The nurse may be able to help the person to grieve for his losses if they are apparent.[9,21,29] For example:

A teenager was depressed because his older brother had left home to work in Alaska. He was just out of school for the summer, and he had not been able to find a summer job. The nurse encouraged him to talk about his brother, how much he missed him, and how much fun they had together. She also encouraged him to talk about school, his friends, and the events of the year. At some point, he began to talk about the summer and how it would seem without his brother around and without school. She listened as he expressed his annoyance and anger with his brother for leaving and with his small home town for the lack of interesting activities and job opportunities available to him. The teenager's depression lifted gradually within a week and he was making plans to work as a farm helper during the summer to earn money.

If the losses are not apparent, the nurse may be able to help the individual uncover what he has lost, but if he is reluctant to discuss this area, it is best left alone. His psychological equilibrium may be dependent upon not facing his losses. Children may best be able to communicate their feelings through play. Puppets work especially well for some children in helping them express themselves.

The nurse may cautiously wish to help the depressed individual to express his anger over his situation.[10,31] As stated earlier, this must be done with sensitivity. The individual may displace his anger on others first. He may see the nurse as a safe target for his anger while others on whom he is more dependent are not. The nurse may eventually be able to help the individual to see that he is displacing his anger. As previously mentioned physical activities may help dissipate anger.

One young mother reacted to angry feelings when her husband drank by becoming irate at her children and making their life miserable, after which she felt guilty. After a nurse intervened, she never learned to direct her anger at her husband but did gain insight into her behavior and coped with his drinking by getting out her iron and pressing everything in sight with vigor before she became depressed. Thus her angry outbursts at her children were reduced.

The depressed patient may be unable to face decisions of complexity and may need the help of the nurse.[10] She must make only those decisions which really need to be made and slowly promote his decision making in appropriate doses to avoid making the patient dependent.

The child or adult may need a gentle nudge to get involved in activities at his own pace.[10,26] This does not mean a strong shove. The individual should be allowed periods of inactivity also. His entire day does not need to be scheduled. Some "worry time" may be beneficial as he faces his problems.

If the patient is expressing guilt, shame, and negative concepts about himself, the nurse must avoid agreeing with him or trying to talk him out of them. To agree with him adds another source of condemnation. To disagree with him implies that one does not really understand how bad he feels and that one does not want to discuss his problems. The nurse may wish to suggest to the patient what she sees to be some of his strengths. This should be done spontaneously as appropriate. Although the patient may deny them at the time, the optimistic thought that someone thinks he has worth will have been planted.

If the patient indicates the appropriateness, he may appreciate talking with a religious advisor. Many individuals have found this of comfort in decreasing their depression because it may decrease guilt leading to depression. If this resource is not available the nurse should be able to talk with patients about their religious beliefs with respect and open-mindedness.

Music seems to directly influence the moods of many people. The adult or child may be able to identify music which will lighten his mood and this can be provided for him.

The nurse may encounter individuals who cope with their depression in a manner that provides only temporary relief and eventually leads to greater depression. These individuals may need to learn healthier methods of coping.

One woman who was alone with two small children in a small apartment for long hours while her husband struggled to launch his own business became depressed on rainy days when the outside world seemed cut off. She would frequently take her children to a large shopping center and her mood would improve as she bought items for herself and her family. But as the shopping trip drew to a close, she would again feel depressed as she realized how much money she had spent and how many other things she would like to have which she couldn't have. By the time she returned home, she was more depressed than before. Her husband seldom was angry with her because he felt guilty over being gone from home so much of the time. A nurse noticed this situation when she met the woman in a prenatal clinic after one shopping trip. Through discussion the woman became aware of her behavior. The mother thought she still would need to get out of the apartment on rainy days but planned to go to places where she would be with other people but would be less likely to spend money, such as the art museum or the airport.

If there is a recognizable environmental situation which is compounding the patient's depression, the nurse may be able to help the patient change the situation.[35] For example, improved housing or a more pleasant job may do much to diminish depression.

The nurse who works with children who are depressed must teach the parents or caretakers of the child to recognize the signs of depression the child is manifesting. The nurse can teach the parents how to intervene.[3] The parents need to learn how to help the child express his anger and communicate his feelings, and how to relate to the child in ways that increase his feelings of self-esteem. It has been found that giving the depressed child a suitable pet has been beneficial to some. A pet is always accepting and never critical.

As the depressed individual improves, the nurse should withdraw slowly.[2] She should be sure she leaves behind resources on which the patient can call if needed. This is one condition in which the nurse should not encourage a long term relationship. This can lead to dependency upon the nurse and return to feelings of helplessness.

If the depressed individual is not improving, she may wish to consider that the individual is receiving more reinforcement from his environment to stay depressed than to improve.[22,29] Depressed individuals often receive considerable secondary gain from their depression. They may be excused from ordinary expectations, pampered, and showered with attention. If this is happening, the nurse needs to rearrange the situation to reward improvement and extinguish depressive behaviors. Guidelines for reducing mild to moderate levels of depression are presented in Table 10-4.

**Table 10-4.** Possible nursing actions for intervening in mild and moderate depression

1. Attempt to form a helping relationship.
2. Validate the presence of depression with the individual.
3. Provide assurance and understanding, not reassurance.
4. Avoid excessive cheerfulness.
5. Help individual grieve for losses leading to depression if possible.
6. Encourage expression of repressed anger cautiously.
7. Avoid presenting person with decisions.
8. Encourage activities.
9. Use communication skills to facilitate adult's or child's expression of feelings.
10. Consider music as therapeutic.
11. Encourage helpful coping methods.
12. Teach parents to recognize and help a depressed child.
13. Terminate gradually.
14. Use behavior modification if warranted.

## Tertiary Prevention

If the nurse is unable to establish a relationship with the patient, if he is becoming more depressed, if she feels he is agitated or suicidal, or if his depression has lasted longer than it should, the nurse should seek additional resources for the patient.

## THE NURSE AND DEPRESSION

Nurses seem particularly prone to developing feelings of depression. As a human being somewhere in the life cycle, the nurse is subject to all the multiple factors which can lead to depression which have been discussed. Because the vast majority of nurses are women and because women are more likely to develop depression than men, she is at high risk. There seem to be some particular factors associated with the nursing profession itself that might make depression likely.

First of all, a nurse may become depressed from contact with the many depressed patients she cares for. Working with depressed patients is often emotionally draining.[11,16] And because improvement is slow, the nurse may feel discouraged and useless.

Secondly, the nursing profession sets for itself very high expectations of performance. In many situations, the nurse is expected to have a great depth of knowledge about nutrition, pharmacology, and medicine so she can participate in the medical treatment, monitor the patient's progress, and do appropriate teaching. She is expected to use management skills and group dynamic skills in working with other members of the health team. In addition, she is to be proficient in the central care of nursing practice which involves helping people in any setting achieve and maintain wellness and cope with large and small alterations in health from birth to death. It is little wonder that every nurse will experience feelings of inadequacy and loss of esteem which may lead to depression as she tries to be all things to all people.

In addition, the nurse is supposed to avoid reacting emotionally in patient care situations. She is rational, empathetic, other-centered, and clinically neutral. She does not express anger, hurt, self-interest, judgment, bias, or rejection. This is very difficult if not impossible. If she does become cognizant that she is acting on emotion she may feel guilty. If she is able to somewhat suppress her feelings, she may be building up anger and ambivalence subconsciously. Either way she may eventually experience depressive feelings.

Failure with some patients and families is inevitable and may lead to guilt and depression. No one has yet learned how to cure poverty and its multitude of emotional and physical manifestations. For the nurse who is committed to dealing with the ills of society, success may rarely occur. Obviously, all nurses will occasionally need ways to cope with depression for personal and professional reasons.

First of all, the nurse should learn to grieve for her own losses. She may need to seek help from colleagues, supervisors, or counselors when facing a loss of significance.

Next, the nurse must strive to lead a life of many interests because narrowness increases the chance for changes and losses to be seen as devastating. She needs to learn to look ahead and plan for the future. One suggestion is to set aside some time and write the names and ages 10 years from now of all family members and significant individuals in her life. When these ages are studied, events that are likely to occur will emerge. For example, for one nurse it might reveal that one or both of her parents will most likely die, all of her children will have graduated from high school, she will probably be a grandmother, the person she is responsible to at work will have retired, her husband will be nine years from retirement, and she most likely will have completed the period of involution. She can then reflect on what she could be doing now to better prepare herself for these possible events.

The effects of aging on our bodies and minds seem to be particularly depressing to most of us. Our society overemphasizes youthfulness and devalues age. The nurse can begin to reorient her thinking to look for and look forward to the advantages and rewards of aging, stop thinking of signs of aging as negative and unattractive, and plan realistically for the aging stage with the same thought she gave to other stages in her life. She can then start helping patients to do the same.

The nurse can learn to search for and express the anger that is bound to arise in the stressful situations in which nurses often find themselves. In the past, the "ideal" nurse may have been thought of as a doormat for the world but that kind of acceptance of abuse from others will hardly lead to emotional health. When she feels twinges of anger, it is an alarm signal to reflect on what provoked her anger and to decide how to express it in that particular situation.

The nurse can begin to watch for any particular pattern of depression which she experiences. Is she always depressed after the weekly staff meeting? Is she regularly depressed after talking with a specific friend? Does her depression seem related to the weather? If a particular incident does seem to repeatedly be associated with feelings of depression, she should try to decide why. Does she lose her "cool" in the staff meetings and say things she later regrets? Does her friend always seem to be excelling when she is in a slump? Do rainy Mondays send her into the dumps? Once she can begin to look for the cause of her depression she is closer to self-understanding.

Usually depression can be related to unrealistic expectations one has of onself.[19] Does she expect herself to be a superwoman? What makes her think she can always get along with everyone she works with? Why should she expect to always have everything done on time? Who says that no one is entitled to a few bad days? Why does she have to perform well in groups when she much prefers to work with only one or two other people? Isn't everyone entitled to a few character flaws? She certainly can work on her flaws but she has a right to have them and still like herself.

Maybe she is trying to ignore things that are making her frustrated and angry. She can try to look for them. If she feels jealous of her friend, she can admit it to herself. Everyone experiences jealousy, anger, hate, revenge, and hostility. How she handles these emotions is the mark of growing maturity. She can try to decide what it is that she is jealous of. Did someone fail to get a promotion and secretly she was glad? We have all felt this way. Why does she think she should always have only kind thoughts about others? Regular practice at allowing oneself to be human can lead to less depression and greater self-awareness. This may lead her to work on changing what she does not like about herself.

In addition to looking for a pattern to her depression, the nurse can try to look for and remember things that make her feel good and feel good about herself. Does she feel good about herself after she has rearranged the furniture, remembered to send a birthday card on time, or spent extra time with a patient who needed her? Is there a particular song which lifts her spirits? Does she have a favorite dress which is comforting to wear? Does she like to walk in the rain? Does she like to go into a nursery and rock babies? The nurse can try to avoid depression by doing things that make her feel good about herself. If she's already depressed, she can try to do things that will make her feel better.

One helpful suggestion for the nurse for improving her self-esteem is to write on a card what she feels are her good points.[22] This may be hard to do at first. Then she places the card where she will see it frequently. She adds to the card as she thinks of good qualities she has. She should memorize her good qualities and remind herself of them when she feels discouraged. This personal inventory helps to provide a feeling of self-esteem and insulates against failures.

We sometimes have learned to repeat self-defeating themes to ourselves such as, "I am always making stupid mistakes," or "My apartment is always a mess." The nurse might try learning some esteem building themes and repeating them to herself in place of others such as, "Everyone makes mistakes but I try to correct mine" or "I may not be the neatest person in the world but I always have time to listen to my friends when they need to talk to me."[22]

The whole purpose of esteem building for the nurse is to fortify herself against depression. When she knows she is a person of value and ability, she will be able to better take the discouragement and failure which goes along with living without deciding that she is totally worthless and hopeless. She may find that certain individuals make her feel better about herself and others regularly lower her self-esteem. The nurse will need to decide what is occurring in these relationships and what to do about it. She can start evaluating all of her life situations. Are they esteem building or esteem lowering?

## A TOOL FOR ASSESSMENT AND EVALUATION

Psychiatrists and others have attempted to categorize depression in various ways. Thus one finds a constellation of terminology in the literature which overlaps and contradicts. There is mention of affective mood disorders, neurotic depression, reactive depression, involutional melancholia, endogenous depression, psychotic depressive reaction, "normal" depression, smiling depression, and masked depression to name only a few forms of depression. It has been shown that the reliability among psychiatrists in placing individuals into these classifications is poor and more related to where they practice and what kind of practice they have than to the symptoms of the individuals.[18] It would seem most useful then to describe only three categories of depressive behavior—mild, moderate, and severe as they exist on a continuum over which there can probably be greater agreement. The assessment tools in Tables 10-5 through 10-7 will guide the nurse in determining if the person she is caring for suffers from feelings of depression and in deciding how severe the depression is if it does exist. Individuals whose depression is severe are at high risk while those whose depression is mild have a good prognosis. These tools may help the nurse to assess her own depression. They can be used to assess the effectiveness of nursing intervention. If intervention is effective, the individual's depression should lessen.

No one individual will perfectly exemplify any one category, but each individual will express his depression in a unique response. Of course, depression does not exist in only these three categories. Rather depression exists on a continuum, and these three categories are points on the continuum. Any one individual may be somewhere between these categories at a given time.

Evaluators should remember that they are assessing *change in behavior* from what was normal behavior for a particular individual. For example, lack of interest in any activities outside of work may be normal for a few individuals but if someone with usual interests in

**Table 10-5.** Assessment tool for depression in infants

| Behavior | Mild depression | Moderate depression | Severe depression |
|---|---|---|---|
| Mood | Happy, curious | Some despair but usually normal | Apathetic |
| Feeding behavior | Hungry, vigorous suck reflex | Some loss of interest in food, nurses less | Resists eating, poor suck reflex, may nurse only if bottle propped |
| Growth | Normal | Normal or slowing | Below normal for length and weight |
| Developmental abilities | Normal | Normal or some delayed development | Abnormal for age |
| Play behavior | Normal with periods of disinterest and detachment | Some increase in listless behavior | Lack of play |
| Self-comforting behavior | Occasional | Frequent | Almost persistent |
| Response to painful stimuli | Vigorous protest | More annoyance than protest | Little response |
| Response to human face | Normal | Normal | Unresponsive or negative |
| Response to separation (when appropriate) | Active protest | Short protest | No response |

other activities loses all interest, it is not normal. Family members often notice depression before an outside observer does.[16]

## Assessment of Depression in Infants

The assessment tool in Table 10-5 for infants 6 months and older is based on speculation and experience. There has been little or nothing written on degrees of depression an infant may manifest except for the studies which describe severe depression in infants.[1,30] The behaviors which might appear in mild and moderate depression in infants are suggested only as a starting point and need to be validated by further research and observation before they are accepted as reliable.

## Assessment of Depression in Childhood

The assessment tool for children in Table 10-6 is again based more on experience and speculation than actual reported observations although some suggestions have been found in the literature.[3,6,17,18,25,29,33] This tool needs also to be validated by further research and observations.

## Assessment of Depression in Adolescents and Adults

Most of the assessment tool for adults in Table 10-7 can be applied to adolescents. This tool is based on criteria reported in the literature.[5,8–10,20,27,29,31]

**Table 10-6.** Assessment tool for depression in children

| Behavior | Mild depression | Moderate depression | Severe depression |
| --- | --- | --- | --- |
| Mood | Appropriate | Periods of sadness | Persistent gloom |
| Play | May show presence of depressive themes | Most play associated with depressive themes | Unable to play |
| Activity level | Normal, mild fatigue, or mild hyperactivity | Fatigues easily, appears tired or very hyperactive | Appears very tired, psychomotor retardation |
| Thought content | Some covert expressions of guilt and worthlessness | Overt expressions of helplessness and hopelessness | Preoccupied with miserable state |
| School performance | Normal | May show waning interest | Deteriorating performance |
| Change observed by parents | None | May feel child is tired or "going through a stage" | Notice marked changes |
| Acting out | Absent | Occasional | May be present |

**Table 10-7.** Assessment tool for depression in adolescents and adults

| Behavior | Mild depression | Moderate depression | Severe depression |
|---|---|---|---|
| Mood | Bored, worried, "down" | Gloom, helplessness | Devastating melancholia, hopelessness |
| Persistence of mood | Fluctuates during day | Mood varies from one day or one week to the next | Mood relatively fixed for weeks |
| Effect on school or work activities | Functions much the same | Manifests some decrease in output | Unable to perform meaningful work |
| Effect on home life | Close observation shows changes | Readily apparent changes in home life | Almost nonfunctional at home |
| Activity level | Fatigues easily, extra effort required for usual activities. Adolescent may show mild hyperactivity | Unable to perform some of usual activities. May be restless. Adolescent may become hyperactive | Psychomotor retardation or agitation |
| Thought content | Expresses realistic worries, guilt absent | Some preoccupation with unhappiness. Blames others for his difficulties | Preoccupation with his miserable state, guilt present |
| Suicidal thoughts or attempts | Rare | Occasional | Frequent |
| Physical changes | None | Some loss of appetite or mild insomnia or overeating | Usually insomnia, anorexia, constipation, etc. |
| Reality testing | Normal | Normal | Impaired, may have delusions |
| Ability for enjoyment | Enjoys some things. Hard to keep optimistic thoughts in mind | Little or no enjoyment found, optimism gone | No enjoyment felt, persistent pessimism |
| Subjective feelings | Doesn't feel good, but doesn't feel terribly bad. States he knows things aren't as bad as they seem at the moment. | May feel ill, may complain of aches and pains | May have hypochondriacal delusions, believes things are as bad as they seem |
| Onset | Abrupt | Abrupt | Insidious |
| Acting out (in adolescents) | Absent | Usually alternates with more "typical" depressive behavior | May be persistent |
| Change noticed by others | Only by close friends | May be apparent to associates at work or classmates | Apparent to distant acquaintances |
| Depressive equivalents | Absent | May have vague headaches, etc., not accompanied by other symptoms | May have persistent unrelenting symptoms which are not accompanied by the more classical symptoms of depression |

# AN EXAMPLE OF NURSING INTERVENTION IN DEPRESSION

The following nursing intervention was undertaken by a nursing student during her experience in caring for children in an episodic setting.

Lisa was a tiny 4-year-old girl brought to the hospital on a Sunday evening because she had a fever and infected sores around her mouth. She was accompanied by her grandparents who stated they did not know where her mother was. The chart stated that both grandparents had apparently been drinking heavily, and that the child was very dirty, dehydrated, and scared.

Lisa lay motionless in her bed. She was heavily restrained because she might attempt to disconnect her I.V. The only responses she made to her environment were to refuse to take medicine by clenching her teeth, to fight feebly when her mouth scores were cleaned, and to turn her head away when her bed was approached. Her small size, her sunken eyes, and her tired expression made her look the picture of dejection. The student who was to care for Lisa on Monday morning had been the last to choose her assignment and had Lisa only because no other student had chosen to care for her. The student was less than eager and was soon looking for her instructor for help. Together they decided that Lisa was probably coping with her environment by withdrawal, regression, and depression and the student was challenged to apply what she had studied about intervening in depression over the next few days.

The first morning, the student performed Lisa's care with slowness and gentleness. She gave her short specific information on what she was doing. Lisa kept her eyes closed and partially resisted physical contact. When the student gave Lisa her medications and cleaned her lesions she talked to Lisa as a way of helping her express her emotions and to show acceptance. "You hate to take this stuff, don't you? You wish we would leave you alone. This hurts, doesn't it? You wish I would go away." After the morning care, the student sat at the bedside and occasionally spoke to Lisa.

At the end of the morning, the team leader announced to the student that Lisa was to be moved to a four-bed ward because the physicians had decided that her infected mouth sores were not contagious. The student objected to the move and convinced the team leader and head nurse that Lisa needed a quieter room and attention from only a few people until she was more responsive. The student wrote her ideas on caring for Lisa on the care plan.

On the second day, Lisa initially appeared much the same. Again the student performed all care slowly and with minimal verbalization. During the bath the student noticed that Lisa opened her eyes and took a quick look at her. Again the student talked to Lisa during the painful parts of the care. After the bath, the student decided to rub some lotion on Lisa's back because Lisa had accepted physical contact. During the backrub the student said to Lisa, "I'll bet you wish you were home with your grandma. You like your bed at home better, don't you?" After the care the student again sat at the bedside. Lisa didn't turn her head away as before. Just before the student left she read one short story to Lisa.

On Wednesday morning, the student proceeded in the same manner. Lisa had her eyes open and watched the nurse with a blank expression. Unfortunately Lisa's I.V. had infiltrated and was to be restarted. During the procedure Lisa surprised everyone by yelling a very loud (and very appropriate) curse word at the physician—the first word she had said since admission. The student responded by expressing her obvious delight and saying, "You can tell us when you are mad." Later in the morning, the student asked Lisa a few one-answer questions but Lisa refused to respond. She did try to give Lisa a pillow doll to hold which she usually rejected and ignored, but Lisa seemed to accept the doll that morning. She asked Lisa if she would like to watch TV and Lisa's eyes seemed to light up. The student then arranged for Lisa to be moved to a room with a TV. There were two other girls in the room who usually were in the playroom most of the day.

The student did not have clinical duties on Thursday but went to visit Lisa for an hour before class. She offered Lisa something to drink and for the first time Lisa sat up and drank from the glass. The student sat beside her on the bed and eventually held her on her lap and read several stories. Lisa looked at the pages. The student noticed that the pillow doll was gone. As the student told her goodbye and mentioned her name again, Lisa abruptly said, "My name's not Lisa, it's Sissy." The student told her how glad she was to know that and said, "You must have been really upset with us for not even knowing your name." As she was telling the nursing staff about the name, a nurse mentioned that she had torn apart the pillow doll and shredded the stuffing. The student suggested to them that this was a sign that Lisa might be ready to express her anger and they decided to try to find some paper that she could tear up. The student visited Sissy again after her classes were over and found Sissy had just awakened from her nap and was crying. She went readily to the student and continued to sob while the student comforted her and suggested to her why she might be crying. Sissy asked for a drink and nodded her head when the student suggested that they go over to look out the window. Sissy pointed at cars and buses but was soon tired. When the student left, Sissy started to cry and refused to wave goodbye or look at her.

The student visited Sissy again on Friday morning. Sissy was watching TV but would not eat her breakfast. The student was told that Sissy had tried to bite a nurse when she gave her some medicine during the night. The student found a baby teething ring and told her she could bite it when she was mad. She also brought Sissy some crayons and some paper and encouraged Sissy to color. Sissy peeled all the paper off of each crayon before she would use it. She answered questions about her home and her brothers and sisters as she colored.

On Friday evening the student found the grandmother sitting beside Sissy's bed. She was talking with other parents in the room about her family and ignoring Sissy who was lying in bed awake. The student talked to Sissy for a while and held her while she asked the grandmother questions about Sissy's behavior at home. From the information she received, it appeared that Sissy was behind developmentally and lacking in appropriate diet and stimulation. According to the grandmother, Sissy spent most of the day sleeping and watching TV. She was not yet toilet trained. The grandmother seemed uninterested in talking about Sissy and kept saying "She gives me no trouble except she's always getting sick." She then complained about her problems with Sissy's older brothers and other boys in the neighborhood. The student felt that the grandmother was not currently able to focus on Sissy so she asked the grandmother if a community health nurse could visit her to talk with her about problems with her family and to see if she could help keep Sissy from being sick as much. The grandmother agreed and the student made the referral, writing a detailed summary of Sissy's hospital stay and the interview with the grandmother. Sissy gave her a hug and a kiss when she left.

Sissy was discharged on Saturday morning. She was responsive, her sores were healing, and she was eating but she was not the enthusiastic or exuberant child she should have been at 4 years of age. The student concluded that a depressive episode in Sissy's life had been resolved but that Sissy was showing evidence that she might become chronically depressed unless her home environment could become more appropriate to her needs.

# SUMMARY

Mild or moderate depression is a common experience. It is felt to result primarily from the feeling of having suffered a loss. Depression can occur to individuals throughout the life cycle and it may take many forms. The nurse is in frequent contact with individuals who are likely to become depressed because of alterations in their level of wellness or life style. The nurse can use primary and secondary prevention to intervene to relieve depression. Nurses too may become depressed and there are ways the nurse can learn to cope with her own feelings of depression.

# REFERENCES

1. Bowlby, J.: "Pathological mourning and childhood mourning." J. Am. Psychoanal. Assoc. 44:500, 1963.
2. Brown, M. M., and Fowler, G. R.: *Psychodynamic Nursing*. W. B. Saunders, Philadelphia, 1971.
3. Chapman, A. H.: *Management of Emotional Problems of Children and Adolescents*. J. B. Lippincott, Philadelphia, 1974.
4. Chappel, J. N., and Daniels, R. S.: "Puerperal psychosis." Hospital Med. 5:26, 1969.
5. Crary, W. G., and Crary, G. C.: "Depression." Am. J. Nurs. 73:472, 1973.
6. Cytryn, L. and McKnew, D. H.: "Factors influencing the changing clinical expression of the depressive process in children." Am. J. Psychiat. 131:879, 1974.
7. Enelow, A. J. (ed.): *Depression in Medical Practice*. Merck, Sharp and Dohme, West Point, Pa., 1971.
8. Enelow, A. J.: *Uncovering Depression in the Anxious Patient*. Merck, Sharp and Dohme, West Point, Pa., 1973.
9. Evans, F. M.: *Psychosocial Nursing*. Macmillan, New York, 1971.
10. Francis, G. M., and Munjas, B.: *Promoting Psychological Comfort*. Wm. C. Brown, Dubuque, 1975.
11. Havens, A.: "Care of a depressed medical-surgical patient." Am. J. Nurs. 70:1070, 1970.
12. Jourard, S. M.: "Suicide: The invitation to die." Am. J. Nurs. 70:269, 1970.
13. Kaplan, H. I.: "Depression," in Freedman, A. M. et al.: *Modern Synopsis of Comprehensive Textbook of Psychiatry II*. Williams and Wilkins, Baltimore, 1976.
14. Kubler-Ross, E.: *On Death and Dying*. Macmillan, New York, 1969.
15. Lee, R. E., and Ball, P. A.: "Some thoughts on the psychology of the coronary care unit patient." Am. J. Nurs. 75:1498, 1975.
16. Limandri, B. J., and Boyle, D. W.: "Instilling hope." Am. J. Nurs. 78:79, 1978.
17. Malmquist, C. P.: "Depression in childhood and adolescence: Part one." New Engl. J. Med. 284:887, 1971.
18. Malmquist, C. P.: "Depression in childhood and adolescence: Part two." New Engl. J. Med. 284:955, 1971.
19. McBride, A. B.: *The Growth and Development of Mothers*. Harper and Row, New York, 1973.
20. Mendels, J.: *Concepts of Depression*. John Wiley and Sons, New York, 1970.
21. Mitchell, R.: "Depression." Nurs. Times 70:1085, 1974.
22. O'Leary, K. D., and Wilson, G. T.: *Behavior Therapy: Application and Outcome*. Prentice-Hall, Englewood Cliffs, N.J., 1975.
23. Peplau, H. E.: "Mid-Life crises." Am. J. Nurs. 75:1761, 1975.
24. Reeder, S. R., et al.: *Maternity Nursing*. J. B. Lippincott, Philadelphia, 1976.
25. Renshaw, D. C.: "Suicide and depression in children." J. School Health 44:487, 1974.
26. Risley, J.: "Nursing intervention in depression." Perspect. Psychiat. Care 5:65, 1967.
27. Robinson, L.: *Psychological Aspects of the Care of Hospitalized Patients*. F. A. Davis, Philadelphia, 1972.
28. Schoenberg, B., et al.: *Loss and Grief: Psychological Management in Medical Practice*. Columbia University Press, New York, 1970.
29. Soloman, P., and Patch, V. D.: *Handbook of Psychiatry*. Lange Medical Publishers, Los Altos, Calif., 1971.
30. Spitz, R.: "Hospitalism, an inquiry into the genesis of psychiatric conditions in early childhood." Psychoanal. Study Child 1:53, 1945.
31. Stockwell, M. L.: "Depression: an operational definition with themes related to the nurse's role," in Zderad, L., and Belchner, H. (eds.): *Developing Behavioral Concepts in Nursing*. Southern Regional Education Board, Atlanta, 1968.

32. Vaillot, Sr. M. C.: "Hope: The restoration of being." Am. J. Nurs. 70:268, 1970.
33. Varley, J. E.: "Depression in children." Nurs. Times 70:1568, 1974.
34. White, C. L.: "Nurse counseling with a depressed patient." Am. J. Nurs. 78:436, 1978.
35. Wicks, R. J.: *Counseling Strategies and Intervention Techniques for the Human Services.* J. B. Lippincott, Philadelphia, 1977.

## BIBLIOGRAPHY

Boyajean, A.: "Fighting despair." Am. J. Nurs. 78:76, 1978.
"Programmed instruction: Helping depressed patients in general nursing practice." Am. J. Nurs. 77:1007, 1977.

# PART 3

## POTENTIAL GROWTH SITUATIONS FOR PATIENTS AND FAMILIES

This section deals with four selected situations which may occur to individuals during their life span. These are situations which are not unique to any particular medical condition or health care setting but transcend diagnostic categories and health care institution boundaries.

These situations are supreme challenges to the individual experiencing them. Each situation has the potential for enhancing or diminishing the functioning of the individual involved and possibly that of those around him. The purpose of this discussion is to alert the nurse to the dimensions of each situation and prepare her to assess and intervene appropriately to promote a favorable outcome and growth of the individuals involved as a result. In addition, the nurse may face each of these potential growth situations and she may benefit from the information given personally. The situations included are crisis, change in self-concept, fatal illness, and parenthood.

# CHAPTER 11

# CRISIS

The nurse often comes in contact with individuals or families who are nearing or are in a state of crisis. Some crises will be more severe than others. The nurse who encounters a family or individual in crisis must intervene intensively to be of utmost benefit. This chapter will present information designed to acquaint the nurse with the concept of crisis and how to assess and intervene in crises her patients encounter. Information will also be given on how the nurse can respond to the personal crises she faces.

## REVIEW OF THEORY

In the most general terms, a crisis can be thought of as an unusually demanding situation which an individual or family cannot resolve easily or quickly. A period of time ensues in which the demands of the situation persist while the individual or family involved struggle to meet them unsuccessfully. This period of time represents a phase in which the usual patterns of life of the individual or family are disrupted.[22]

## The Anatomy of a Crisis

A crisis is believed to occur in response to a certain series of events. The stages listed below represent these events in a simplified manner.

1. The individual or family is in a steady state.
2. A hazardous event occurs.
3. The situation is perceived as a threat or danger.
4. The usual methods of coping are tried and fail to reduce the threat.
5. A disruption of usual mental and emotional functioning occurs.
6. A period of disequilibrium occurs with an increase in discomfort, anxiety, or depression.
7. A solution is found or severe personal disorganization occurs.[1,2,4,22,31]

## Hazardous Events

A crisis is initiated by the occurrence of a hazardous event. One faces many hazardous events during one's lifetime and may be in precarious situations often, but usually one copes and seldom is a true state of crisis reached.[15] It is impossible to give a comprehensive list of events which are likely to produce a crisis for all individuals. There are some situations which are likely to produce a crisis for all individuals such as the death of a close friend. There are other situations which are likely to lead to crisis for some but not for others.[24] For example, the birth of a premature baby may send one family into crisis but not another. The meaning of a hazardous event is unique to each individual or family.[25]

How the individual or family interprets the event is a key factor. Hazardous events which are interpreted as a threat will usually lead to predominant anxiety. Those events which involve a loss often lead to depression. If the hazardous event is interpreted as a challenge, there may be a helpful mobilization of resources.[24]

The hazardous event does not always lead immediately to a crisis. There is often a period of days or weeks before the individual or family becomes uncomfortable enough to seek help. As unbelievable as it may seem, the individual or family in crisis does not always know specifically what the hazardous event was which precipitated the crisis. Therefore, recognizing the hazardous event is one goal of intervention.[15]

One point to be emphasized is that the actual nature of the hazardous event is not as important as the perception of the hazardous event which the individual or family has. It is believed that coping is better and crisis more likely avoided when the hazardous event is perceived realistically. Unrealistic or distorted perception of the hazardous event leads predictably to crisis.[1]

Hazardous events can occur in clusters so that the effect of each one is magnified or compounded. The event which finally leads to crisis may be difficult to determine in this situation.

## Types of Hazardous Events

It has been mentioned that crises are the result of hazardous events which are unusually numerous or troubling or for some reason appear to be so to the individuals involved. Some theoretic speculation has been done on the types of hazardous events likely to lead to crisis.

### ROLE CHANGE

Much attention has been given to events involving role change as important causes of crisis. Crises do seem to be frequent during times which involve many role changes such as during adolescence, marriage, parenthood, and retirement, for example. The theory is that crisis occurs when the individual is unable to make the role change.[33] The stresses on the individual or family related to role changes can involve many factors.[28,33,34] The person or family may not want to make the role change but may feel pressure from others to do so. This might occur when a younger sibling is expected to take over the role of an older sibling who dies. Or the opposite may be true in that the role may be desired by the person involved but others may be hesitant to let him assume the new role. This might explain the crisis prone adolescent years. An individual or family may experience difficulties making a role change because of a lack of certain skills necessary to successfully perform the new role. This may be due in part to a lack of experience, education, or proper role models. For example, a man coming from a family where there was much disharmony and few examples of compromise and problem solving may encounter a crisis in his own marriage in assuming the role his wife expects and he desires. Another situation related to role change involves the loss of an important role. This might explain crisis which occurs following death of a spouse, at retirement, or after menopause.

When the nurse identifies a crisis state, she may be able to offer concrete help if she determines if the individual or family has experienced or are experiencing a role change. Valuable data may be obtained by determining from the family if there was preparation for the change, how much disparity exists between the new role and the old one, if there was dissatisfaction with the old role, and how reinforcements or punishments being given by others are affecting the old and the new role. It is important to remember that even if the role change is highly desired it can still be crisis producing.

## LOSS

Loss can be viewed as a cause of crisis. An examination of most crisis situations will demonstrate that a loss has occurred.[12] Loss of a loved one can occur through death, desertion, divorce, or separation. Loss of self-esteem can occur because of changes in physical appearance, control or functioning, status, and pattern of employment, among others. The loss of an important role can occur because of retirement, college graduation, or disabling illness. Loss of social supports can occur because of moving, loss of friends, loss of a job, and children leaving home. Even losses which result from changes in the environment such as a loss of familiar possessions, home, or community structures can lead to crisis. Loss of faith in others or a personal loss of faith can lead to a crisis.

Each crisis situation should be assessed in terms of what losses the individuals involved are experiencing. Severe grieving over losses can resemble a crisis.

## THREATS

Threats to an individual may lead to a crisis. These can include threats to bodily integrity such as occur during surgery or physical illness, or threats to the self system as would occur following any situation where one's self-esteem is put in jeopardy. Examples of this include going into debt, losing a pregnancy, or an unsuccessful attempt to assume a new occupation.

In summary, many events can lead to a hazardous event and result in a crisis, including events which involve role change, loss, and threats to the individual.

## Methods of Coping

After experiencing a hazardous event, the individual or family will subconsciously attempt to reduce anxiety or solve the problem by their normal coping mechanisms. This attempt may fail in some circumstances for several reasons.

First of all, the hazardous event facing the individual or family may be more complex or stressful than any they have previously experienced so that their familiar coping methods are ineffective. This might occur when one family member experiences a major illness. Secondly, the methods usually available to cope with stressors may have become unavailable. For example, a young woman who coped with adverse situations by excessive reliance on her parents developed a crisis when she went to another state to attend college and she could no longer depend as exclusively on her parents to solve her problems. Thirdly, in some situations the individual or family may be under such stress that they do not remember methods of coping which were effective in the past.

As many abortive solution attempts are made and fail, the individual experiences increasing anxiety which he expresses in various ways through control behaviors. Once coping methods have failed, the individual may begin to rely on defense mechanisms. Some feel that crisis begins at the point where coping mechanisms fail and predominantly defensive mechanisms are used.[19] Coping mechanisms are basically attempts to solve the problem and therefore crisis is less likely to ensue. Defense mechanisms are more related to attempts to avoid the problem and crisis is more likely to result. Table 11-1 examines some differences between control behaviors used as coping or defense mechanisms. Using this information, the nurse can examine the behaviors the individual is using to see if they are coping or defense mechanisms. Note that some control behaviors could be healthy or unhealthy depending on how they are being used at the time in a particular situation so that one cannot label behaviors as absolutely healthy or unhealthy. If the behaviors being used by an individual to face a crisis predominantly resemble those characteristics of coping mechanisms, crisis is unlikely. However, if his behavior predominantly resembles the characteristics of defense mechanisms, crisis is likely.

**Table 11-1.** Some characteristics of control behaviors used as coping mechanisms as contrasted to control behaviors used as defense mechanisms

| Coping mechanisms | Defense mechanisms |
| --- | --- |
| Behavior promotes awareness of present situation | Behavior lessens awareness of present situation |
| Reality orientation is maintained | Distortion of reality occurs |
| Present situation is accurately evaluated | Present situation is distorted in terms of the past |
| Behavior conserves energy | Behavior consumes energy to be maintained |
| Behavior allows continuation of important relationships with others | Behavior impedes important relationships |
| There is balance among actions | One behavior used repeatedly |
| Behavior is dropped when hazardous situation ceases | Behavior continues after situation ceases |
| Use of the behavior controlled by the individual | Behavior controls the individual |
| Behavior favors solution of the problem | Behavior favors denial of the problem |
| Growth of the person is possible | Growth is unlikely |
| Behavior results logically from the situation | Behavior results because of experiences in the past[8,19,30] |

These two examples illustrate the use of predominantly defense behaviors by one person and the use of predominantly coping behaviors by another.

> Mrs. Smith and Mrs. Jones were both shocked to learn that their 16-year-old daughter was pregnant.
>
> Mrs. Smith reacted with anger towards her daughter. She blamed her daughter's friends and the school she attended. Mrs. Smith had herself become pregnant out of wedlock and had been forced into a marriage by her parents which ended in divorce. She saw this situation as proof that she had failed as a mother. She avoided her friends, quit her bridge club, and ceased going to church. She insisted that the pregnancy be kept a secret. She could not support her daughter or plan for her health care because of her own emotional response. She became increasingly more despondent. Her daughter avoided home more and more. Mrs. Smith was brought to the emergency room late one night by her daughter. She had apparently taken an overdose of sleeping pills.
>
> Mrs. Jones was also angry initially at her daughter, her daughter's friends, and the school. She remembered that one of her closest friends had been through the same situation a few years earlier and she sought her out. She also told her friends at the next bridge game. Her friends listened to her and offered their sympathy and support. She took her daughter to their family physician. He was aware of her emotional turmoil and assured her that an out-of-wedlock pregnancy was difficult for everyone involved but that it happened frequently and most families were able to survive the experience. Mrs. Jones and her daughter went home and began the first of several long conversations on how to handle the daughter's situation. She was able to see how fearful and ashamed her daughter was. Mrs. Jones told her friends that she was bitter that the whole thing had happened but since it had, they might as well make the best of a bad situation.

## Period of Disequilibrium

The presence of a period of disequilibrium in which the individual or family does not function normally is a hallmark of crisis.[16] This period results after coping has been ineffective. It is described by the individual in crisis as a state of great emotional turmoil and upset. It is during this stage that the individual may seek help. Anxiety, depression, anorexia, tension, anger, withdrawal, guilt, restlessness, and confusion are characteristic symptoms.[6] This stage of acute disequilibrium cannot last long and usually is over in four to six weeks.

If a solution has been found to the crisis problem, the individual or family may emerge from the period of disequilibrium at the same level of functioning which existed before the crisis or even at a higher level. If no solution or a poor solution has been found, the individual or family may emerge at a lower level of functioning. Examples of solutions which in certain circumstances are evidence of reaching a lower level of functioning include solving the problem through use of alcohol, drugs, other types of chemical abuse, family dissolution, suicide attempts, successful suicide, homicide, or the development of a frank mental illness.

There are two important reasons why one should recognize when individuals or families are in a period of disequilibrium. First, the family or individual at this point is very likely to be helped significantly if a helper can work intensively with the persons involved. The potential for growth and change in a positive direction is high.[16] Without help, adverse responses are likely. Secondly, at the time of disequilibrium, other related problems are likely to emerge and can be dealt with constructively.[22,24] For example, Mrs. Smith in the previous example reacted to her daughter's pregnancy with emotional responses somewhat colored by her own previous pregnancy out of wedlock. With the appropriate help, Mrs. Smith might have gained some ground in resolving this much earlier problem as the present crisis was solved.

## Classification of Types of Crises

There have been many attempts in the literature to classify crises. Some of the more useful ways of representing crises are presented below.

### SITUATIONAL AND MATURATIONAL CRISES

Crises are sometimes separated into situational and maturational types. Maturational crises are those that occur during transition periods from one stage of development to another during the normal course of life. Erickson has defined eight stages of development and described the challenges inherent in each stage. These stages range from infancy to old age and are potential crisis periods because when one must make the transition from one phase to another, new ways must be substituted for old ways of functioning.[7] Examples of individual maturational crises include the identity crisis of the adolescent and the crisis of the menopause. Family maturational crises could be identified as marriage, the first pregnancy, and the "empty nest" period. Maturational crises occur gradually and are common. These are now commonly thought of as not necessarily crises but rather as crisis prone periods. Thus one can anticipate needs and give special help to individuals or families facing transition periods in development and in family life.

Situational crises on the other hand occur because of unexpected, unusual events which are not necessarily common to all individuals or families. Examples of situational crises include death of a spouse, destruction of one's home by a tornado, and the birth of a premature baby. Situational crises are sudden, and because they are uncommon, few individuals are familiar with them or prepared for them.

Many crises cannot be definitely separated into either category but belong partially to both. For example, the crisis associated with school entry is partly developmental and partly situational.

### EXTRAFAMILIAL AND INTRAFAMILIAL CRISES

Another way to classify crises is by determining whether the crisis arises from inside or from outside of the family.[11] Crises which arise from within the family tend to be more potentially disintegrating to the family. Examples include divorce, illegitimacy, illness of a member, and alcoholism. Crises which arise from extrafamilial causes may be more likely to solidify the family. Examples of extrafamilial crises include war, destruction of the family home, and loss of employment. This framework provides some ideas about how the crises may be perceived by the family.

### INTERNAL AND EXTERNAL CRISES

Still another classification system for looking at crisis centers on the nature of its cause.[20] When one is unexpectedly fired or a loved one dies, an externally caused crisis can occur. An internally caused crisis arises when one begins to question one's view of the world and one's role in relation to it. Internally caused crises are more disruptive and complicated because they demand personal change. Examples of internally caused crises include deciding to seek divorce, deciding to change careers, or deciding to go against cultural standards.

Use of the foregoing classification systems may help the nurse put the crisis into perspective. Thus she can determine whether the crisis was expected or unexpected, associated with maturation or situation, arising from within the family or from outside, and caused by external events or change within the person.

## Crisis Proneness

In order to explain why some individuals or families experience a crisis while others facing the same situation do not, proneness to crisis must be considered. Several factors affecting proneness to crisis have been identified.[11,16]

1. Crisis prone life style. Some families face numerous crisis provoking events which may occur because of their life style in that they are frequently exposed to losses, threats, and role changes. The cumulative effect of frequent events can lead to an increased number of crises.

2. Failure to achieve developmental tasks. Individuals or families who have unresolved individual or family developmental needs are believed to be more poorly prepared to cope with hazardous events. For example, the young couple who conceive before wedlock and then have a premature baby may not have had sufficient time to develop their marital relationship so they can support and sustain each other through the situation and crisis may be more likely.

3. Lack of supportive relationships. Other individuals who may be helpful to families or individuals facing a crisis are relatives, neighbors, friends, clergy, physicians, and other professionals. Individuals or families who are removed from their extended family and isolated from other sources of help may be more prone to experience crises. When assessing the supportive relationships available to a family or individual, one should look at both quantity and quality of the relationships. One true friend may be more valuable than 25 nodding acquaintances.

4. Lack of coping skills. A number of individuals have developed faulty coping skills for a number of reasons and may react to a crisis situation with the development of defensive behavior because of unresolved needs, conflicts, or because excessive anxiety is preventing problem solving.

5. Lack of resources. Money, wellness, space, religious faith, energy, heredity, intelligence, rituals, creativity, perseverance, and ingenuity are some of the resources which families or individuals may or may not possess. Resources which one individual or family has may reduce the threat of a crisis while another individual or family without the same resources may be incapacitated.

> Bob and Bill were both in their middle 50s when they suffered identical car accidents. Bill had taken good care of himself by exercising regularly, eating a balanced diet, and wearing his seat belt when in a car. His family had a comfortable savings account. He recovered from the injuries he sustained promptly.
>
> Bob, however, was not in as good a state of health. He was overweight, out of shape, hypertensive, a heavy smoker, and had significant coronary artery disease. He suffered more severe injuries because he wasn't wearing his seat belt. His family had practically no savings in the bank at all. His recovery was complicated by his less robust physical condition and he and his family experienced a crisis because of the prolonged and costly medical care involved and his lengthy loss of income.

6. Inaccurate perception of the hazardous event. Those who look at events and situations from a distorted perspective are more likely to misinterpret a hazardous event and are more likely to experience a crisis. This is likely caused by a distortion of the present because of unresolved problems from the past so that the present is seen in terms of some past event which may not be relevant.

7. Crisis prone family characteristics. Hill has described the crisis prone family as one which is highly mobile, small, poorly structured, possesses few economic reserves, and attempts self-sufficiency. Favorable family characteristics are adaptability, integration, affectionate relations, social activity, democratic control, good marital adjustment, companionable parent-child relationships, and previous successes with crisis.[11]

These factors can help the nurse predict those whom she works with who may be most in need of help when a hazardous event occurs.

## Intensity of Crises

Crises can vary in intensity from mild to severe. Everyone has probably experienced a mild crisis sometime during his life where for several minutes or hours his attention was totally absorbed by a situation and he was functioning at a very minimal level. Later one may have looked back at the situation and wondered why he coped so poorly. The more severe crises which involve weeks of disequilibrium are less frequent. The intensity of the crisis can be assessed by noting the amount and the length of the period of loss of functioning which occurs to the individuals involved. Thus a mild crisis lasts for a short period of time and involves less loss of usual functioning. A severe crisis involves profound loss of normal functioning and lasts weeks.

## The Value of Crisis

What has been presented so far may lead one to believe that hazardous events are to be avoided at all possible costs. However, if one did attempt to lead his life in a manner which avoided all possible chances of loss, threat, or role change, his existence might be very mundane. Crisis situations are potential turning points in life and provide challenge. For those who enter the crisis situation well equipped and emerge the better for it, crisis situations sometimes provide the spice of life. Crisis situations then are not synonymous with illness or maladjustment. What is important is that the individual facing a crisis be helped towards the most optimal conclusion possible while experiencing the least amount of disorganization possible.

## The Role of Culture

Another factor which affects how an individual or family faces a crisis is cultural expectations.[12] The influence of culture may help to define if a particular event is or is not a crisis. For example, a pregnancy out of wedlock is acceptable and understandable in some cultures and highly unacceptable in others. Other aspects of the culture may support or increase the threat during a crisis. The nurse will need to be alert to how the individual's particular cultural expectations influence his perception of his situation. If her values and attitudes are different from his, she may make erroneous conclusions about the cause of the crisis and the proper solution. For this reason, she needs to learn about other cultural and subcultural expectations besides those she holds. She should realize that her lack of knowledge about other ways of life can limit her effectiveness with those whose life values are different from hers.

# MANIFESTATIONS OF CRISIS THROUGHOUT THE LIFE CYCLE

Although crisis is frequently written about in the literature, little has been described about how crisis affects individuals in various phases of the life cycle. The following sections offer some speculations based on normal growth and development.

## Young Children

Even young children probably have the potential for experiencing crisis situations. Examples of role changes which may occur to a young child include being replaced as the "baby" by a new sibling and being progressively forced to accept responsibility for control of bodily functions and impulses. Threats to self-esteem include feelings of insecurity and failure. Threats to bodily integrity can include medical treatment and accidental injuries. Losses which can threaten the young child include losses caused by separation from those significant in his life.

Little has been written about how young children experience crises. Because coping mechanisms are immature, the young child is likely to handle a crisis by denial, repression, projection, and regression.[26,30] These behaviors are commonly seen after the birth of a younger sibling and during illness. The young child who is in a family in crisis is prone to unsuccessful crisis resolution because he is likely to be unaided by the adults in the family who themselves are functioning at a low level. Therefore children in the family in crisis need particular attention. Harm to the child's personality is not likely if the situation does not last too long. It is known that children have the ability to weather devastating crises well.[9]

## School-aged Children

Older children experience a major role change in school entry and a crisis is likely to occur in some children.[14] Threats to bodily integrity can include medical treatment, mutilating injuries, and fatal diseases.[30] Threats to the self system can include failure to achieve or excel, peer rejection, and criticism for inappropriate sex role linked behavior.[23] Losses can be symbolic such as loss of status or self-esteem after parental divorce or actual losses such as loss of a parent, sibling, grandparent, or a pet.

The school-aged child responds to crisis with the same defenses as the younger child used with more effectiveness. The school-aged child may evidence the period of disequilibrium through declining school performance, withdrawal from peers and family, regression to earlier behaviors, and somatic expression of anxiety. The school-aged child in a family in crisis will have some strengths of his own to deal with crisis but he may need help from others because of the inability of the adults involved to focus attention on his needs. Children of this age and younger often draw considerable support from their siblings even though they may not appear to do so. For this reason, it is usually best to advise parents not to separate their children when a crisis occurs. In fact, if the whole family can manage to stay together, the outcome is enhanced.

## Adolescents

Role change is one of the primary tasks of the adolescent and the difficult and necessary transition from child to adult is likely to be accompanied by a crisis in identity for a large number of teenagers. Other role changes can occur when the adolescent finishes school, marries, becomes employed, or becomes a parent. For some teenagers, many of these role changes may occur quite rapidly and crisis proneness is accentuated by a lack of resources in some cases.

Threats to bodily integrity can occur over rapid body changes, illnesses, medical treatment, and accidental injuries. Threats to the self system can revolve around rejection by peers, conflict with parents, achievement failure, and self-concept alteration. Losses the teenager may experience include loss of parents, siblings, friends or symbolic losses such as loss of status, reputation, or faith.

Teenagers possibly react to crises with adultlike coping methods. Anxiety may lead to hyperactivity or acute anxiety episodes. Disequilibrium is sometimes difficult to differentiate because it may be assumed to be some of the usual behaviors of teenagers such as daydreaming, periods of apathy, moodiness, and escape sleeping.

## Young Adults

Role changes associated with young adulthood are usually numerous as one assumes work or career roles, marries, and becomes a parent. Role confusion is likely as one tries to balance work responsibilities, family obligations, relationships between the family of origination and procreation, and needs for personal accomplishment. Usually role models are prevalent and patterning oneself after others, even parents, may grant the young adult some role security. Threats to bodily integrity and threats to the self system are numerous. Losses are usually not as crisis provoking as they will be later but they may occur.

The young adult's proneness to crisis will be unique for each individual and family group according to their circumstances. A lack of resources is a common problem for many young families. Periods of disequilibrium are usually easy to determine and will manifest themselves as disturbances of functioning at work and at home. More subtle signs may include loss of interest in sexual relationships and a withdrawal from the community.

## Middle-aged Adults

Role changes faced by middle-aged adults may be more troublesome in this stage of development. Losses or changes in employment can be threatening. Divorce or death of a spouse and the resulting role changes can be crisis provoking. Other role changes are likely as children leave home. Threats to bodily integrity may increase as physical complaints and illnesses become more noticeable and aging begins in earnest. Threats to the self system can include an awareness of aging, and realization that one has not accomplished all that was intended. Losses are likely to become more numerous including the loss of parents, friends, and sometimes spouses. Symbolic losses likely to occur include loss of youthfulness, parental role, respect, and loss of health. All of these together probably account for the renowned "mid-life crisis." Because of all the possibilities described, crises might be likely to occur abundantly in the middle years except there is often a balancing factor involved. The middle-aged adult may have more resources and may have found more effective coping methods to deal with hazardous events. He may have had successful experiences with previous crises to fall back on. Supportive relationships may be plentiful and of high quality. Children, now mature, may be seen as a positive factor.

## Older Adults

Role changes as one reaches older adulthood become prominent. Losing a spouse, retirement, relocation, and increasing dependency may require considerable role adaptations. Threats to bodily integrity can include failing vision, hearing, and deterioration of general functioning. Threats to the self system can include a lack of recognition, respect, and status. Losses can include loss of youthfulness, self-respect, value, worth, resources, and supportive relationships. Some older individuals may suffer from a pervasive feeling of loss. Sometimes another loss occurs before grieving for the last loss is complete.[5]

The elderly, then, are likely to experience crises because of the increasing number of hazardous events they confront combined with dwindling resources and supports. On the positive side, they have much more experience than younger individuals to fall back on including memories of times when they overcame hazardous situations.[5]

The disequilibrium an older individual may experience in a state of crisis may not be recognized but assumed to be behavior caused by senility such as withdrawal, decreased functioning, and somatic representations of anxiety through bodily complaints which are common in the elderly.

# NURSING INTERVENTION IN CRISIS

## Primary Prevention of Severe Crises

Primary prevention in this instance will focus on preventing unnecessary crises or major severe crises. Preventing all crises is not possible or even desirable. For example, becoming a parent can lead to a crisis for many individuals, but no one would suggest absolute prevention by advising everyone not to become a parent. Realistically, primary prevention would focus instead on educating individuals for parenthood so that crisis, if it occurs, would be mild. The goal of primary prevention, then, is seen as preventing crisis if possible and desirable or preventing intense crisis.

There are many events in the lives of individuals which have a high probability for producing a crisis for a significant portion of the population. Many of these are predictable such as school entry, adolescence, marriage, parenthood, mid-life, and retirement. The nurse can promote education to individuals approaching and reaching these periods including services such as counseling, support groups, published information, and programs in churches, community centers, and schools.[19,24,25,33] This type of anticipatory guidance helps build coping skills.[35]

Some possible crisis provoking events are more unpredictable, such as home destruction, widowhood, relocation, illness, loss of employment, premature birth, divorce, and death of a family member. Primary prevention of excessive crisis states for these individuals would consist of early identification and intervention before the individuals involved are in crisis or are still in a mild crisis. This calls for different kinds of programs than those mentioned above. For example, one community has an emergency service for families who lose their homes because of fire. The program was started by a family who lost all their possessions and their home in a fire themselves.

Another approach to primary prevention of intense crises would be to identify individuals who are more prone to developing a crisis and provide them with resources to turn to in times of need. Specifically ego support is needed to help the individuals develop coping skills to deal with new experiences.[35] In one city, a number of elderly individuals and families were forced to leave their homes for an urban renewal project. Many of them moved into a government owned high rise apartment building in another part of the city. A collegiate school of nursing in the city opened a counseling center in an unused space in the building because they recognized that this particular population might be temporarily reduced in terms of supportive relationships, resources, and coping skills. It was probable that the individuals involved were experiencing role changes, threats to self, and many losses. The students and their instructors received a matchless opportunity to practice crisis prevention.

Actions of the nurse related to primary prevention are summarized in Table 11-2.

**Table 11-2.** Possible nursing actions to prevent unnecessary or severe crises

1. Promote efforts to prepare individuals and families for situations which may predictably lead to crises.
2. For crisis situations which cannot be predicted, provide early intervention before crisis occurs.
3. Develop resources for individuals and families who are crisis prone.

## Secondary Prevention in Crisis

Secondary prevention in crisis centers on finding individuals in crisis early and offering them help to restore equilibrium as soon as possible. In general, intervention in a crisis situation should be done as early as possible while the individuals involved are very susceptible to help and be done quickly and intensively. The focus is on the immediate situation and reaching the previous or a higher level of functioning. Complicated psychological classifications of the individual's problem are not necessary and may slow down intervention. Certain principles of intervention can guide the nurse in providing the necessary help.

1. *Define the problem.* The first activity with the patient or family in defining the crisis is to determine if possible what caused the crisis.[1] The nurse may feel that she already knows but it is beneficial to get the patient's perspective. The patient may be able to specifically delineate the hazardous event such as, "Having the stillbirth has really left me upset" or "My wife says she wants a divorce and I'm falling apart." Some patients cannot specifically pinpoint the event or events and may say, "I don't know what went wrong" or "Everything is going wrong. I can't cope anymore." Determining the cause if possible is important and sometimes requires special techniques. Sometimes the situation can be put in perspective if the nurse and the patient draw a time line for the past few days and mark events on the time line.[17] The nurse should try to pinpoint the exact time when the patient's functioning changed and seek out the events that happened just before. The patient may have repressed the event which was the most upsetting. Specific direct questioning may help.

> Mrs. Twomey was in a state of disequilibrium and unable to care for her home or children. She went to see her physician for a checkup at her husband's insistence. The nurse in the physician's office recognized the crisis state and began intervention. Mrs. Twomey could not identify any specific reason for her current state. A time line showed that she had begun her present behavior on a Sunday night 10 days previously. The nurse worked backwards from there. The nurse found out that on a Thursday night Mrs. Twomey had gone to a kindergarten open house where her oldest son was a pupil. The nurse asked, "What happened there?" and Mrs. Twomey recalled that she had been upset to learn that her oldest child was the slowest in the kindergarten group and the teachers were asking her to keep him back from first grade for a year. As this situation was discussed, Mrs. Twomey began to express more and more emotion, and soon it became apparent that this incident was highly significant in her present crisis. It was notable that she had not told her husband about the incident because she felt that he would blame her for their son's supposed intellectual slowness. Mrs. Twomey began to express other worries about her son's intellectual abilities and her worth as a mother. The nurse concluded that this threat to Mrs. Twomey's self-esteem was instrumental in causing her crisis.

Children may be able to communicate only in indirect methods such as through play activities or drawings. If any one specific event cannot be identified within a reasonable period of time, the intervention may have to proceed without an identified hazardous event.

After determining the hazardous event which led to the crisis, the nurse should explore the meaning of the event with the patient. Is it seen as a loss, a threat, or a role change? Is it a situational event or one related to normal growth and development? Has it arisen from outside of the family or within? Does it relate to a crisis from within the individual himself or was it caused by an external factor? These questions and their answers guide the nurse in understanding the crisis and how it has affected the family or individual.

Next the nurse should determine if the adult or child has an intellectual understanding of the problem.[1] She may venture her interpretation if she feels it is accurate without waiting for the patient to arrive at one.[13] She might say, "So you were told that your work has been unacceptable and this has resulted in your present state" or "Your husband has started drinking again. You have become depressed as a result because you just don't think you can take it anymore but yet you don't feel there is anything you can do." The important aspect is for the patient to see his present state as a result of the events that have happened to him. This makes the crisis more understandable, less frightening, and thus easier to cope with. The nurse's interpretation should be offered tentatively and with obvious concern expressed for the patient.[13] Often clarifying the situation and the patient's response is enough to lead to resolution of the crisis by the patient himself.[24]

In this stage of the intervention, it is not necessary to collect vast amounts of background data or deal with underlying problems.[32] The focus should be on the immediate problem and the information obtained relevant to it. Defining the problem should be done quickly during the first contact.

2. *Assess the situation of the patient or family.* After the problem area has been defined, the nurse should collect some pertinent information about the family's current situation. Specifically she needs to know what other hazardous events are present in the situation, where the individual or family stands in relation to developmental tasks, what supportive relationships are available, what the coping skills of the individuals involved are, what resources are present, and what the characteristics of the family are. This information does not need to be exhaustive but collected quickly and precisely. This information will help her focus the plan she develops and the help she gives so that it will do the most good in the shortest amount of time. Next she needs to estimate the intensity of the crisis. This information will help her to estimate the amount of help the family or individual may need.

3. *Provide an opportunity for expression of feelings.* After the problem has been defined and the patient's situation evaluated it is helpful to give the patient a chance to ventilate his emotions if this has not already occurred.[1] This may occur very naturally as the patient talks if the nurse picks up on cues the patient gives her or the nurse may need to initiate the discussion. She can do this by saying, "This must be a very difficult time for you" or "You must be feeling many things related to this situation." Children may best express their feelings in play activities. A chance to unburden pent up emotions may make the patient feel subjectively better immediately. The nurse can give permission to the patient to feel the way he does. She may need to say, "I can understand why you would feel helpless" or "Your anger at your sister is understandable to me."

4. *Generate a plan.* The nurse and sometimes the patient together can develop a plan to decrease the crisis situation. The nurse may need to be very directive if the patient is nonfunctional.[1] She herself may need to carry out most of the plan but it is best to allow the patient and family to do as much as possible depending on the circumstances. If the patient or family is in mild crisis she may only need to suggest alternatives and allow them to pick. The nurse may do things for the patient or family in crisis which she would normally want the patient to do for himself in other circumstances.

> Mr. John Libby came into the emergency room of a hospital. He was highly anxious and distraught. John had long suffered from ulcerative colitis, had recently lost a considerable amount of blood, and was extremely weak. He refused to be admitted because there was no one else to care for his two daughters. He had not been able to work for the past week. He told the nurse something had to be done because he could not cope any longer. The nurse arranged for a homemaker to go to John's home. Then she told John that he could be admitted since his daughters would be taken care of by a competent and careful woman. She drove John to his home to talk to his daughters and pack his belongings for the admission. The homemaker arrived as they were leaving. John kissed his daughters goodbye. The homemaker assured him that they would be well taken care of. John fell asleep in the car on the way back to the hospital.

5. *Offer concrete help.* It is important at the first contact to offer the patient some concrete help with the immediate problem. During a crisis, the nurse should not worry about creating dependency in the patient. If the patient could solve his own problem with his resources, he would have done so.

Help may take many forms. An important focus is to provide help with the common activities of living so that the patient can be free to focus on the problem he is facing.[3]

> Betty Blackman had called the community health nurse. She was desperate. Her husband had been gone for three weeks. She had not been able to find him. She had no money or food and one of her three children

appeared to have a strep throat. The nurse found some emergency funds, took the ill child to the clinic, filled a prescription at the drugstore, and took Mrs. Blackman to the court house to get food stamps and left her at the neighborhood grocery. When the community health nurse checked back the next afternoon, Mrs. Blackman was in a much better frame of mind. Her family had had two decent meals, a good night's sleep without interruptions from the sick child, and she was now ready to figure out how to cope with her situation.

An important part of this step is to infuse hope into the patient.[5] This is done by approaching the situation optimistically with visible confidence that the patient will be capable of solving his problem.[21] Reminding the individuals involved of situations they have handled well in the past and of their personal resources can aid hopefulness.[5]

6. *Set up supportive networks.* An important part of intervening in crisis situations is supplementing supports for the individual or family.[1] The person in crisis often feels isolated so one helpful measure is to reduce isolation. A good place to start is by finding persons already present in the patient's environment who can help and arranging for them to help. This information can be obtained by asking the patient who he talks to when he is troubled or who he can go to with his problems. Often supportive relationships are available which the patient in his crisis state had not considered.

If supportive relationships do not already exist within the environment, the nurse may be able to create supports. Neighbors or relatives can be asked to visit the patient and perform various services. Sometimes professionals must be used to create a supportive network. Communications with all involved individuals are important to assure continuity.

Mrs. Greely was 78 when her husband died. She had been very dependent on him due to her advanced arthritis and failing vision. Her precarious situation combined with her grief reaction to her husband's death led to a crisis state. No supportive relationships could be readily elicited. Money was one ample resource. The nurse arranged for a twice weekly housekeeper and for a visiting nurse to perform exercises and general health care. "Meals on Wheels" were delivered daily. In addition, a volunteer telephone service that checked daily on elderly individuals was given Mrs. Greely's name for a call each day. A high school teacher came in once a week to pay bills and manage Mrs. Greely's finances. Mrs. Greely's minister, who was trained in counseling techniques and familiar with the family, began visits in Mrs. Greely's home to help with the grieving process and the crisis. The nurse who had discovered the crisis coordinated all efforts but was not actually involved with Mrs. Greely herself.

7. *Consider the entire family.* Crisis rarely affects only one individual in a family because a crisis for one family member may tie in with a crisis for another.[10] For example, a change in one member's role will affect the other members' roles as a result.[34] For this reason, the nurse working with an adult or child must assess the effects on all family members of the patient's crisis. Each member will perceive of the crisis from a unique viewpoint and may need different forms of help. Young children in the family are particularly vulnerable because in the confusion of the crisis, their reactions and needs may be overlooked. Most important is to keep the family members together if at all possible.[11]

8. *Concentrate on strengths.* As the nurse works with an individual or a family in a crisis situation, she may be overwhelmed by some of the immense problems of those she is working with. There are some individuals and families who seem to be always emerging from one crisis or entering another one. If the nurse looks for strengths of the individual or family and builds on them, she may be more helpful in a short period of time than if she dwells on all the problems present.[13]

Mr. and Mrs. Johnson were well known to the community health nursing agency. Mrs. Johnson, who was blind, was perpetually pregnant. Mr. and Mrs. Johnson were of different races and both of their families had severed ties with them. They lived in a small crowded house in a deteriorating neighborhood. Their neighbors were hostile towards them because the older boys were suspected of minor vandalism and the house and grounds were the disgrace of the neighborhood, and because of the biracial marriage. Mr. Johnson worked only during the summer months of each year. The current crisis centered on Mr. Johnson's admission to the county hospital with a gunshot wound in June. Mrs. Johnson was near term with her pregnancy.

The community health nurse on her first visit identified the following major problems:

1. Help needed with laundry, housekeeping, cooking, shopping, and supervision of the children.
2. Loss of income because Mr. Johnson was planning to work all summer.
3. Care of the children while Mrs. Johnson was in the hospital for delivery.
4. Health and dental care for all children was lacking and several children had obvious health needs.

There was also a great number of lesser problems. The community health nurse knew there were no quick answers to their problems and she knew she must deal first with the current crisis. Looking at the family's strengths she concluded:

1. The Johnsons had survived many crisis situations—most without help.
2. The older girls were reliable and capable of much help but needed direction.
3. The older boys could help if provided with some limits and specific responsibilities. They would obey their father who usually coordinated family activities.
4. Mrs. Johnson was a gentle and loving mother with her children.
5. Mrs. Johnson had easy deliveries and recovered rapidly.

The nurse and Mrs. Johnson developed their plan around positive facts about the family. The plan which evolved was unique to the Johnsons and included the father calling regularly several times a day from a phone at his bedside to direct activities at home, written lists for each child, a home delivery for Mrs. Johnson with a nurse midwife in attendance, and emergency funds from the township trustee.

In many families in crisis the nurse cannot hope to solve all of the long-standing problems in existence. She should focus on facilitating appropriate coping and on returning the individual or family to at least the previous level of functioning even if to her it seems built on an unreliably fragile foundation.[5]

9. *Promote coping behavior.* The nurse needs to assess how the individual or the family is coping and promote behaviors which are related to ultimate problem solving and growth in the crisis situation. Thus, she serves as a support for the patient's or family's coping attempts.[19]

One way the nurse can accomplish this is by gently presenting reality in doses the patient can tolerate.[3,18] This helps to reduce tendencies to deny or repress problems and keeps the problem as the focus. This requires tact and good timing.

Another way the nurse promotes coping is by providing emotional support.[21] Her support through use of the helping process allows the patient to focus his energy on problem solving.

Another way of promoting coping is to help the patient work through emotions which interfere with problem solving such as guilt, anger, hostility, and so forth. She does this by listening nonjudgmentally, understanding, and accepting the patient and his feelings. It is probably useful to restrict the patient's tendency to blame others or to be destructive.[3,18] With children, the use of planned touch often communicates support and acceptance best.

It may be possible to promote the use of healthy coping mechanisms by helping the person in crisis to identify with another person who is using healthy coping behaviors.[29] For example, a mother of small children who is suddenly without a husband may benefit from joining a group of other mothers raising their children by themselves. Sometimes watching a particular TV series, a movie, or reading a story or book might be helpful. Teenagers may benefit from discussion groups with others who share their problems. Patients sometimes feel that the actual stories of one who has been through the situation are very valuable. Lay self-help groups such as La Leche, Reach for Recovery, Alcoholics Anonymous, and Parents Anonymous often have been credited by individuals with providing immense help in times of crisis. Nurses should be familiar with resources such as these for the particular patient population they have contact with. The patient may also identify with the nurse's way of approaching his problems and her use of problem oriented strategies may influence the patient towards healthy coping.

Another source of helpful coping behaviors may be the past. If the patient can be helped to recall a healthy way he handled a difficult situation in the past, he may be able to apply that behavior to the present situation.

Healthy coping is promoted by summarizing the situation periodically and commenting on what progress has been made. This promotes cognitive mastery of the situation and favors coping versus defensive behaviors.

If the individual persists in using unhealthy coping mechanisms, the nurse may need to refer the patient to someone with more knowledge in helping individuals who are coping with a crisis in an emotional unhealthy way.

10. *Utilize knowledge of special situations to plan intervention.* In many situations, the patient and family may be experiencing a crisis caused by a common hazardous event about which there is known concrete information the nurse can use. For example, a sudden, unexpected death can cause a crisis and the main feature is likely to be disequilibrium caused by grief reactions of the family members. The nurse working with this family can use information on grieving and the appropriate nursing intervention as the basis for intervening in the crisis. More and more common and specific situations and nursing intervention are being described in the nursing literature. Examples include, in addition to grieving, premature birth, birth of a defective child, fatal illness, hospital admission for children, chronic disease, the menopause, marriage, and retirement. The nurse can adapt this general information to the unique needs of the child or adult she is working with. If she works in a specialized area, the nurse should be familiar with the areas of general information which are likely to be applicable in her practice. For example, if the nurse works in a neonatal unit, information related to the reaction and needs of parents of premature infants and defective children and information on the grieving process would be relevant and useful for crisis prevention and intervention.

11. *Intervene to reduce excessive anxiety or depression.* High levels of anxiety with or without depression are common accompaniments of a crisis because of the reaction of the patient to unsuccessful attempts to solve the problems he is facing and often his lack of comprehension of what is occurring.[1] Special nursing measures can be taken as described elsewhere in this book to reduce anxiety and depression. It is beneficial to leave the patient with enough anxiety to facilitate problem solving, however.

12. *Use the crisis situation to promote further growth.* After the crisis has abated, the individuals involved can often profit from the situation they have been in if appropriate action is taken. This includes summarizing what has occurred, delineating what has been learned, determining how a similar crisis situation could be prevented or better handled in the future, and determining further action if needed.[1,13] If the patient arrived at a new coping behavior which proved effective, special recognition of the behavior may be helpful. If previously troublesome problems emerged during the crisis which are not resolved, the patient may now be ready to deal with them. This may necessitate referring the patient to more comprehensive helping services. The individual's ownership of his life and how he can take charge of his life can be emphasized.[27]

Measures for the secondary prevention of crisis are summarized in Table 11-3.

## *Tertiary Prevention in Crisis*

Tertiary prevention in crisis situations would involve helping individuals who have emerged from a crisis at a level of functioning which is lower than their previous level of functioning. This implies that they have become mentally ill or solved the crisis through use of chemical

**Table 11-3.** Possible nursing actions for individuals and families in crisis

1. Define the problem by determining the hazardous event and its meaning and describe verbally what is happening to the one in crisis.
2. Collect information about the current circumstances of the crisis situation to assess help needed.
3. Promote expression of feelings.
4. Develop a plan to remedy the current problem.
5. Offer concrete help especially with normal daily activities so the individual or the family can focus on their problems.
6. Mobilize supportive resources in existence or create new ones.
7. Assess to see if other family members need help.
8. Avoid becoming overwhelmed by long present problems by focusing on the current problem and strengths.
9. Promote coping behaviors rather than defense mechanisms.
10. Use nursing theory of common nursing problems in intervention if appropriate.
11. Reduce excessive levels of anxiety and depression.
12. Look for opportunities to promote growth.

agents, suicide, suicide attempts, homicide, or other "nonsolutions." In these cases, knowledge is needed beyond the scope of this book and the nurse should seek specialized resources for the patient.

## THE NURSE AND CRISIS

In general, nurses are as subject to crisis provoking events as are all individuals. In particular, nurses may experience some specific hazardous events which might lead to crisis.

Role change in nursing is a continual phenomenon. Nurses are now sharing some roles commonly believed to belong to other professionals. Role changes of this type can challenge the nurse's adaptability and problem solving skills.

Threats to bodily integrity can become very real when nurses are exposed to contagious organisms, radiation hazards, and other environmental dangers. Fortunately, these hazards are not usually at crisis provoking levels, but a crisis can occur. For example, one nurse experienced a crisis when he developed hepatitis while working with kidney dialysis patients. The resultant loss of income and the grave illness caused a crisis in his young family who were dependent on his income and participation in the family.

Threats to self-esteem can occur when nurses experience feelings of failure and frustration. Nurses may experience frustration when their work environments do not permit them to practice as they feel qualified to practice because of control by others of their practice.

Losses can occur when patients die or improve and nursing care is terminated. The nurse frequently shares the losses that her clients experience such as being given a fatal diagnosis or suffering bodily mutilation.

Each nurse should assess her professional and personal life to determine what role changes, threats, and losses are present or possible. In addition, each nurse can assess her proneness to crisis. The following questions are designed to aid this goal.

1. What potentially hazardous events do I face? How plentiful are they? How likely to occur?
2. Have I achieved my age-appropriate and family developmental tasks? How could they be more successfully resolved?
3. What supportive relationships exist? What professional helpers are available to me in time of need? What could be done to increase or improve supportive relationships?

4. How do I cope with difficult situations? Do my efforts usually result in problem solving? Am I flexible in responding to challenges?
5. What personal resources can I count on in time of need? What areas could be expanded? In what areas do weaknesses exist? What could be done about them?
6. Do I perceive events clearly and realistically? What factors and problems from the past might be influential in distorting my perception of events around me? What can be done to reduce distortion?
7. What characteristics exist within my family which relate to crisis proneness? What changes could be made?

The nurse can remember that experiencing crisis in itself is not unhealthy, but one can sometimes develop a life strategy which allows them to balance crisis provoking situations with preparedness.

What can the nurse do when she herself is in a crisis situation? One resource in the literature addressed itself to how individuals can help themselves when faced with crisis situations. Some of the suggestions given will be adapted and applied to nurses.[20]

First of all, the nurse must recognize that crises of some degree are part of normal life. They are opportunities to experience personal growth. Having a crisis is not a sign of emotional ill health or instability. It is a sign that one needs or wishes to change something in one's life.

Second, one should learn to recognize when one is in crisis. The characteristic signs of crisis are anxiety, depression, and disequilibrium. These can be recognized by assessing oneself or by being alert to indications from others that one is not functioning as usual.

Third, the nurse should strive to go into the crisis rather than go away from it. This involves experiencing the crisis fully and determining the true nature of the crisis. There is usually a "crisis question" which should be explored. Going into the crisis involves centering attention on the crisis and making it a priority.

Fourth, the nurse in crisis should realize that there will not be a quick or easy solution to her crisis. She should not make any snap decisions but allow time to evaluate her decisions fully. Invariably in a crisis situation, she will have to change and try something different. This may involve trying a new coping behavior or a new life style.

Last and of utmost importance, the nurse should find someone to talk to during the crisis. If there is not anyone already present in her environment, she should seek out a professional counselor or similar person to talk to.

## A TOOL FOR ASSESSMENT AND EVALUATION

The factors in Table 11-4 can help the nurse in determining if the patient or family is adapting well in a crisis situation. It may also suggest whether the interventions of the nurse are helpful in improving the crisis state. The following factors have been drawn from the literature and from speculations based on clinical experience.

## AN EXAMPLE OF NURSING INTERVENTION IN CRISIS

Jeff was a 17-year-old high school student in the school where Connie was employed as a school nurse. Jeff was usually an above average student. All of this changed when his father had a heart attack. Jeff came to see Connie a few days later because of an upset stomach. After talking with him for a few minutes, Connie began to see that Jeff was in a

**Table 11-4.** Tool for assessment in crisis

| Behavior | More optimal | Less optimal |
|---|---|---|
| *Hazardous event* | | |
| Cause of the crisis | Easily identified | Unknown |
| Nature of the event | Event was expected | Event was unexpected |
| Severity of event | Major event caused crisis | Minor event caused crisis |
| Perception of event | Seen realistically | Distorted by the influence of the past |
| Actual threat to self | Identified | Vague or unknown |
| Acknowledgment of event | Faced realistically | Ignored, escaped |
| *Coping* | | |
| Control behaviors used | Coping mechanisms predominate | Defense mechanisms predominate |
| *Period of disequilibrium* | | |
| Length | Short duration | Long duration |
| Effects of discomfort | Motivates individual to action | Immobilizes individual |
| Outcome | Old unresolved problems are revived | Old problems remain buried |
| Intensity | Minor dysfunction occurs | Major dysfunction occurs |
| Level of anxiety | Kept at a minimum | Anxiety dominates |
| *Use of supportive relationships and resources* | | |
| Use of resources | Seeks out help | Waits to be helped or withdraws from helpers |
| Acceptance of dependency | Tolerated temporarily | Cannot permit dependency |
| Reaction to offers of help | Accepts | Rejects |
| Availability of resources | Available in present environment | Unavailable |
| Availability of supportive relationships | Available in present environment | Unavailable |
| *Solutions found* | | |
| Focus of solution | Geared to problem | Not focused on problem |
| Family reaction | Increase in solidarity | Polarization or disintegration |
| Community participation | Renewed involvement | Withdrawal continues |
| *General* | | |
| Previous success with crises | Past successes | Past failures |
| Recovery | Occurs quickly | Occurs slowly |
| Psychological functioning after crisis | Normal functioning | Development of neurosis, psychosis, maladaptive behavior[11,18,24] |

state of crisis. Connie could distinguish symptoms of despair and confusion in Jeff's conversation. In Jeff's own words, "Nothing is the same since Dad's heart attack." Further conversation with Jeff revealed that Jeff knew that he was in a crisis and he knew that it was largely related to his father's illness but there seemed to be other dimensions to his problem.

Connie knew that Jeff's situation demanded intensive intervention so she put everything else aside and devoted her full attention to Jeff. As he talked, more elements of the situation began to emerge. Jeff blamed his mother for his father's heart attack. His parents, it appeared, had been going through a difficult period in their marriage with frequent arguments. Jeff was afraid that the tensions at home had led to the heart attack. Jeff was very close to his father and usually spent much time with him discussing his activities. He was very afraid that his father was going to die. Jeff was also resentful of his mother's limitation of his activities since his father was hospitalized. His mother refused to let him go anywhere with his friends who were very important to him and she insisted that he be home each evening with his younger sisters while she went to the hospital. He characterized his relationship with his mother as never good and not getting better.

After 30 minutes of conversation during which Jeff talked readily, he appeared to have described most of the elements of the current situation. Connie felt that she had some degree of understanding of Jeff's current crisis and his coping behaviors, resources, and supports. Jeff too knew that his difficulties were initiated by his father's illness and that the restlessness, lack of sleep, and loss of interest in school could not go on much longer. Connie decided that there were a few things she should say to Jeff to increase his understanding of what he was going through. She said, "Your father's heart attack has been a big worry to you. You are very worried about him and yet there seems to be little you can do for him. This has made you anxious and depressed and explains why you are having trouble sleeping and studying. You usually discuss your problems with your dad or your friends but now you are limited in talking with them." Jeff nodded in agreement. "I don't know how to get hold of myself. If this goes on my grades may fall and I may not be accepted at college." Connie assured Jeff that what he was going through was understandable and that there were things they could do to improve the situation.

Next Connie gave Jeff a chance to talk more specifically about his feelings. Jeff described in more detail his confusion and hostility towards his mother. Connie expressed acceptance of his feelings without agreeing.

Connie and Jeff began to develop a plan to help immediately reduce some of the problems in Jeff's current situation. One immediate area of concern was related to Jeff's coursework. The semester was almost over and several papers were due which Jeff knew he could not write. In these courses, Connie proposed that he talk with the teachers and ask for an extension so that the papers could be handed in after Christmas vacation. Jeff agreed. There was also one course which Jeff was taking as an extra course. Jeff asked Connie if he could drop this course, and Connie arranged for the deletion of the course from his schedule.

A second area of concern was that Jeff did not get to see his father and he probably interpreted his physical condition as worse than it was. Jeff badly wanted to go to the hospital to see his father and he came up with the idea of asking one of his girlfriends to come stay with his younger sisters one night so he could go to the hospital. Jeff decided to present the idea to his mother that night in the hopes that it could be arranged for the next night.

Jeff also planned to try to get his mother to discuss with him more about his father's condition which was not presently being done.

Since some of Jeff's usual supports were missing, Connie suggested that he come in to see her each day for a while at a specific time so they could evaluate the action taken and continue to plan for coping with the present situation. Jeff agreed. Connie thought that one positive coping behavior of Jeff's was seeking help in the first place so she commented to him as he was ready to leave, "I think it was beneficial that you could recognize that you had a problem and take action to solve it." Jeff left walking with a little more assurance in his step than when he came in.

Connie knew that Jeff was likely not the only member of the family in crisis. She called the school health nurse at the grade school where the sisters attended to inform her of the situation. She also called Jeff's mother, Mrs. Stevens, and explained that she had heard of her husband's admission to the hospital and would like to come talk to her about how the children might be helped through the experience. Mrs. Stevens told Connie she would be glad to see her so a conference was scheduled for the next morning.

Connie found that Mrs. Stevens appeared to be coping appropriately with her situation. She had a close circle of friends whom she spent most of the day with. She did not appear close to any of the children. She stated that she knew the situation must be "rough on the children" but she could not be more specific. Connie surmised that Mr. Stevens had long provided the major share of interest and support for the children. Connie discussed some of the things the children might be feeling in general and Mrs. Stevens listened attentively. Connie suggested that Mrs. Stevens and the three children might benefit from a time set aside to discuss how everyone was feeling about their father's illness and what they each could do to help each other. Mrs. Stevens seemed interested.

Jeff came in to see Connie again that afternoon. He stayed 45 minutes and had much to talk about. He was relieved to have one less class to go to and had been able to use the extra time to prepare for other classes. He had presented his plan to his mother to go to the hospital with her the next night. She had at first been negative about the idea but had finally agreed. Jeff was happily anticipating the opportunity to see his father. Connie talked to him for a few minutes about what he might see in the coronary care unit to prepare him. Jeff's friends wanted him to go to a race with them on the weekend and he was planning to ask his mother if he could go. He seemed only mildly interested in going but Connie encouraged him to go because it would be a chance to be with his friends. He had talked with most of his teachers and had been given time extensions for handing in work.

Connie told Jeff that she had visited his mother and tentatively approached the subject of increasing his understanding of how his mother's behavior towards him might be related to her worries over his father but Jeff was not yet receptive to discussing anyone else's problems.

Jeff returned the next afternoon. He had been encouraged by his visit to see his father who did not appear as ill as he expected. Jeff's father must have realized Jeff's concern because he reassured him about his progress and talked with him about school and such. Jeff had asked his father with his mother there if he could go out with his friends on the weekend and his father had agreed. He was getting more interested in going. Connie commented to Jeff that he seemed less depressed and Jeff agreed. He told Connie that he was sleeping better too.

Connie did not see Jeff again until the next Monday afternoon. He came in to report that he had had a good time with his friends and was glad that she had encouraged him to go. He was excited that his father had been moved out of the coronary care unit to a regular unit and now had a telephone which he used to call home and talk to Jeff, his sisters, and their mother. Jeff was able to study at school during free periods and reported studying somewhat better at home although he still felt he could not concentrate well.

The next time Jeff came in was Thursday of the same week. He had been going to the hospital regularly with his mother who now decided that the sisters could come along and wait in the lounge. He said that his mother was not yelling at him as much and talking with him more. He continued to talk to his dad on the phone before bed. Jeff was now asking his dad for permission to go out and his father was apparently coaching the mother in how much freedom to allow him. Jeff was doing better in his school work and had started one paper which he thought he could finish on time. He was devoting some extra time to helping his sisters with their studies. Connie asked Jeff if he thought things were almost back to normal and he agreed that they were.

Connie asked Jeff what he had learned from the situation he had been in. He replied that he should have come to talk to Connie earlier before things got so bad and that his mother was not as bad as he thought to get along with. Connie commented that she was probably very worried about his dad herself and he agreed. He was also pleased with how nice the teachers had been to him about making up his work later and he thought next time he would have gone to them sooner. "I guess," he said, "I sit and worry too much when I should get out there and do something about my problems." Connie believed that Jeff was nearly out of the crisis situation and had learned a little lesson about himself as a result. She only saw Jeff one other time when he came in to tell her that his father was coming home. He was smiling and relaxed and with a new girlfriend.

## SUMMARY

A crisis can occur when an individual or family is overwhelmed with a particularly troublesome situation which leads to disequilibrium and which for some reason they cannot cope with at that particular time. Losses, role changes, and threats to the psychological and physical self are believed to be events which may initiate crises. Crises can be classified as maturational, situational, extrafamilial, intrafamilial, internal, or external. Some individuals and families are more prone to experience crises than others. Individuals throughout the life cycle may experience situations which can lead to crisis. Intervention focuses on preventing unnecessary crises and on intervening quickly, forcefully, and aggressively in existing crises. The nurse may at some time in her life experience a crisis and she should learn to recognize a personal crisis and seek help.

## REFERENCES

1. Aguilera, D. C., and Messick, J. M.: *Crisis Intervention: Theory and Methodology.* C. V. Mosby, St. Louis, 1978.
2. Bloom, B. L.: "Definitional aspects of the crisis concept," in Parad, H. J. (ed.): *Crisis Intervention: Selected Readings.* Family Service Association of America, New York, 1965.
3. Cadden, V.: "Crisis in the family," in Caplan, G. (ed.): *Principles of Preventive Psychiatry.* Basic Books, New York, 1964.
4. Caplan, G.: *Principles of Preventive Psychiatry.* Basic Books, New York, 1964.
5. Ebersole, P.: "Geriatric crisis intervention in the family context," in Hall, J. E., and Weaver, B. R. (eds.): *Nursing of Families in Crisis.* J. B. Lippincott, Philadelphia, 1974.
6. Edinburg, G. M., Zinberg, N. E., and Kelman, W.: *Clinical Interviewing and Counseling: Principles and Techniques.* Appleton-Century-Crofts, New York, 1975.
7. Erikson, E.: *Identity, Youth and Crisis.* W. W. Norton, New York, 1968.
8. Freud, A.: "The role of bodily illness in the mental life of children." Psychoanal. Study Child 7:14, 1952.
9. Haas, A.: "How youngsters survive trauma." Indianapolis Star Mag. May 30, 1976.
10. Hall, J. E., and Weaver, B. R.: "Crisis: A conceptual approach to family nursing," in *Nursing of Families in Crisis.* J. B. Lippincott, Philadelphia, 1974.
11. Hill, R.: "Generic features of families under stress," in Parad, H. J. (ed.): *Crisis Intervention: Selected Readings.* Family Service Association of America, New York, 1965.
12. Hitchcock, J. E.: "Social and psychological crises," in Kalkman, M. E., and Davis, A. J. (eds.): *New Dimensions in Mental Health-Psychiatric Nursing.* McGraw-Hill, New York, 1974.
13. Hitchcock, J. E.: "Crisis intervention: The pebble in the pool." Am. J. Nurs. 73:1388, 1973.
14. Klein, D. C., and Ross, A.: "Kindergarten entry: A study of role transition," in Parad, H. J. (ed.): *Crisis Intervention: Selected Readings.* Family Service Association of America, New York, 1965.

15. Kuenzi, S. H., and Fenton, M. V.: "Crisis intervention in acute care areas." Am. J. Nurs. 75:830, 1975.
16. Messick, J. M., and Aguilera, D. C.: "Crisis," in Clark, A. L., and Affonso, D. D.: *Childbearing: A Nursing Perspective*. F. A. Davis, Philadelphia, 1976.
17. Mitchell, C. E.: "Identifying the hazard: The key to crisis intervention." Am. J. Nurs. 77:1194, 1977.
18. Murray, R., and Zentner, J.: "Crisis intervention: A therapeutic technique," in Murray, R., et al.: *Nursing Concepts for Health Promotion*. Prentice-Hall, Inc., Englewood Cliffs, N.J., 1975.
19. Oehrtman, S. E.: "Assessment and crisis intervention: A model for the family," in Hall, J. E., and Weaver, B. R. (eds.): *Nursing of Families in Crisis*. J. B. Lippincott, Philadelphia, 1974.
20. O'Neill, N., and O'Neill, G.: *Shifting Gears*. Avon Books, New York, 1974.
21. Parad, H. J.: "Preventive casework: Problems and implications," in *Crisis Intervention: Selected Readings*. Family Service Association of America, New York, 1965.
22. Parad, H. J., and Caplan, G.: "A framework for studying families in crisis," in Parad, H. J. (ed.): *Crisis Intervention: Selected Readings*. Family Service Association of America, New York, 1965.
23. Pothier, P. C.: *Mental Health Counseling With Children*. Little, Brown and Company, Boston, 1976.
24. Rapoport, L.: "The state of crisis: Some theoretical considerations," in Parad, H. J. (ed.): *Crisis Intervention: Selected Readings*. Family Service Association of America, New York, 1965.
25. Schulberg, H. C.: "Picking up the pieces: Intervening in disaster situations." Omega 5:77, 1974.
26. Scipien, G., et al.: *Comprehensive Pediatric Nursing*. McGraw-Hill, New York, 1975.
27. Shields, L.: "Family crisis intervention." J. Psych. Nurs. Mental Health Ser. 7:222, 1969.
28. Spiegel, J.: "The resolution of role conflict within the family," in Bell, N., and Vogel, E. (eds.): *A Modern Introduction to the Family*. Free Press of Glencoe, Glencoe, Ill., 1963.
29. Veeder, N. W.: "A stress-strength model for nurse-social worker collaboration." Mental Retard. 12:39, 1974.
30. Waechter, E. H., and Blake, F. G.: *Nursing Care of Children*. J. B. Lippincott, Philadelphia, 1976.
31. Walkup, L. L.: "The concept of crisis," in Hall, J. E., and Weaver, B. R. (eds.): *Nursing of Families in Crisis*. J. B. Lippincott, Philadelphia, 1974.
32. Wicks, R. J.: *Counseling Strategies and Intervention Techniques for the Human Services*. J. B. Lippincott, Philadelphia, 1977.
33. Williams, F. S.: "Intervention in maturational crises," in Hall, J. E., and Weaver, B. R. (eds.): *Nursing of Families in Crisis*. J. B. Lippincott, Philadelphia, 1974.
34. Williams, G. F.: "Intervention in situational crises," in Hall, J. E., and Weaver, B. R. (eds.): *Nursing of Families in Crisis*. J. B. Lippincott, Philadelphia, 1974.
35. Wise, D. J.: "Crisis intervention before cardiac surgery." Am. J. Nurs. 75:1316, 1975.

## BIBLIOGRAPHY

Barrell, L. M.: "Crisis intervention: Partnership in problem-solving." Nurs. Clin. North Am. 9:5, 1974.
Berliner, B.: "Nursing the patient in crisis." Am. J. Nurs. 70:2154, 1970.
Brose, C.: "Theories of family crisis," in Hymovich, D. P., and Barnard, M. U. (eds.): *Family Health Care*. McGraw-Hill, New York, 1973.
Bruce, N. M., and Dawson, A. E.: "The school—its relationship to health services," in Kalafatich, A. J. (ed.): *Approaches to the Care of Adolescents*. Appleton-Century-Crofts, New York, 1975.
Byrne, M., and Thompson, L.: *Key Concepts for the Study and Practice of Nursing*. C. V. Mosby, St. Louis, 1972.
Fink, S. L.: "Crisis and motivation: A theoretical model." Arch. Phys. Med. Rehab. 48:592, 1967.
Henning, E. D.: "Crisis intervention theory applied to nursing," in Clark, A. L. (ed.): *Parent-Child Relationships: The Role of the Nurse*. Rutgers University Press, New Brunswick, N.J., 1968.
King, J.: "The initial interview: Basis for assessment in crisis intervention." Perspect. Psychiat. Care 9:251, 1971.
Maloney, E. M.: "The subjective and objective definition of crisis." Perspect. Psychiat. Care 9:258, 1971.
Rapoport, L.: "Working with families in crisis: An exploration in preventive intervention," in Parad, H. J. (ed.): *Crisis Intervention: Selected Readings*. Family Service Association of America, New York, 1965.
Schmidt, L. J., and Evans, D. F.: "The crisis intervention nurse in community mental health practice," in Reinhardt, A. M., and Quinn, M. D. (eds.): *Family-Centered Community Nursing: A Sociocultural Framework*. C. V. Mosby, St. Louis, 1973.

# CHAPTER 12

## CHANGE IN SELF-CONCEPT

The images one has of oneself have a pervasive influence on all aspects of one's life. Self-concept might be thought of as composed of several elements. Most basic is the *existential self* which would be stated as, "I am" or "I exist." Second, there is an element of *physical self* or body image which contains all of the individual's conscious and unconscious beliefs and thoughts about his body—external and internal. Some of these might be, "I am tall," "I am female," or "I am aging." Third, the self-concept contains an element which could be described as the *psychological self*. In this element one possesses attitudes about oneself such as, "I am intelligent," "I am capable," or "I am friendly."

It is not difficult to imagine that situations which bring individuals into contact with nurses may well be ones that may challenge a patient's self-concept. The patient's psychological self may be threatened ("Can I master this?"), his physical self ("Is my body intact?"), or his very existence ("Will I survive?"). The nurse needs an understanding of the many aspects of self-concept in order to help patients recognize and cope with threats to their self-concept.

The nurse will experience threats to her own self-concept and this will be explored.

## REVIEW OF THEORY

### Formation of Self-Concept

Theories on how an individual develops his self-concept are speculative. It is likely that the existential self develops first. It is speculated that the infant determines that he exists by first noting that his actions such as crying or smiling have an effect on others. This information is dependent on receiving feedback in relation to his actions.[28] He probably learns who he is as he differentiates that parts of the world around him are "me" and parts are "not me."[36] He might decide that his fingers are part of him because he can almost always find them and he receives sensations when he sucks on them which are different from those received when he sucks on his blanket. He may decide that mother is not part of him because he cannot always find her. The infant could conceivably begin differentiating himself from other objects *in utero.*

Studies confirm that even young infants have a rudimentary ability to identify themselves and therefore a self-concept. Infants at four months of age were found to be particularly fascinated with their images in mirrors and smiled at themselves more than at motion pictures or slides of other infants.[38] The infant at eight months of age has acquired the idea that objects can exist even when out of sight, thus he may be able to grasp that he has permanence. It can be seen that the identification of self as described is dependent on intact sensory equipment and appropriate environmental stimulation.[49]

As the child continues to mature, many circumstances combine to influence his beliefs about his self. How others relate to his body and the continuing messages he receives from his body lead to knowledge of his physical self. His abilities to use his body to influence others in his environment may lead his psychological self to conclude that he is cared about by someone.

It is believed that the concept of self is never static. Throughout life it is continually altered and expanded to adapt to changes of the self and changes in the environment. The following illustrates the complex information which results in a self-concept.

1. *What one is.* The infant does not know his sex or his race but he will be certain in a few years. The individual continuously surveys himself visually and tactually and listens to internal and external sensations. In this manner he collects information that he exists and about his physical and psychological self.

2. *What one thinks others think he is.* In addition to what one is, an individual is very influenced by his perceptions of what the thoughts and beliefs of others are related to him. Parents are felt to be primarily influential in deciding and communicating to the child that he exists and what the characteristics of his physical and psychological self are. Peers and siblings are probably next in importance.

3. *What one thinks one should be.* Another important perception is related to what an individual perceives others to be and how he compares. Unfortunately, man frequently compares himself with the highest ideals possible. He compares his physical self with the young, strong, and the beautiful, and his psychological self with the intelligent and the competent.

4. *What one thinks he is.* This last perception represents the conclusions one arrives at after considering what he is, what he thinks others think he is, and what he thinks he should be. The potential for inaccuracies abounds. Therefore, all individuals function with some distortions of their self-concept.

## *Self-Esteem*

This last perception, what one thinks he is, is also referred to as self-esteem. It is commonly assumed that one can hold himself in a certain amount of self-esteem such as high or low esteem. Threats to an individual are described as threatening one's self-esteem or how one feels about himself.

Distortions in one's self-concept are probably formed in order to maintain equilibrium in self-esteem. For example, if an individual has decided that he is "just average" he may distort accomplishments of lesser or greater merit so that he sees them as average in order to maintain his self-esteem.

Self-esteem has been found to be highest when an individual was brought up in an environment where he experienced acceptance, respect, and defined limits and where his parents themselves had high self-esteem.[7]

## Sex Role Identity

It would be erroneous to give the impression that self-concept develops in the same ways for males and females. The first question parents ask is, "Is the baby a boy or a girl?" and from that point on males and females develop and are socialized very differently which has implications for their self-concept formation. Maleness or femaleness becomes one of the primary ingredients of self-identity and is probably of more importance in determining the future of the child than his race, intelligence, or social class. Sex role development does not refer only to sex or reproduction but to the whole constellation of behaviors considered appropriate for each sex by society. Because of the importance of sex role identity in self-concept formation, it will be examined in some detail.

To begin with differences between male and female infants are being demonstrated in studies. Newborn male and female infants appear to differ in relation to hearing capabilities, attending to visual cues, sensitivity to tactile stimulation, pain threshold, crying and sleeping behavior, and gross and fine motor movements.[22,29,33]

An interesting investigation has been done on fetally androgenized females who were identified and treated successfully. When these girls were assessed a few years later they were found to be less interested in babies, jewelry, hairstyles or makeup, slower to date, likely to engage in outdoor physical play, and were referred to as tomboys more than their sisters who were used as controls.[13] There is the possibility that differences in temperament between the sexes and the wide range of behavior differences among individuals of the same sex may be influenced by subtle prenatal hormone levels. Although these differences in biology exist, it is of importance to note that man is the only animal in which biology is not necessarily destiny.

Another factor to be considered in addition to biologic differences concerns parental differentiation of responses to their male and female children. Mothers of 3-week-old infants imitated the vocalizations of females more and used greater amounts of stimulation with boys and more stressing of musculature such as holding the infant in a standing position.[33] Another study showed that mothers of girls touched and vocalized to their young infants more than mothers of boys. At 13 months the same girls talked to and touched their mothers more than the boys touched or talked to their mothers.[19] In one of the most comprehensive studies ever attempted on child rearing, Sears, Maccoby, and Levine found that mothers treated their sons and daughters quite differently. For example, sons were expected to stay and fight back in a conflict situation while their sisters were expected to withdraw and come home.[45]

The effects of these differential responses possibly combined with biologic differences are apparent in other examples of children's behavior. Girls of 7 to 19 months were more frightened by male strangers than boys. Girls responded to a barrier between themselves and their mothers by sitting in the middle and crying. Boys responded to the barrier by attempts to go around it at the edges. At 13 months, girls played with toys which required more fine than gross muscle coordination and with toys with faces. Boys played more with toys requiring gross motor activity, explored the environment more, and played more with environmental objects that were not toys (i.e., doorknobs, light plugs).[19]

It is hypothesized that girls learn appropriate sex role behavior by identifying with their mothers. Boys instead must identify with a cultural stereotype of maleness because their fathers are less available physically and psychologically and it is, therefore, not as easy to observe what males do. The female learns to restructure what her mother does and thus learns by imitation. The boy learns to be masculine by learning not to be feminine and therefore learns by abstraction.[30] This may contribute to differences in cognitive abilities later and explain why men have been found to be more proficient in problem solving.

Another equally important consideration in addition to biologic differences between the sexes and differential parental behavior is the influence of models. Children observe their parents as models of "maleness" and "femaleness" and also note the contrast between them. Children raised without the father present in their early years have been shown to exhibit some specific characteristics. Girls were found to have difficulty in heterosexual relationships and boys were found to be less aggressive.[21] Older siblings also serve as models to younger ones. Girls who have an older brother tend in general to be more likely to be referred to as "tomboys" and boys with an older sister are in general more likely to engage in less "masculine" activities than boys with older brothers.

The peer group provides another source of models for sex-appropriate behavior and it is interesting to note that the differentiation in sex roles correlates with the appearance of cooperative play. Children's relationships with their peers are different from their relationships with their parents and it seems likely that the peer group extends the sex typing process.[20] It is believed that peer groups usually demand conformity to more rigid stereotypes of appropriate male and female behavior than do parents.[20] Thus, the boy and girl who see both their mother and father work outside of the home and share in home chores will still most likely learn in the peer group that only boys go to work and only girls belong in the kitchen.

The influence of the peer group may help account for some of the reasons why boys and girls behave differently in school. Boys make three times as many unfriendly approaches toward the teacher as compared to girls. Girls make twice as many friendly approaches. Boys receive more disapproval and are passed less frequently.[26] At recess, boys run around in large noisy groups in unpredictable activities utilizing large amounts of physical space. Girls play in very small groups nearer the teacher and engage in less physical and more predictable repetitive activities such as skipping rope.[18]

Other models of appropriate sex role behavior are provided to boys and girls by television and written materials. One survey of books written for children in elementary schools showed that the model of female behavior presented in the literature represented women and girls as silly, inactive, dull, easily frightened, and menial laborers. Men and boys were the subject of twice as many stories and were active, adventuresome, important, leaders, thoughtful, and intelligent. In the illustrations, women and girls were nonexistent or peripheral while men and boys were central. Even in a story of Madame Curie, the accompanying illustration showed her husband and another man actively talking while Madame Curie peered passively from the background![23]

How these factors of biologic differences, parental differentiation, and available models combine to produce differences in mature male and female behavior is difficult to determine. Girls show more varied and later sex typing than boys which could be accounted for by hypothesizing that genetically females have a wider range of behavior potential, parents allow girls more variation in sex role behavior than boys, or girls see more varied models while boys see very discrete models.[35] All of these may be true. In any case, male and female behaviors vary considerably in our culture and self-esteem is closely related.

How desirable is it to be a female in our culture? Studies have shown that the characteristics assumed to be "male" such as assertiveness and logical thinking are those identified as indicative of mental health for both men and women. These characteristics assumed to be "female" such as submissiveness and emotionalism are those described as indicative of poor mental health for both men and women.[5] Thus, it would appear that all females with typical "feminine behaviors" are by definition mentally unhealthy. Or, it might be said that man is the norm and the female is an emotionally unhealthy male.[46] In fact, in one study, when asked to choose among adjectives which describe themselves, women chose terms which described themselves as less adequate, more negligent, more fearful, and less mature than did men.[3] Both men and women rate men as more worthwhile than women.[31] Both women and men prefer to have male children.[10] Women were found to be more unhappy with their body image than men regardless of illnesses.[44]

One could conclude possibly that women are socialized into a role of low self-esteem from birth. The implications may be most obvious for women but there are implications for men also. If male self-esteem is based on differentness from and dominance of a less desirable group—women—it is perilous at best. Obviously, sex role identity must be considered as an important factor in the development of self-concept and in self-esteem.

## The Crucial Nature of Body Image

Although body image is only one of the elements of self-concept, it occupies a very prominent position. Our society is very concerned with physical appearance. The young are impressed early with the importance of appearance. Storybooks often portray villains as ugly, disfigured, very poor or very rich, and non-Caucasian. Heroes are handsome, white, and middle class.[25] Villains frequently have handicaps such as Captain Hook.

It is not surprising, therefore, that studies repeatedly confirm that more physically attractive individuals receive the more favorable responses from others in numerous situations. For example, college students were given descriptions of children's unpleasant behavior randomly paired with pictures of attractive and less attractive children. In each case, regardless of the behavior, the most attractive child was judged as more honest, pleasant, and less likely to repeat the unpleasant behavior than the less attractive child.[11] Another study of nursery school children showed that even at that age, children attributed the most negative social behavior to their less attractive peers.[12] In yet another study, ' 'young, idealistic" student teachers were given short teaching assignments and told that certain white and black high school students were gifted and that others were normal in intelligence. In reality, all were of average IQ and were randomly assigned to groups. Interaction records showed that the black students were given less attention, ignored more, praised less, and criticized more than the white students. The supposedly gifted black students were treated even more negatively.[42] Subconsciously, the child quickly becomes aware of the importance of his physical self related to social acceptance and the correlation continues throughout life.

The ideal body image in our society has been said to represent youth, beauty, vigor, intactness, and health. There are a limited number of individuals who can meet this ideal and for only a short length of time. There is likely to be a resulting decreased self-esteem, insecurity, and anxiety among those who deviate significantly from this ideal.[23] It is believed that a decrease in the value of one aspect of the self leads to a decreased assessment of the self in general. For example, the individual who feels physically deviant will likely feel he is also psychologically deviant and, therefore, less capable and less intelligent.

The nurse will have contact with many individuals whose body image does not meet the cultural ideal. She should be alert to resulting generalized loss of esteem.

## Events Which Can Alter Self-Concept

Many events have the potential for affecting an individual's self-concept. This can occur because of altered appearance, functioning, or control. A few examples of events in each category will be mentioned; a complete listing would cover all events known to man. It should be realized when discussing how an individual reacts to an alteration that his previous self-concept integration is influential. Thus the individual who enters adulthood insecure in his abilities and displeased with his appearance is more vulnerable to disruptive reactions to events than an individual who accurately perceives and accepts himself.

A disturbance in self-concept can occur in any situation in which an individual must reintegrate his self-concept in a new fashion to agree with new information about himself. A distorted self-concept occurs when the reintegration is inaccurate or when reintegration was not done to account for the new data.

### ALTERED APPEARANCE

Innumerable events happen to individuals which result in a change in their physical appearance. Some of these events can be gradual or chronic such as the development of obesity or arthritis or some occur acutely such as the injuries experienced in a car accident. Some alterations are mostly temporary such as a bruise and some are permanent such as a leg amputation.

Serious prolonged alterations in physical appearance which occur to children can have profound effects on their development. Studies with children show that the disabled are listed lower in desirability as friends.[39] And the disabled are assumed to be different in personality and attitudes.[54] When asked to rank pictures of children with defects in terms of who they would most like to play with, girls were more intolerant of children with disabilities which would affect the child socially and more tolerant of disabilities which affected the child functionally. Boys showed the opposite pattern. Differences in attitudes toward disabilities were also seen related to the child's ethnic background.[39] It is assumed that children learn negative attitudes toward the disabled from their peers and parents. It is likely that these attitudes are incorporated into the self-image of the disabled person himself. Boys with handicaps were found to refer to themselves negatively in 45 percent of their self-references while boys without handicaps had only 15 percent negative self-references.[40] Studies reiterate that children with handicapping conditions do seem to be less well adjusted psychologically and cognitively than their physically normal counterparts.[49] It may all start from the incorporation of the negative appraisal they are given by others. There is little reason to believe that negative attitudes toward the self developed in the formative years by individuals with disabilities are not carried over into adulthood.

Even less severe alterations in physical appearance can be threatening, depending upon the meaning an individual attaches to his appearance. Consider the impact on the appearance conscious teenager of acne. The fact that it is common and temporary is of little consolation.

It is difficult to predict how an individual will react to a change in physical appearance because one is not always aware of the special significance of the change. It is possible that individuals themselves are not always able to anticipate how they will react to a change in physical appearance. For example, many women report being unprepared for the intensity of their reactions after a mastectomy.

As a general rule, an individual who has a chance to prepare for a change in body image such as might occur in surgery more easily incorporates the change into his self-concept than an individual whose body image alteration occurs without warning such as with an accidental burn. However, it is very difficult for anyone to visualize how his body might appear when changed so that even a person who has reflected on a change in appearance may experience profound shock when the change does occur.

It should not be surprising that the reason for the change in body image is also significant in how well one adjusts to it. The individual who loses his hair in the course of chemotherapy for cancer may accept the hair loss more easily than one whose loss was accidental.

The nurse will encounter individuals who choose a preserved body image over life itself. In these cases, the individual's physical self-concept, "I am intact" is much more important to him than his existential self-concept of "I exist." An example of this situation might be a patient who refuses a bowel resection for carcinoma because he would rather die than live with a colostomy. These situations can be difficult for the nurse to accept because she may feel that a colostomy is a small price to pay for a chance for survival. If the nurse can understand that the patient's focus at this time is more on preserving appearance than existence, she will be more likely to help the patient.

Occasionally the nurse may erroneously assume that an individual is not concerned with his physical appearance because he falls short of the culturally defined ideal appearance. It is probably safest to assume that all individuals are sensitive to changes in their physical appearance. Thus, the 45-year-old man who pays little attention to weight and personal grooming may be just as distressed over the appearance of his abdominal incision as a 21-year-old beauty queen and will need as much intervention.

In addition to the points already discussed, the impact of an alteration in physical appearance is somewhat dependent on its bodily location. The face and especially the eyes are endowed usually with more significance than other body parts. The individual's reaction to an alteration is colored by his perception of how apparent the alteration will be to others, and how easily camouflaged.

Other underlying factors may potentiate the effect of an altered appearance on an individual. For example, a woman reluctantly approaching menopause may be more vulnerable to increased concern over appearance. She may experience severe distress over another simultaneous body change such as a mastectomy.[53]

Each individual reacts in a unique way to changes in his physical appearance based on the meaning of the change to him. Healthy reactions include incorporating the change into his self-concept in an accurate manner. Denying the alteration or overemphasizing it are less satisfactory reactions.

## ALTERED FUNCTION

Other events may or may not cause changes in physical appearance but threaten an individual's self-concept primarily because of perceived or actual changes in function. One example of this type of alteration is a hysterectomy. As an event, hysterectomy signals the end of a function which many women consider their primary reason for existence so that a lowered self-esteem is likely. A hysterectomy is also seen by some women as altering their sexual functioning so that it bears a dual threat.

Events which lead to changes in self-concept because of altered function may be more difficult to appreciate because they are subtle and less obvious than changes in body image. For example, a man and women who are infertile may experience a threat to their self-concept because they are incapable of a normal function. Giving birth to a premature or defective infant may threaten self-concept because the individual involved experiences a deviation in a normal function. The patient with an ulcer has to alter his diet and other functions which may threaten his self-concept.

Immobility is probably one of the most profound changes in function an individual can experience. Normally, the individual uses his body to facilitate his life as he goes about economic, social, and various other pursuits. In these activities he figuratively transcends his body. When an individual is immobilized, he can no longer escape from his body in the same fashion and becomes essentially a prisoner of his body boundaries as his territory and experiences shrink to the confines of one or a few rooms. An overconcern with bodily discomforts and processes is likely to occur as a result.[41]

Some changes in function can be purely psychological and yet the potential for disrupted self-concept is great. For example, divorce means the individual involved no longer functions as a husband or wife; therefore, divorce is frequently associated with a sense of lowered self-esteem.

Events which have an element of both altered physical appearance and altered function may be more problematic for an individual than events with only one type of alteration. For example, a laryngectomy alters an individual's appearance and function. In situations where both appearance and function are altered, it is helpful for the nurse to learn from the patient how he feels about the two. For example, one patient with an amputation may be more concerned about learning to walk with his prosthesis than about his altered appearance while another patient may feel just the opposite concerns. The nursing approach to these patients might vary because of this knowledge.

In general, altered function may cause one to change his psychological self with resulting changes in his self-concept. Conclusions such as, "I'm not the man I used to be" or "What good am I if I can't have children" are indicative of a lowered self-esteem because of the altered function. Healthier adaptation is shown when one recognizes the change in body function without also ascribing negative connotations to the self-esteem in general. This might be demonstrated by "I'll have to change my eating habits now because of my diabetes but I can handle it."

## ALTERED CONTROL

In some situations, an individual may experience altered control of his body which leads to changes in his self-concept. Normally, one's body interferes little in his life and requires little attention. Even a slight illness such as an upset stomach suddenly places the demands of the body in the forefront and limits to some degree the normal activities of the individual. Some individuals experience this situation as threatening to their self-concept because their body is now controlling them and occupying their attention. The pregnant woman who is experiencing morning sickness, frequent urination, heartburn, fatigue, and breast pain may feel distressed by her inability to perform her usual tasks and her inability to consciously limit the symptoms she is experiencing.

An inability to perform even trivial tasks that were previously done with little conscious attention can result in the feeling of lost control.[41] Similarly, the stroke victim who cannot write with his hand or the patient with Parkinson's disease who cannot tie his shoe experiences feelings of frustration and uselessness. Even small losses can lead to large changes in how an individual thinks of himself. The need for a urinary catheter or an enema implies that one has lost control of some aspect of his body. Procedures which invade the body such as venipuncture, surgery, or x-ray may imply loss of control of entry to the body.

The depression an individual experiences when diagnosed as having cancer may be due to feelings of loss of control. He may describe his feelings as having a harmful enemy within his body which no one may be able to control and which may eventually control him.

Neurologic impairments frequently contain an element of altered control. The individual with seizures is humiliated when he has a seizure in a place and at a time that he cannot control. The patient with aphasia may be overwhelmed by his inability to communicate normally and control what he says. Many other neuromuscular impairments leave the individual involved with feelings of altered control such as multiple sclerosis and muscular dystrophy.

Anesthesia and some drugs lead patients to experience a loss of control. The individual who has a chemical addiction to drugs or alcohol has lost the ability to control whether or not he uses the substances.

The individual who has experienced a physical attack was at that time not in control. Rape victims frequently report a loss of self-esteem for having "yielded" to the rapist's demands.

Pain may be experienced as a situation of altered control because the pain controls an individual's activities and attention.

Some illnesses are likely to produce guilt and lowered self-esteem in the individual experiencing them. Pregnancy out of wedlock may lead to a decreased self-esteem for some individuals because it signifies that they were not in control of their emotions or in control of their fertility. The obese individual may feel that others have a right to despise him and that others consider him lazy or lacking in self-discipline.[8] The heavy smoker who develops lung cancer or emphysema, the heavy drinker who develops cirrhosis, or the "workaholic" who develops an ulcer or myocardial infarct may feel similarly unworthy because their conditions may be attributed to a lack of control over themselves. This may be unwittingly reinforced by health care workers who remind them continuously of their contribution to their condition. Almost any illness has some potential for eliciting guilt.

Failure to live up to an expected standard may symbolize loss of control to some individuals. A woman who hopes for natural childbirth to be a meaningful experience may instead experience guilt and shame over her inability to concentrate and perform as the women in the childbirth movies did and as her husband and physician expected her to.

It is possible for an individual to experience altered appearance, function, and control in response to the same event. The patient with an ileostomy has a stoma on his abdominal wall, his bowel function is altered, and he has no control over the secretions that emerge from the stoma. The nurse will need to recognize all of these possible alterations and what they mean to the person involved.

It should be obvious by now that a tremendous variety of events have the possibility for altering an individual's appearance, function, or control and therefore his self-concept. The nurse can help patients recognize and cope with many of these events.

## SELF-CONCEPT AND THE LIFE CYCLE

### Infants

As mentioned previously, the development of one's self-concept begins either during fetal life or early in infancy. As the child passes through infancy, he will have tentatively decided if his body is a source of pleasure or pain. It is believed that he decides that his body is good if his bodily sensations have been satiated promptly before they were overwhelming. Because body image is believed to be basic to identity formation,[50] it is very important at this time and probably exists at the feeling level.[4] Disabilities which limit the infant's abilities to experience his environment and differentiate himself may lead to a distorted self-concept.[49] The infant may turn his attention inward. It may be difficult for a caretaker to initiate and maintain an effective relationship with a disabled child which may contribute further to the problem.[49]

### Toddlers

The toddler expands his knowledge of himself through self-exploration. It is believed that most of what he has incorporated into his self-concept is based on what his parents have communicated to him regarding his place and importance in the world and the value and acceptability of his body. He is very troubled by the differences between bodies which demonstrates his cognitive ability to distinguish normal from abnormal appearance and function.[36] The toddler's increased physical skills at this time lead him to experience satisfaction from sheer physical activity, therefore restrictions in physical activity may change his image of himself. Toilet training which occurs during this time is a potentially dangerous situation. The child who experiences failure may perceive that his body is shameful and that he is a disappointment to his caretaker. The child who experiences success will develop the desirable attitudes that his body is good and that he is competent. The young child is believed to experience a threat to self in a generalized undifferentiated manner. Thus a scraped knee is an insult to his entire being.[47] The concept of being a boy or a girl is becoming established.

### Preschoolers

The preschool child is interested in increasing mastery of his body in activities such as jumping, cutting, and riding toys. He is fearful of bodily mutilation.[48] And at this age, in concert with his increased language ability, the child becomes more aware of body parts. Physical disabilities at this time can threaten his self-esteem.

As the preschooler becomes increasingly aware of his playmates, he becomes interested in differences, especially genital differences.[36] He is very curious and this leads him to be concerned over any "defect" he or others may possess. For the toddler, peer interactions are crucial in self-concept development.[20] Illness at this time may reduce his opportunities to develop social skills in interaction with peers so that later attempts to play with peers lead to rejection or uncertainty and a feeling of "I am not lovable." Disabilities will become very apparent to the child and his peers and may signify punishment.

The preschooler's self-identity is still very diffuse as evidenced by the ability of the child to pretend to be someone or something else without difficulty.[1] Because the child is so dependent on his parents, their appraisal of him is incorporated readily into his self-concept. If they are unaccepting of his appearance or of a defect such as a limp, he will be acutely sensitized.[7,32]

## School-aged Children

During the early school years acceptance by peers and success in school acquire paramount importance. Performance in school subjects is reportedly a direct determinant of self-esteem. The child's self-esteem is dependent on how well he lives up to what he perceives is expected of him. An increasing emphasis on physical appearance appears. While the preschool child is eager to just see himself in a picture, the school-aged child becomes focused on how he appears.[4] The school-aged boy's prowess in physical activities is directly related to his popularity. The girl's appearance becomes increasingly important. The slow to develop, poorly coordinated, or physically impaired are left out and illnesses which restrict opportunities to participate in the peer group may lead to decreased self-esteem. Male and female behavior is now firmly differentiated.

## Adolescents

During adolescence a rapidly changing body and the appearance of new sensations of an erotic nature channel the teenager's interests inward upon himself.[24] The teenager becomes extremely appearance conscious—not only of himself but of all others too. His body is likely to fall short of the cultural ideal, which causes him undue anguish and attempts at rectification through clothes and hairstyle. Attempts to gain peer group acceptance may place him in conflict with his parentally instilled values. Hopefully, the teenager will emerge from this stage with an accurate image of his body which typifies feelings of "I am acceptable" and "I have many good points."

The teenager with illnesses is deeply vulnerable during this stage to disrupted self-esteem. In addition to coping with normal rapid changes, he must incorporate his altered self. The teenager who is not as accepted as he wishes may use his body as an excuse.[9] "I'm not popular because I'm too short." To be different is to be inferior and being obese or short is being different.[9] The slow to mature adolescent and the one who cannot succeed in school may engage in behavior which brings negative sanctions just to be noticed.[43]

## Adults

Self-concept does not remain static during adulthood but continues to be revised as one's body and insights are changed by life experiences. Hopefully, the adult accurately and realistically adapts to changes in his physical and psychological self.

During adulthood, the process of aging requires periodic changes in one's self-concept. During periods of rapid changes in physical appearance, particular attention may be focused on a changing body image. This might occur around the menopause for a female, for example. Rapid changes in body image are difficult to incorporate without experiencing some periods of disequilibrium. Other changes in physical appearance during the growth process may occur so gradually that one is hardly aware of them. In our culture, youthfulness is more highly valued than aging so most individuals will consider changes perceived as related to aging as unpleasant and undesirable. Each individual copes with changes brought about by aging differently. Some may attempt to deny the aging process by efforts at preserving the youthful appearance of the body. Others may allow the fact that their body is aging to unjustly alter their self-concept.

In addition to altered appearance, changes in functioning occur with aging. For example, there are frequently changes in digestion and sleep pattern and these may lead the aging adult individual to experience a feeling of altered control as he must change dietary habits and adjust to shorter periods of deep sleep during the night.

It is unfortunate for the individual to conclude, "I'm getting old and, therefore, I am becoming useless." Hopefully, the individual accepts his aging body without allowing the change in his physical self to unduly influence his conception of his psychological self. Currently, there is much emphasis on trying to see aging as more positive than negative so that an individual might experience awareness of aging with an increased self-concept. For example, one could conclude: "I am getting older and, therefore, I am becoming a more mature, knowledgeable, and experienced person."

Alterations in psychological function occur also. It is likely that women are threatened differently by aging than men because a woman's self-concept may be more dependent on functions that are undermined by aging. For example, a man whose self-concept is dependent on competence in goal directed behavior is less likely to see the aging process as threatening than his wife whose self-concept is based on attractiveness, childbearing, and childrearing. And in reality, women, more so than men, have been found to experience loss of self-esteem during adulthood.

Some distortions of self-concept are likely as an individual strives to maintain a stable self-esteem. Some conclusions an individual made about himself as a child or teenager may remain operative from the individual's frame of reference although they are not now relevant. For example, the adult who as a child incorporated a "sickly" role into his self-concept may continue to distort situations to maintain his self-concept of ill health. The obese woman who was very slender and beautiful when younger may continue to dress and act as if she was still slender and beautiful. These situations occur because the individual has not revised his self-concept to fit new information.

Another factor deserving of attention is that, especially during adulthood, certain parts of the body are endowed with more importance and significance than others. The child is equally threatened by an appendectomy and a craniotomy. The adult, however, has assigned more importance to some bodily structures and capabilities than others. These values are peculiar to each person and are, therefore, difficult to anticipate without exploring the situation with the person himself.

Even though the adult has more changes to adapt to, he may have more resources to cope with disruptions in his self-concept. A threat to his body image, for example, may be somewhat counterbalanced by his intellectual, social, or spiritual resources.

# NURSING INTERVENTION IN ALTERED SELF-CONCEPT

## Primary Prevention

There are a number of actions the nurse can engage in to help prevent self-concept disturbances.

One obvious primary prevention measure involves undertaking efforts to make society in general more tolerant and accepting of variations in appearance, function, and control. An example of one such effort under way is integrating children with handicaps into the public school system. It remains to be seen if these efforts will achieve success. When individuals with alterations are accepted more readily, the hazardous effects imposed on their self-concept by the negative reactions of others will be lessened. The nurse should initiate, promote, and support efforts such as these.

Another primary preventive measure involves helping parents and educators to promote the most positive and accurate self-concept possible for all children. Theoretically, an individual with a positive self-concept would not be as devastated by an alteration suffered as a child or adult as an individual who has a more negative self-view. Parents and teachers who berate a child continuously may adversely affect a child's self-concept.[32] Parents and educators need an understanding of the factors involved in the development of self-esteem and male and female self-concepts and the effects their negative and positive feedback can have on the child.

The nurse should promote efforts to reduce the prevalent overemphasis on physical appearance in our culture. She can especially work to help individuals prepare for and accept the physical changes of aging in the hopes that an individual's self-esteem does not diminish because of aging.

There is a tendency for some individuals in our society to engage in altercasting of those who deviate in appearance.[51] For example, obese individuals are frequently cast into the role of being "jolly," and strong, muscular, athletic men are suspected of lacking intelligence. The nurse can use opportunities available to her to correct opinions consistent with altercasting. She can show by her example that an individual should not be judged solely on the basis of his appearance.

Careful preparation of individuals for events in which one's self-concept will be changed can be useful. A nurse can think of many ways to help the patient grasp what will be changed. For example, a child who is going to have a tonsillectomy may appreciate looking at his throat with a mirror and flashlight and seeing where his tonsils are. Many children have gross misconceptions about how and why their tonsils are being removed. Similarly, a patient facing divorce might benefit from listening to others discuss divorce.

Primary preventive nursing actions are summarized in Table 12-1.

**Table 12-1.** Possible nursing actions to prevent self-concept disturbances

1. Promote an increased tolerance for individuals whose functioning or appearance is deviant from normal.
2. Promote positive and accurate self-concepts in children.
3. Decrease emphasis on physical appearance.
4. Work to reduce altercasting based on physical appearance.
5. Prepare individuals for changes in self-concept.

## Secondary Prevention

The goal of nursing intervention with patients who have an altered self-concept is to help the patient to incorporate the alteration he has experienced into his self-concept accurately. A patient adapts to a change in self-concept slowly. The length of time involved depends on the meaning of the change to each individual. There is little mention in the literature of the time necessary to adjust to events, but subjective observations would suggest that adjustment to adaptation to a major event such as a chronic illness, a mastectomy, or an amputation requires many months and possibly years. The earliest days after the alteration seem very important in relation to the degree of adaptation which results. The nurse must remember that the patient's perception of the actual event is more important than the reality she sees.[34]

Initially, the nurse should collect information on the patient's previous self-concept and self-esteem. Previous unsuccessful adaptations to disruptions are predictive of a graver significance for the present threat. Also, the nurse needs to determine if the patient is experiencing his event in relation to altered appearance, control, and/or function. The nurse should assign priority to dealing with the factor which is most important to the patient.

Several authors have described distinct stages an individual passes through in reaching acceptance of an alteration.[14,15,52] These stages are based on frameworks related to crisis, stress, and grieving. An understanding of these stages is necessary in order to engage in appropriate nursing intervention. The following represents a combining of elements of several frameworks adapted to the case of an individual facing a change in self-concept and the related nursing action.

## SHOCK

In this phase the individual is helpless and numb. He passively accepts what is being done to him. The nurse, during this stage, provides personalized competent physical care as needed. The patient is not ready to face his alteration or to discuss it.

## DISBELIEF

At this time, the patient escapes reality by refusing to believe that the alteration has occurred. He may use fantasy or denial. The nurse allows the patient to persist in his denial but she does not encourage or participate in the denial. For example, a nurse could tell the patient that she is going to change his ureterostomy bag but she does not force him to look at it or discuss it. More information on intervention with the patient who is denying is found in Chapter 7.

## AWARENESS

Eventually, the reality of the situation becomes so great that the patient's defenses against believing that the alteration has occurred break down and he becomes intermittently aware of what has happened. This is a very difficult stage because the patient vacillates between disbelief and awareness. The patient may engage in considerable emotional expression such as anger, hostility, and blame. The child may lack all behavioral controls.

The nurse should facilitate the patient's expression of his feelings at this time because it is very helpful in promoting awareness and it is important for his awareness to increase and his disbelief to decrease. The child may express his emotions indirectly through fantasy or play activities. The nurse can present pieces of reality to the patient at this time to help him toward awareness. She should proceed cautiously because overwhelming the patient may lead to stronger denial. For example, a patient who has been burned is not ready to survey all of his burned areas or to discuss grafting, scarring, and rehabilitation, but the nurse might begin during this stage to get the patient involved by having him assist in dressing changes by holding items. This probes him gently into awareness. It is possible for the patient to become arrested in this stage.

A perplexing occurrence in some individuals after the removal of a significant body part is the appearance of "phantom" sensations. Some patients experience painful or prickling sensations which appear to originate from a part of their body which is no longer there. Explanations for this phenomenon vary from purely physiologic to purely psychological. The consensus seems to be that phantom sensations are largely due to a psychological discrepancy between the new body image and the previous body image.[16,17,27] It is suggested that the degree of perception of phantom sensations is directly related to the degree of body image disruption. Some patients are disturbed by the phantom sensations and are relieved to learn why they are occurring and that they have been reported frequently by others.

It is appropriate at this time to help the patient to become aware of what specifically has happened to him. He may have distorted his alteration and overgeneralized the parts of his body that have been involved.

## ACKNOWLEDGMENT

When the patient experiences increasing periods of awareness and less denial of the existence of his alteration, he has reached the stage of acknowledgment. During this stage, the full impact of the alteration is realized and the individual grieves for what has been lost. The individual's behavioral controls are not at their usual level and he still experiences active and prolonged periods of anger, depression, hostile behavior, and manipulative behavior which the nurse should accept empathetically. He will begin to have longer periods of behavioral control. He needs to see how his alteration affects him in general and how it is related to what has not been altered.

The nurse will continue to provide most of the patient's care at this time but she now orients the patient increasingly to his alteration, keeping the focus on the here and now and not the future. If the patient has rapid mood swings as frequently occurs, the nurse may find herself particularly challenged to adjust to these moods.

The nurse needs to be cognizant of the fact that she is providing the patient with much information about how he will be seen by others and he may watch her intently to see if she is repulsed or avoids him. Her touch and interest convey acceptance. The patient at this time is often challenging to work with as he struggles to recoil from his stress. The nurse should seek support from others as she deals with her feelings and reactions to the patient.

## ADAPTATION

As the individual regains behavioral controls, his attention turns toward mastering the situation he is in and resolving his losses. The nurse must realize that adaptation to a change in self-concept does not mean necessarily that the adult or child involved enjoys the alteration or accepts it completely. He will emerge from this stage with a new identity which has been altered to fit his alteration—hopefully accurately. The patient engages in activities which show an increased awareness of his environment and a decreased self-absorption. For example, he may begin reading the newspaper, worrying about other family members, and talking with others. The child begins to use every opportunity for play. The emotional expressions of the patient are very appropriate and he is in control of them.

The nurse at this time begins to prepare the patient for complete independence in care if possible and encourages the patient in focusing on the future. The patient may experience setbacks as the demands imposed on him increase. It is necessary at this time for the patient to be somewhat unaccepting of his alteration and any accompanying limitations and incapacities. This lack of tolerance for his alteration provides the patient with the incentive to strive for something better.[41] The patient who is too accepting may never reach for the optimal functioning possible and continue to live with unnecessary limitations. Thus his physical self may have been successfully rehabilitated but not his psychological self. This form of disability may be the most common.[6]

Males are particularly distressed when they are forced into a role considered appropriate in our society only for women.[6] This might include being confined to home or rendered passive or dependent. Thus the male may experience not only an alteration in his physical, psychological, or existential self but also an alteration in his perceived sex role identity. Disability may be less threatening to the female not subject to these forms of distress.

The patient must now test the effect of his alteration on others not connected with the medical world. The nurse can provide support as he does this.

The family of an individual reacts in much the same manner as does the individual experiencing the change. The nurse can intervene with them as they progress from shock to adaptation. Several points need to be highlighted.

1. The patient and the family may not be at the same stage of adaptation at the same point in time. Even family members may differ in their progression towards adaptation. The nurse may have to relate to each person differently because of this.
2. Failure to consider the family can undermine progress by the patient. For example, a child patient may be ready to strive for independence but if his parents have not been helped to adapt to his alteration, they may keep him unnecessarily dependent.
3. It is believed that parental responses to alterations in their children are crucial in determining how the child responds. Thus parents need particular nursing intervention.[2]
4. The nurse can serve as a vital role model for the family in how to relate normally and positively to the patient.

Nursing actions to promote the adaptation of children and adults to changes in self-concept are summarized in Table 12-2.

**Table 12-2.** Possible nursing actions to help adults and children adapt to changes in self-concept

1. Assess individual's previous self-concept, self-esteem, and the meaning of the alteration to him.
2. Provide appropriate physical care to individual in state of emotional shock without forcing confrontation of reality.
3. Allow individual to deny change but do not promote or engage in denial.
4. As individual develops awareness, facilitate expression of emotions and present current reality as the individual is ready.
5. Explain phantom sensations if appropriate.
6. Help individual see change in self-concept accurately.
7. Promote appropriate grieving response as individual acknowledges changes.
8. Keep focus on the present until the individual is ready to face the future.
9. When the individual strives for adaptation, promote full recovery from any disabilities rather than passive acceptance of unnecessary limitations.
10. Promote focus on the future to encourage optimal adaptation.
11. Provide support as individual contacts the outside world.
12. Remember to consider the family and intervene appropriately.

## Tertiary Prevention

Tertiary prevention is indicated when assessment indicates that an individual after a considerable length of time has not adapted optimally to an alteration in self-concept. This may be because he has not completed the process of adaptation or because his alteration has been distorted.

Initially, the nurse should try to determine the stage attained by the individual in relation to his adaptation to the alteration. Most individuals who do not adapt successfully to their alteration are fixated in the stage of partial awareness. The nurse tries to intensify the appropriate intervention in that stage so that denial is decreased and awareness facilitated. Most patients who have not adapted to their alteration have developed considerable resistance to adaptation for various reasons. One particularly difficult factor to overcome is behaviors by the family of the patient which contribute unintentionally to the denial of the alteration by the patient.

Suzy was a 13-year-old who had never had to accept her diabetes. Her mother gave her the insulin injections, tested her urine, and nagged her into eating the proper diet. When Suzy's mother had to be away for a prolonged period of time, Suzy was quickly out of control and in the hospital. She showed little interest in learning why she had gone into acidosis or in how to prevent it. Her mother had "owned" her condition for her and she had almost totally ignored it. Suzy had tremendous resistance to assuming her care and perceived that if she ignored the problem it would go away. She also was adept at manipulating her father, who had diabetes, into overconcern. A community health nurse followed Suzy after discharge and eventually employed some rather drastic measures to prod Suzy into acknowledging that her diabetes would not disappear. One of the most effective interventions of the nurse was to work with Suzy's father to permit Suzy a period of time in which she was to do totally as she pleased about her insulin, urine testing, and diet. As Suzy became progressively more ill, the nurse and father did not rush to her rescue until she herself asked for help. After the second admission in acidosis, Suzy's denial defenses were weakening. Unfortunately, the progress the nurse had made was undermined when Suzy's mother returned and was unable to see that her understandable desire to "help" Suzy was prolonging her denial. The mother apparently gained much secondary benefit from Suzy's dependency.

The individual who has distorted his alteration presents as great a challenge as the patient who has not adapted to his change. Distortion has occurred when the individual lets the alteration affect his life more than is reasonable and relevant. In this situation, the patient has reached the stage of adaptation but has become overly concerned with the alteration and has not gained mastery over his alteration or returned to an appropriate external focus. In this situation, nursing intervention involves attempts to correct the distortion by putting the alteration in its proper perspective.

> Mr. Ralston was a 6th grade elementary teacher with rheumatoid arthritis which had been discovered when he was in college. Mr. Ralston had allowed his illness clearly to become the focus of his life. He communicated to others that he expected little from himself and his pupils. Although he was only in his early 50s his conversations and outlook already evidenced a focus on the past that would have been typical of a much older individual. The school nurse where Mr. Ralston taught became interested in Mr. Ralston who persistently sought her out to complain about his health. She had noticed that he was preoccupied with his inabilities at work although his home life seemed very active for a man who professed such restricted activity. The nurse used behavior modification techniques to reward Mr. Ralston with attention when he appeared future or present oriented and active and ignored him when he appeared tired or complained about his health. After a few months, the nurse told the principal about the program and she became quite interested in participating. Although the data used to evaluate the success of their intervention are not overly reliable, over the next year Mr. Ralston's attitude and activities inside and outside of the classroom at school appeared to change. In addition, the scores his students made on standardized achievement tests were higher in the next year than they had ever been.

Although this is a rather unusual example of nursing intervention, it illustrates the idea of helping the patient to put his alteration in the proper perspective.

One of the largest blocks to correcting the patient's distorted self-concept is that he may be getting considerable gain from maintaining his distortion. Again, the family is often unwittingly reinforcing the patient's distortion. A good time to intervene is often when a change in family relationships occurs or when another threat to self-concept is likely so that a realignment of self-concept appears imminent. Obviously, it is much easier to prevent self-concept disturbances than to remove denial or distortions which have become firmly incorporated in an individual's life style.

Possible nursing actions in tertiary prevention are summarized in Table 12-3.

**Table 12-3.** Possible nursing actions for individuals who have not achieved optimal adaptation to a change in self-concept

1. Determine the stage attained by the patient in the adaptation process and promote advancement to the next stage.
2. Promote corrections of perspective if alteration has been distorted.

## THE NURSE AND SELF-CONCEPT

One of the most important things a nurse can do is to become aware as much as possible of her self-concept. She can reflect on the comments she remembers her parents and others making about her appearance and abilities. She should try to recognize and define her ideal self. Looking at these factors can make her more aware of how distorted or accurate her self-concept is.

Next, the nurse should assess the influence on her thinking of the factors that form her sex role identity. How do these influence her feelings about herself and her performance in the roles she engages in?

The nurse should assess the influence on her attitudes of physical appearance. If she is like most Americans, she is somewhat uncomfortable around the disabled and the physically impaired. An awareness of this fact is the first step in learning to place physical appearance where it belongs—as only one element among many which she should consider. Nurses understandably prefer initially to care for those who do not deviate from normality but the nurse can work to reduce her resistance to the abnormal by self-reflection and conscious efforts to see each patient as an individual with many facets.

The nurse can assess how she regards the normal changes associated with aging. She can work to increase her acceptance of the aging process and reduce her overreaction to signs of physical aging. Many feminist organizations are supporting efforts aimed at promoting acceptance of aging.

One interesting way to reflect on one's self-concept is to write down as many completions of the statement "I am . . ." as possible. This summary can be kept, added to, and revised periodically.

The nurse who experiences a change in her self-concept can reflect on the stages she is passing through and seek help from others to assure optimal adaptation.

## A TOOL FOR ASSESSMENT AND EVALUATION

The tool in Table 12-4 is proposed to aid the nurse in assessing how well an adult, child, or family member is adapting or has adapted to alterations in appearance, function, or control. The patient who has just experienced an alteration will most likely evidence a few signs of less optimal adaptation but will show movement away from them toward more optimal adaptation if adaptation is progressing well and nursing intervention has been appropriate. Each item may not be relevant for all individuals depending on the alteration they have experienced. Any individual who evidences primarily less optimal behaviors should be considered as a high risk for maladaptation to an alteration in self-concept.

## AN EXAMPLE OF NURSING INTERVENTION IN SELF-CONCEPT DISTURBANCE

The following example of nursing intervention was chosen to represent an intervention which has been necessarily quite prolonged and the elusive nature of adaptation. The individual involved experienced altered control and altered function which threatened her self-concept although her appearance was never affected.

Florence Hansen was a pleasant, poised 57-year-old woman whom the nurse, Judy, first met when Mrs. Hansen appeared for an appointment with a neurologist. Mrs. Hansen had been referred to the neurologist after her family physician suspected an inner ear disturbance. As Judy collected Mrs. Hansen's history, she discovered that Mrs. Hansen had been physically well until a few months before when she had experienced an attack of vertigo and acute dizziness at work. She had been unable to stand or sit and she had lain down on the floor until she was driven home by a friend. Mrs. Hansen related to Judy that she had been very embarrassed by the attack. She was a college professor and chairperson of the home economics department in a small state college. The attack had occurred while she was teaching a class and her students had been frightened. Mrs. Hansen had felt completely recovered by the next day and returned to work.

Four weeks later Mrs. Hansen began to have tinnitus and a severe headache which lasted for several days. Shortly thereafter she had another attack at home and was unable

**Table 12-4.** Tool for assessment of altered self-concept

| Behavior | More optimal | Less optimal |
|---|---|---|
| Use of disability | Is not used to receiving special treatment | Uses alteration for personal gain |
| Dependency needs | Normal dependency on others | Exaggerated dependency on others |
| Social interaction | Adult interacts normally, child plays appropriately with peers | Withdrawn or isolated |
| Place in family | Assumes a normal place | Becomes center of family attention or is excluded |
| Self-references | Mostly positive | Increased negativity |
| Self-portrait or self-description | Accurately indicates alteration | Distorts to deny or overemphasize alteration |
| Generalization to other areas | Does not allow alteration to interfere with unrelated aspects of life | Alteration interferes with other unrelated areas |
| Self-esteem | Restructures around other abilities | Allows alteration to result in overall lowered self-esteem |
| Risk taking | Predicts success in new situations and willing to try | Predicts failure in new situations, unwilling to try |
| View of future | Realistic | Sees future as ruined or as unchanged |
| Mourning over alteration | Normal mourning process | Does not mourn or engages in prolonged mourning |
| Depression | Feelings of depression may occur but dissipate | Prolonged state of depression |
| Emotional components | Initially may be present but dissipate | Blames others; anger, shame, guilt prolonged |
| Attempts at recovery | Seeks to learn new information, techniques, willing to discuss, accepts help | Refuses to listen, doesn't attend or intellectualizes. Refuses help. |
| Group identification | May seek to help others in same situation | Avoids others with same alteration |
| Phantom sensations | Occasional | Severe and prolonged |
| Personal identification | Unchanged | Begins to refer to self by derogatory names or terms |
| Planning | Plans life around alteration | Refuses to plan or makes unrealistic plans |
| Life style | Realistic changes | Tries to maintain exact life style or makes unnecessary alterations |
| Response to required changes | Incorporates new demands | Ignores precautions or neglectful of care related to alteration |
| Humor | Can describe something humorous related to alteration | Humorless about alteration |
| Interest in bodily functions | Normal | Preoccupied with functions |
| Fantasy life | Normal | Vivid fantasy life |
| Reactions to other stresses | Can summon adaptive capacities | Decreased capacity to cope with other demands |
| View of causation | Sees change as caused by logical circumstances | Sees change as punishment or caused by illogical circumstances[4,17,34,37,49] |

to go to work for three days. This had given her the impetus to contact her physician. She related to Judy that she was worried over what was happening to her. She had always prided herself on her strong "constitution" and ability to shrug off common illnesses such as colds. She told Judy that she assumed she had a "cold in her ears" and was anxious to get it treated.

As the neurologist examined Mrs. Hansen and conducted several audiometric tests, Judy noted that Mrs. Hansen wanted to know the details of all that was being done and wished information which was understandable. After the examination, the physician counseled Mrs. Hansen that he suspected Meniere's disease and described briefly the significant features of the disease to her. He prescribed changes in her diet and several medications. She was told that she would need to return frequently as he checked the appropriateness of the treatment. Judy explained to Mrs. Hansen that she routinely made home visits to see all new patients who would like her to come, and Mrs. Hansen and Judy made their first appointment for later in the same week.

Judy planned on the first visit to assess how Mrs. Hansen was adjusting to her condition, diet, and medications, and to learn more about her as an individual which would be helpful in planning her care. One of the first things she learned was that Mrs. Hansen was resourceful. She had talked to nursing faculty members at the college where she taught and read in their textbooks about her condition and about the prescribed medications. She told Judy that she had not particularly liked what she had read. Judy discovered that she was particularly bothered by the unpredictable nature of the disease. Judy speculated that Mrs. Hansen might react to her condition with feelings of loss of control and that this might eventually lead to problems with self-esteem. The fact that Mrs. Hansen had read about the condition alerted Judy to the fact that she must have some beginning acceptance of the diagnosis but Judy felt that Mrs. Hansen might remain somewhat skeptical of her condition for a while if her symptoms did not become more severe.

Judy discovered that Mrs. Hansen led a very busy life. In addition to being a departmental chairperson and teaching a full schedule of courses, she served on many college committees and was active in her church. She was married and was the sole source of family income. Her husband had been injured in a car accident several years before and had not worked since then. Mrs. Hansen described him as having had some brain injuries and added that he was on numerous medications "to keep him calm." Mrs. Hansen appeared to have planned her life carefully, but this illness did not fit in with her plans.

Judy determined that Mrs. Hansen had some awareness of what was ahead but at this time was coping with her diagnosis through the belief that by following her diet, taking her medications, and concentrating she could will away any more attacks. Judy allowed her this belief but did not reinforce it. Judy decided that Mrs. Hansen would be likely to adhere carefully to medical care even while partially denying her illness and that her intellectual approach to her condition was a method of coping with the unknown by making it seem more known.

Over the course of several months, Mrs. Hansen at first experienced some relief from her condition only later to experience the resumption of symptoms and a third and fourth attack in rapid succession. Judy went to visit Mrs. Hansen after each attack. Mrs. Hansen's initial command of the situation seemed very threatened as she developed awareness. Judy discovered that Mrs. Hansen was very afraid of not being able to continue teaching until she was 65. She had devoted much of her life to her profession and was unwilling to step down. She told Judy how difficult it was to do her work with the persistent headache and tinnitus. She found herself becoming irritated with students and coworkers. She was finding it very difficult to drive during heavy traffic periods and was, therefore, leaving for work earlier and arriving home later. She found the usual hassles of her job such as coping with a decreasing budget almost overwhelming. Finally, Mrs. Hansen discussed with Judy her worst fear which was being confined to home. She confessed that she would find continual contact with her husband all day long very trying. Judy provided herself as an accepting nonjudgmental listener.

At this time Judy concluded that Mrs. Hansen was facing some alterations in her usual functions which were a challenge to her self-concept and at this time she was channeling her energies into trying to go on with her usual functions as close to previous levels as possible. Judy decided that Mrs. Hansen was coping by focusing on preserving function and was not ready to talk about the future and changing her life more drastically and altering some of her present functions. She was most likely in the stage of awareness or acknowledgment.

After a few more months Mrs. Hansen appeared in many respects to be mourning for what she had lost or was losing. She seemed particularly perplexed over her inability to diminish her symptoms through diet, medication, or willpower. This feeling that she was losing control was very difficult for Mrs. Hansen because she was by nature inclined to be the master of things around her. For Mrs. Hansen, altered control seemed as much of a problem as altered function at work. Judy concentrated on teaching Mrs. Hansen information which might help her achieve more control. For example, Mrs. Hansen learned to move her head very slowly, how to reduce drug side effects, and how to administer her own subcutaneous injections to help abate attacks once they had begun. Judy also attempted to help Mrs. Hansen to focus on the areas of her life which were not affected by her condition. As Mrs. Hansen showed interest in learning more about her condition specifically, Judy presented more information.

During this period of time, Judy tried to discover if there were other sources of support available to Mrs. Hansen. Mr. Hansen was not able to grasp his wife's problems, and her children lived too far away to be of help. Mrs. Hansen described her relation with her fellow faculty members as pleasant but she did not want to discuss her health problems with anyone connected with school. Mrs. Hansen's greatest support seemed to be a personal friend who had long been her confidante and she continued to share her problems with her during this new development.

Contacts with Mrs. Hansen continued in home visits and in the office. During periods of remission, Mrs. Hansen continued her life much as before but the periods of increased symptoms became more numerous and her hearing loss became progressively more severe. Eventually, Mrs. Hansen began to mention more concern for what might happen in the future so Judy concentrated efforts on facilitating Mrs. Hansen's efforts at planning her life style to complement her impairment. Mrs. Hansen arrived quite unexpectedly at the decision to relinquish her chairmanship of the department and coped with her disappointment by making elaborate plans for orienting her successor to her duties. She apparently arrived at this decision when she began to suspect that her functioning was being too greatly affected by her condition. She began discussing selling her home and moving to an apartment but she was never able to come to action on this issue. Judy expected that living in a smaller area was particularly threatening to her because she and her husband had individual territories in their home. One significant adaptation was that Mrs. Hansen was finally able to stay home when she was particularly bothered by symptoms without forcing herself to go to work only to have a terrible day. Judy interpreted this as real progress in adaptation because it indicated that she was beginning to accept the fact that there were times when she had to give in to her disease.

Mrs. Hansen did experience some loss of self-esteem after resigning as department chairperson and she confided to Judy that it was very difficult to give up some of the privileges she had experienced because of her status such as a large, pleasant office and attending policymaking meetings and board meetings. She noticed that people did not pay as much attention to what she had to say as before. Judy encouraged Mrs. Hansen to talk and to reflect on other esteem building themes.

While Mrs. Hansen seemed to reach the stage of adaptation, Judy still experienced difficulty in getting Mrs. Hansen to plan for other areas of the future which she felt were going to be difficult. Mrs. Hansen was very persistent in going on as usual until events forced her to face the need for change. Judy eventually decided to support this pattern because Mrs. Hansen was able to face each problem and take appropriate action as the time came. She suspected that Mrs. Hansen did have some plans for the future but could not face actually putting them into words.

At the present time, Judy is especially concentrating her efforts on helping Mrs. Hansen continue at work even though Mrs. Hansen has had to resort to a part time class load. For Mrs. Hansen, self-esteem is heavily tied to her work, and so preserving a meaningful work role is extremely important. It remains to be seen how she will cope when she must relinquish her work altogether and find a more manageable home.

## SUMMARY

Self-concept, which is developed in early childhood and refined throughout life, is composed of three parts: the existential self, the physical self, and the psychological self. Almost every event which happens to an individual has implications for affecting that individual's self-concept such as events which alter an individual's appearance, function, or control. An alteration in any area has the potential for causing a generalized effect on self-esteem.

The nurse can act to prevent self-concept disturbances, intervene to aid optimal adaptation to changes in self-concept, and work to correct distortions of self-concept or incomplete adaptation. She will be most effective with others if she herself has an accurate self-concept.

## REFERENCES

1. Allport, G. W.: *Becoming: Basic Considerations for a Psychology of Personality.* Yale University Press, New Haven, 1955.
2. Arneson, W. W., and Triplett, J. L.: "How children cope with disfiguring changes in their appearance." Matern. Child Nurs. J. 3:366, 1978.
3. Bennett, E. M., and Cogen, L. R.: "Men and women: Personality patterns and contrasts." Genet. Psychol. Monogr. 60:101, 1959.
4. Blaesing, S., and Brockhaus, J.: "The development of body image in the child." Nurs. Clin. North Am. 7:597, 1972.
5. Broverman, I., et al.: "Sex-role stereotypes and clinical judgments of mental health," in Bardwick, J. (ed.): *Readings in the Psychology of Women.* Harper and Row, New York, 1972.
6. Christopherson, V. A.: "Role modifications of the disabled male." Am. J. Nurs. 68:290, 1968.
7. Coopersmith, S.: *The Antecedents of Self-Esteem.* W. H. Freeman, San Francisco, 1967.
8. Craft, C. A.: "Body image and obesity." Nurs. Clin. North Am. 7:677, 1972.
9. Dempsey, M. O.: "The development of body image in the adolescent." Nurs. Clin. North Am. 7:609, 1972.
10. Dinitz, S., Dynes, R. R., and Clark, A. C.: "Preferences for male or female children: Traditional or affectional." Marriage Fam. Liv. 16:128, 1954.

11. Dion, K. K.: "Physical attractiveness and evaluation of children's transgressions." J. Personality Soc. Psychol. 24:207, 1972.

12. Dion, K. K., and Berscheid, E.: "Physical attractiveness and peer acceptance among children." Sociometry 37:1974.

13. Ehrhardt, A. A., and Baker, S. W.: "Fetal androgens, human central nervous system differentiation, and behavior sex differences," in Friedman, R., and Wiele, V. (eds.): Sex Differences in Behavior. John Wiley and Sons, New York, 1974.

14. Engel, G. L.: "Grief and grieving." Am. J. Nurs. 64:93, 1964.

15. Fink, S.: "Crisis and motivation: A theoretical model." Arch. Phys. Med. Rehabil. 48:592, 1967.

16. Fishman, S.: "Amputee needs, frustrations, and behavior." Rehabil. Lit. 20:322, 1959.

17. Francis, G. M., and Munjas, B.: Promoting Psychological Comfort. Wm. C. Brown, Dubuque, 1975.

18. Freedman, D. G.: "The development of social hierarchies," in Levi, L. (ed.): Society, Stress, and Disease. Volume 2. Childhood and Adolescence. Oxford University Press, London, 1975.

19. Goldberg, S., and Lewis, M.: "Play behavior in the year-old infant: Early sex differences." Child Devel. 40:21, 1969.

20. Hartup, W. W.: "Peer interaction and the behavioral development of the individual child," in Schopler, E., and Reichler, R. J. (eds.): Child Development, Deviations, and Treatment. Plenum Publishing, New York, 1976.

21. Hetherington, E. M., and Deur, J. L.: "The effects of father absence on child development," in The Young Child: Reviews of Research. Volume II. National Association for the Education of Young Children, Washington, D.C., 1972.

22. Hutt, C.: "Sex differences in human development." Human Devel. 15:153, 1972.

23. Jourard, S. M.: "Body image, spirit, and wellness," in The Transparent Self. Van Nostrand, Princeton, N.J., 1964.

24. Kalafatich, A. J. (ed.): Approaches to the Care of Adolescents. Appleton-Century-Crofts, New York, 1975.

25. Key, M. R.: "The role of male and female in children's books—dispelling all doubt." Wilson Library Bulletin, October, 1971.

26. Lee, P. C., and Wolinsky, A. L.: "Male teachers of young children: A preliminary empirical study." Young Child. 28:342, 1973.

27. Leonard, B. J.: "Body image changes in chronic illness." Nurs. Clin. North Am. 7:687, 1972.

28. Lewis, M., and Brooks-Gunn, J.: "Self, other, and fear: The reaction of infants to people," in Hetherington, E. M., and Parke, R. D. (eds.): Contemporary Readings in Child Psychology. McGraw-Hill, New York, 1977.

29. Lipsitt, L. P., and Levy, N.: "Pain threshold in the human neonate." Child Devel. 30:547, 1959.

30. Lynn, D. B.: "Sex-role and parental identification." Child Devel. 33:555, 1962.

31. McKee, J. P., and Sheriffs, A. C.: "The differential evaluation of males and females." J. Pers. 25:356, 1957.

32. Missildine, W. H.: "Self-devaluation—Part I. Its beginnings in childhood." Feelings and Their Medical Significance (Ross Laboratories) 9:1, 1967.

33. Moss, H. A.: "Sex, age, and state as determinants of mother-infant interaction." Merrill-Palmer Quart. 13:19, 1967.

34. Murray, R. L.: "Principles of nursing intervention for the adult patient with body image changes." Nurs. Clin. North Am. 7:697, 1972.

35. Mussen, P., and Rutherford, E.: "Parent-child relations and parental personality in relation to young children's sex role preferences." Child Devel. 34:589, 1963.

36. Nahigian, E. G.: "The preschooler—3 to 5 years" and "Effects of illness on the preschooler," in Scipien, G. M., et al.: Comprehensive Pediatric Nursing. McGraw-Hill, New York, 1975.

37. Norris, C. M.: "Body image: Its relevance to professional nursing," in Carlson, C. E., and Blackwell, B. (eds.): Behavioral Concepts and Nursing Intervention. J. B. Lippincott, Philadelphia, 1978.

38. Rheingold, H. L.: "Some visual determinants of smiling in infants." Unpublished manuscript, University of North Carolina, Chapel Hill, 1971.

39. Richardson, S. A., et al.: "Cultural uniformity in reaction to physical disability." Am. Soc. Rev. 26:241, 1961.

40. Richardson, S. A., et al.: "Effects of physical disability on a child's description of himself." Child Devel. 35:893, 1964.

41. Rubin, R.: "Body image and self esteem." Nurs. Outlook 16:20, 1968.

42. Rubovitz, P. C., and Maehr, M. L.: "Pygmalion black and white." J. Pers. Soc. Psychol. 25:210, 1973.

43. Schonfeld, W. A.: "Body image in adolescents: A psychiatric concept for the pediatrician." Pediatrics 31:845, 1963.

44. Schwab, J., and Harmeling, J.: "Body image and mental illness." Psychosom. Med. 30:51, 1968.

45. Sears, R. R., et al.: *Patterns of Child Rearing.* Row, Peterson, Evanston, Ill., 1957.
46. "Self image and identity as women," in *Focus on Women—1975.* Leadership Conference of Women Religious, Milwaukee, 1975.
47. Smith, E. C., et al.: "Reestablishing a child's body image." Am. J. Nurs. 77:445, 1977.
48. Steele, S.: "Children with amputations." Nurs. Forum 7:411, 1968.
49. Waechter, E. H.: "Developmental correlates of physical disability." Nurs. Forum 9:90, 1970.
50. Waechter, E. H., and Blake, F. G.: *Nursing Care of Children.* J. B. Lippincott, Philadelphia, 1976.
51. Weinstein, A.: "Altercasting and interpersonal relations," in Secord, P., and Bachman, C. (eds.): *Readings in Social Psychology.* Prentice-Hall, Englewood Cliffs, N.J., 1967.
52. Weiss, R., and Payson, H.: "Gross stress reaction," in Freedman, A. M., and Kaplan, H. (eds.): *Comprehensive Textbook of Psychiatry.* Williams and Wilkins, Baltimore, 1967.
53. Woods, N. F.: "Psychological aspects of breast cancer: Review of the literature." J. Nurs. Assoc. Am. College Obstetr. Gynecol. 4:15, 1975.
54. Wright, B. A.: *Physical Disability—A Psychological Approach.* Harper and Row, New York, 1960.

# BIBLIOGRAPHY

Baumrind, D.: "Socialization and instrumental competence in young children." Young Child. 26:104, 1970.
Barscheid, E., et al.: "Body image, The happy American body: A survey report." Psychol. Today 7:119, 1974.
Brunner, L. S., and Suddarth, D. S.: *Textbook of Medical-Surgical Nursing.* J: B. Lippincott, Philadelphia, 1975.
Burgess, A. W., and Holmstrum, L. L.: "Rape trauma syndrome." Am. J. Psych. 131:981, 1974.
Corbeil, M.: "Nursing process for a patient with a body image disturbance." Nurs. Clin. North Am. 6:155, 1971.
Crate, M. A.: "Nursing functions in adaptation to chronic illness." Am. J. Nurs. 65:72, 1965.
DeNoble, M.: "The self and crisis during the late adult years," in Hall, J. E., and Weaver, B. R. (eds.): *Nursing of Families in Crisis.* J. B. Lippincott, Philadelphia, 1974.
Dyche, M. E.: "Pelvic exenteration: A nursing challenge." J. Obstet. Gynecol. Neonat. Nurs. 4:11, 1975.
Finney, R.: "Identity and the self system," in Clark, A. L., and Affonso, D. D.: *Childbearing: A Nursing Perspective.* F. A. Davis, Philadelphia, 1976.
Fujita, M.: "The impact of illness or surgery on the body image of the child." Nurs. Clin. North Am. 7:641, 1972.
Gergen, K. J.: *The Concept of Self.* Holt, Rinehart and Winston, New York, 1971.
Iffrig, Sr. M. C.: "Body image in pregnancy." Nurs. Clin. North Am. 7:631, 1972.
Johnson, M. M.: "Fathers, mothers, and sex typing." Sociol. Inquiry 45:15, 1975.
Kalkman, M. E., and Davis, A. J.: *New Dimensions in Mental Health-Psychiatric Nursing.* McGraw-Hill, New York, 1974.
Kolb, L. C.: "Disturbances of the body-image," in Arieti, S. (ed.): *American Handbook of Psychiatry, Volume I.* Basic Books, New York, 1959.
Kowalsky, E. L.: "A lost life style." Am. J. Nurs. 78:418, 1978.
MacBryde, C. M.: "The diagnosis of obesity." Med. Clin. North Am. 48:1307, 1964.
MacIntyre, J. M.: "Adolescence, identity, and foster family care." Children 17:213, 1970.
McCary, J. L.: *Human Sexuality: A Brief Edition.* Van Nostrand, New York, 1973.
Riddle, I.: "Nursing intervention to promote body image integrity in children." Nurs. Clin. North Am. 7:651, 1972.
Schilder, P.: *The Image and Appearance of the Human Body.* John Wiley and Sons, New York, 1950.
Shapiro, A. L.: *Psychoepistemology and Sex.* LeGrand, Inc., Santa Barbara, 1980.
Tudor, M. J.: "Family habilitation: A child with a birth defect," in Hymovich, D. P., and Barnard, M. U. (eds.): *Family Health Care.* McGraw-Hill, New York, 1973.
Warrick, L. H.: "Femininity, sexuality, and mothering." Nurs. Forum 8:212, 1969.

# CHAPTER 13

# FATAL ILLNESS

Nurses in various health care settings often encounter individuals who are dying. The nurse has an opportunity to intervene so that the dying individual and his family adapt to the situation in the most optimal manner possible. In order to do this, the nurse needs to understand what it is like to live with a fatal illness. This chapter will focus on discussing intervention for the patient and family facing a terminal illness. This information might be useful for the nurse herself in learning more about her reactions to and attitudes about death and dying. Chapter 9 discusses the grieving process and contains additional information of relevance.

## REVIEW OF THEORY

### Death in American Society

An exploration of the nurse's role in working with families threatened by death must begin with an examination of the predominant cultural views on death in our society. It is no secret that death is a greatly feared and unpleasant topic in current American society.[27] Most adults avoid using the word "dead" or "death," rarely think of their own death, tend to avoid reminders of death such as cemeteries and funeral homes, and unconsciously believe that they are immortal.[37]

It may be surprising to realize that this fear and avoidance of death has not always been true. Many of the stories and poems of earlier times speak of death quite openly and naturally. Even material for children, such as stories and nursery rhymes, openly mentioned death. Paintings sometimes showed a death bed or a funeral. The death of at least one child in a family was probably common. Deaths as well as marriages and births were frequent common occurrences and occasions for family gatherings. What has happened then to increase the horror of death in our current thinking?

A multitude of events is believed to account for how we feel about death today. First of all, many individuals now reach adulthood without having experienced a death of personal meaning. In earlier times, it was more common for grandparents, parents, or siblings to die at home and when children were still young so that as one matured, one was familiar with the presence and inevitability of death in human life. Large, extended families also increased the probability of contact with a meaningful death during childhood. Increasing longevity, reduced child mortality, and the pattern of smaller, more nuclear families have decreased the likelihood of familiarity with death. Therefore, what one is less familiar with may have become far more frightening. This may account in addition for a desire to remove anyone even remotely suggestive of death from awareness.[5] Thus the elderly, the handicapped, the ill, and the dying are kept away from view.

Second, improved health care, the ability to prevent and treat previously serious or fatal illnesses, and stories of individuals being successfully resuscitated after near death may have caused many to unconsciously believe that death itself is also preventable. Some would suggest that in actuality many an individual behaves as if he will never die and that death, if it does occur, is in many situations an unfortunate accident which should not have occurred. In truth, death is certain and inevitable for everyone. All that is uncertain is how, when, and where one will die.

Third, not only has death been pushed from sight, but the grieving process has been devalued and edited. Individuals suffering losses are expected to "bear up," at least in public. The bereaved may be denied socially approved outlets for their grief.[2] The rituals once associated with grieving such as wearing black, observing a period of mourning, and death wreaths on the front door are passing from common occurrence. Some cemeteries can now provide a service to automatically decorate graves on appropriate occasions for families. The result is that one may reach adulthood without knowledge of or a model of grieving.

Fourth, the American culture is decidedly achievement and future oriented. Individuals are valued largely in terms of what they accomplish. This emphasis can lead to developing near panic, when faced with death, over what one has not achieved.[48] When this is combined with a tendency to live in the future, the fear of dying becomes more marked as one focuses on what one has not yet done rather than reflecting on what has been.

All of these factors contribute to determining one's reaction to death. From them evolves a prevalent tendency to avoid death and also the dying, an inability to consciously think of one's own nonexistence, a death denying way of life, exaggerated fears associated with dying, and a lack of preparation for accepting death. These behaviors create problems not only for individuals with a fatal illness and their families, but also for the health care professional who works with them. Often the individual with a fatal illness is deprived of the support he needs as a result.

## Living and Dying with a Fatal Illness

As medical knowledge increases, it is becoming more and more likely for an individual to live for several years with a condition which will eventually be fatal. This prolonged period of living is, at the same time, a prolonged period of dying. Some of the concerns and challenges facing families under these conditions will be explored.

At the time of diagnosis the family and the patient will probably react with shock and disbelief. Attempts may be made to find a more favorable diagnosis from another physician. In other instances when the individual has been plagued with annoying symptoms, there may be some relief associated with at last having a diagnosis, even if it is unfavorable.

As the family and the patient gain awareness of the situation, methods of coping such as anger, hostility, guilt, depression, withdrawal, and denial can become predominant. The family and the patient at this time may feel in limbo between hope and fear. When the patient improves they may intellectually admit that there is a life threatening illness but emotionally they may find belief in and hopes for a cure paramount. Eventually, if the patient's condition begins to show less responsivity to treatment, a reawakening of awareness occurs. Most individuals will still maintain some hope even during the most difficult stages. Hope may become not hope for recovery but hope for one more holiday or one more period of remission.

Eventually when death is imminent, the family may find themselves torn between wishes that the patient will die quickly with no more suffering and wishes for the patient to survive. When the patient does die, their sorrow is mixed with relief that the ordeal is over. Family members may feel very guilty about having hoped that death would come soon and feeling relief when it does come. If they have already grieved over the coming loss, the reaction at this time is still painful but less so than if the death had been unexpected.

As the family grieves and enters the phase of restitution, there are usually feelings of loss along with feelings of freedom as they realize that there will no longer be the difficult trips to offices and clinics and the agonizing waits at the bedside. Some situations will have developed where family units have been strengthened because of the ordeal but all too often family members will discover that relationships within the family will have become less secure and family dissolution may occur.

The nurse who is aware of these dynamics within the family may be able to help family members and the patient through various crucial periods and increase family cohesiveness.

## Anticipatory Mourning

There are numerous situations when the death of another is predicted before the actual death occurs and the grieving process may occur in a special manner before the loss.

Chapter 9 discussed the grieving process in relation to the period following a loss. Anticipatory mourning is a process which occurs before or as a loss occurs.

When anticipatory mourning occurs, the individual may be at first numb and shocked. Then follows a period of grief work including preoccupation, anger, and anguish. Finally, the individual begins to partially resolve the approaching loss. When the death does occur, the reaction is somewhat less intense than the reaction to an unexpected loss would have been and the individual usually experiences each stage in the grieving process again.

It is possible for the grief process to be so effective that the loss is actually resolved for the family before the actual death occurs.[25]

> Nancy was a 6-year-old with an inoperable brain tumor. After her initial surgery and diagnosis, she lived at home for almost a year before being admitted to a medical center inpatient unit. In a few months, Nancy was continuously comatose. Her parents visited on weekends only as they lived many miles from the center. Nancy came from a large and active family and her parents, who were initially distraught over her situation, became gradually detached and emotionless as they visited. Nancy was hardly recognizable as the lively, bright, and cheerful daughter they had once known. Eventually Nancy's father was offered a promotion if he would accept a transfer to another part of the country. For the sake of the rest of the family it seemed best to accept the transfer. Nancy's parents reluctantly moved after tearfully visiting their unconscious daughter for the last time in all probability. The head nurse offered her support to them and promised to write frequently about Nancy's condition.
> The nursing staff of the unit had difficultly accepting the behavior of the parents whom they felt to be

uncaring. The head nurse explained that their mourning had been complete so that the loss of their daughter was resolved. How could they be blamed that their grief process did not perfectly match the length of Nancy's dying?

Another example of anticipatory mourning involves the middle-aged person who realizes that his parents are aging rapidly. He may begin to mourn their loss and resolve his grief process before they die.

Anticipatory mourning can also occur in the individual facing his own death. The individual facing his own death must adapt to several losses also. Most obviously, he may feel that he is losing his future. He may feel loss of independence as he becomes more dependent on others to care for him and as his activities become limited. If he is hospitalized, he experiences loss of his previous surroundings and intimate interactions with his family and friends. He may experience loss of self-esteem as others begin to assume the roles he played. As he becomes more seriously ill, he is frequently increasingly isolated and feels loss of human contact. These all combine to precipitate anticipatory mourning.

Elisabeth Kübler-Ross has described five stages an individual can potentially pass through in accepting his death, based on her clinical experiences with dying patients.[36] These are:

1. Denial. This is described as shock and numbness and refusal to believe that death is possible.
2. Anger and hostility. This stage is characterized by bitterness towards, and envy of, others.
3. Bargaining. Usually, this is a short stage which is manifested by attempts to deal with God or the health care staff for one more holiday or one more year in return for good behavior or faithful adherence to treatment.
4. Depression and despair. Symptoms of depression such as psychomotor retardation and feelings of worthlessness predominate in this stage.
5. Acceptance. This stage is evidenced by behaviors such as withdrawal from others and a lack of emotional displays such as fear.

While these stages seem reasonable, others have not been able to detect their presence by objective research methods. Research efforts now seem to suggest that the individual does at first experience shock and disbelief but then adapts a characteristic response which typifies his behavior until death.[52] It is likely that an individual's pattern of adaptation is based on how he has perceived and adapted to losses he has faced as he matured. Three predominant patterns have been described which typify how patients respond to a fatal diagnosis.[61]

1. Withdrawal from others, expression of fear, and predominant depression.
2. Rejection of help combined with anger, acting out, restlessness, and annoyance at others.
3. Quiet acceptance which seems reflective of inner resources.

The first pattern is believed to be the most frequently encountered method of adapting found among individuals facing their own approaching death. Acceptance was rarely found. Some reasons for the commonness of depression in addition to the psychological reasons might be explained by the fact that many individuals approaching death are receiving large doses of many medications which may promote depression, they may have a heightened awareness of their condition brought on by increasing symptoms, and they may note their failing capabilities to comprehend the environment.[52] In addition, the physiologic course of many fatal diseases may produce depression because of effects on the body chemistry. Both depression and anxiety have been found clinically to increase in the two weeks before death.[28] Patients may occasionally change from one of these three patterns of coping to another one but it is believed that one of them would consistently predominate for a particular individual.

Adherence to the five stage progressive adaptation theory of Kübler-Ross would lead the nurse to work toward acceptance for patients as the optimal adaptation to fatal illness but from what is presently known, it would seem more likely to support patients in the pattern of adaptation they manifest and to expect depression from most and acceptance from only a few.

Anticipatory mourning is believed to represent a helpful response because it prepares the family and patient to deal with loss.

## FATAL ILLNESS AND THE LIFE CYCLE

Information on how individuals of various ages view death and how they may grieve for a loss is presented in Chapter 9. Discussed here will be how individuals of various ages may view their own death.

### Infants and Toddlers

It seems unlikely that a child under three can understand the concept of death. He cannot, therefore, think of his own death and would probably have little fear of death. He would be sensitive to the emotions of those around him, however, and parental anxiety and concern would be reflected by the child facing death.

### Preschoolers

The child of three has difficulty conceiving of his own death primarily because he lives so decidedly in the here and now. He cannot miss his future because he has difficulty conceptualizing what it is. He is, like the younger child, very sensitive to the emotions of others, however. The seriously ill child of three and one-half to four years of age may not openly talk of his own death, but he has been found to evidence symbolically in stories or drawings that he is preoccupied and aware of how seriously ill he is and that he is going to die.[45,57] He may interpret his parent's attempts to spare him from knowledge of his condition as indifference and feel alienated, isolated, and helpless.[57] The child's knowledge of his fatal condition was found even when elaborate and deliberate attempts had been made to shield him from the truth.[23] Preschool children were sometimes found to begin to talk openly about their death only when and if their parents reached a period of acceptance.[37]

### School-aged Children

The school-aged child who is fatally ill almost always is aware of the seriousness of his condition despite careful efforts by others at subterfuge. Like the younger child, he has difficulty realizing what loss of his future actually means although the child of 10 or 11 years of age will feel more of a sense of loss. Since he now has a grasp of the nature of death, his own approaching death will hold more sense of fear of the unknown for him than for the younger child. Boys may be more likely to act out when they feel anxious about their approaching death while girls may more likely become depressed.[45]

## Adolescents

The teenager with a fatal illness is very aware of his future being cut short and he mourns for his unfulfilled hopes and dreams.[50] Fatal illness which interferes with his appearance and, therefore, his peer acceptance can be especially painful to his ego. Also, illnesses which force him to remain dependent on his parents place him in conflict over his strivings to be independent. The adolescent who is in a profoundly future oriented family may experience higher degrees of anxiety than the teenager in a family which more highly values the present and the past.[50] Teenagers are likely to sentimentalize their situation[50] and may express themselves best in art and by composing poetry or songs. It is understandable that many fatally ill teenagers feel resentful and bitter.[3]

## Adults

It is impossible to classify the many ways in which adults view death. By adulthood individuals have developed varying attitudes related to death. For most adults in this culture, death is greatly feared. Some suggest that much of one's fear of death is actually instinctual rather than learned. Others contend that death is so greatly feared because it is often so closely associated with pain.[55]

For whatever reasons, death is often seen by the adult as an overwhelmingly frightening prospect and he may engage in various behaviors to overcome or cope with his fear of death. He may attempt to prove himself immune to death by successive risk taking behaviors. He may subscribe to religious teachings which promise the conquering of death through a life after death. He may attempt to structure his world so that death is an excluded subject. He may attempt to reorient himself so that death is seen as a glorious fulfillment of life. Through these methods he may feel less fear.

Another likely reaction is to equate death with punishment. While children are expected to equate illness with punishment, one is seldom aware that this view persists in adulthood. Health care professionals may promote an association when they comment, "Smoke and you'll get lung cancer," "Eat animal fats and you'll get atherosclerosis." This reinforces the belief that illness can be a punishment. The association between illness and punishment is evidenced in the common statement, "I knew I was going to come down with something the way I've been pushing myself." Similarly the patient with a fatal illness may consciously or unconsciously relate his illness to punishment. This contributes to feelings of loss of self-worth and depression. As others begin to avoid him, his guilt is reinforced.

Some adults with a fatal illness find most difficult of all their inability to live without a future. Every day may seem more meaningful and richer but the lack of a future causes a feeling of being in limbo and difficulties with planning.[31] Other adults may fear punishment after death.[14] For most the greatest fear is probably that of the unknown because no one really knows what awaits him after death. Other more personal worries may plague the dying patient, such as fears associated with leaving young children or an elderly spouse behind.[37]

## Older Adults

The elderly individual faces his own death in ways characteristic of his life experiences. The common assumption that all older individuals peacefully accept their own death is not true. Many fear their death as much as younger persons. However, death is often more conceivable and less frightening for an older adult.

## INTERVENTION IN FATAL ILLNESS

The nurse often has many opportunities to work with individuals or families facing fatal illness and death. She can intervene to help assure an optimal outcome if she is aware of actions that can be taken.

In general, at the time of diagnosis, the family will experience shock and disbelief even if they had some suspicion about the nature of the illness. Disbelief can be seen in several reactions. The family may feel that the physician has made a mistake. They may offer their own interpretations about the real condition. It is best to allow the family and patient to continue in their denial at this time but not to encourage it.[8]

In order to reduce denial, it is helpful if the health care professionals state the diagnosis with certainty when warranted rather than raising hopes that there could have been error.[47] It seems advantageous to have as many members of the immediate family present as possible when the diagnosis is discussed so that all members hear the same thing at the same time. Those who get their information second hand may more likely deny the truth. If the patient is a child, it is believed to be advisable to have the grandparents present because it has been noted that they sometimes persist in denial of the condition which can be very difficult for the parents.[47]

The nurse may want to spend time with the family after the diagnosis has been given to answer any questions that develop or to provide a method to see that their questions are answered. Families and patients who are helped to verbalize may cope better as this establishes a pattern.[25,33] What can be talked about can more likely be coped with. The presence of the nurse can remind the patient and family of the reality of the situation.

It may be helpful to instill a few central ideas at this time even if the family has not brought up certain questions. These ideas, if truthful, may include the following:

1. Nothing could have been done to prevent the illness.
2. The length of time it has taken to discover the condition will not significantly affect the outcome.
3. The family and patient should avoid their natural tendency to alter their lives drastically and should make every effort to continue usual patterns and activities as much as possible.
4. Research in the area is going on and the results are widely disseminated, so the health care team will take advantage of any new developments as they become available.[49]

These ideas may prevent the family from experiencing excessive guilt, running from one health care facility to another, and may offer some hope. Neither the patient nor the family will comprehend much of what is being said so that instructions which must be given at this time about medications, treatments, return appointments, and contacting help should be written as well as covered verbally. The family must at some time discuss how they will answer the questions of others. Practicing what they will say may help to make the situation easier.

The nurse should stay closely in touch with the family and patient during the early stage or provide someone through referral. She should assess how they are reacting to the situation and how they are likely to cope. She will be able to determine which family members are most likely to be able to support the patient and which ones will probably be completely immersed in their own struggles to cope. She can assess the factors that may influence the family mourning such as the significance of the loss and whether or not it was expected.

As the family and patient develop awareness of the state of affairs, the nurse can assist them in expressing their feelings through use of the helping process. Degrees of anger, guilt, despair, and hostility may begin to emerge as the situation becomes less deniable. These feelings may be reduced after being shared repeatedly with an understanding listener. The nurse may note various ways of coping used by different family members or the patient himself. Some may use intellectualization about the situation. This is very common in individuals with a medical or paramedical background. Others may use religious teachings and beliefs as comfort. Still others may withdraw or regress so that they are no longer able to make decisions they once did. Some tend to become aggressive and hostile. Some may persist in denial which can be detected by noting disregard for treatment measures and unrealistic planning for the future.[26] It is important to realize that adjustments in how each person copes will be made continually because adjusting to a fatal illness is not a once-and-for-all matter but rather a process.[3]

If the patient has a condition which is genetically linked such as cystic fibrosis, the family may be immobilized by guilt and this may interfere with their ability to require compliance from the patient for necessary care.[30] The nurse must provide extra time to help them come to grips with their guilt so they can turn their attention toward the patient.

At this time, a "dying trajectory" is envisioned by the family, patient, and health care workers which represents the anticipated course of the patient's dying.[21] This influences the manner in which the patient and family grieve. The accuracy and congruence of each person's dying trajectory can vary. The nurse should attempt to discover each person's dying trajectory and its accuracy.

The nurse can help the family and patient sustain hope and optimism. She cannot say, "You can be cured," but hope can be provided through implied messages such as, "I will help you when you can no longer help yourself."[7] Patients frequently gain much confidence from association with a prestigious medical center or physician so that they feel, "If anybody can help me, these people here can." This can be promoted by avoiding degrading statements about the treatment and using statements such as, "We will do everything possible to help you here."[7,32]

Pain and side effects of medications can be promoted as signs that the treatment is working and also contribute to hope.[7] Treatments which produce no specific identifiable effects may need to be explained more carefully. As death becomes imminent, hope may take the form of, "Maybe something will be learned which may help another person."[10] This helps the patient and family feel that the patient is somehow extended into the future. It is one way to maintain hope in a hopeless situation.[45]

In situations where the patient feels much improved after the initial treatment is begun, the patient and family secretly wonder if perhaps a mistake has been made in diagnosis even though they may continue to follow the treatment regimen. The nurse can accept this ambivalence as a necessary part of long term dying.[26] As the patient again becomes more acutely ill, the family's doubts and his own will almost disappear. In conditions where remissions and exacerbations reoccur, the patient and family can swing psychologically back and forth from hope to despair. This can last for years and be very exhausting emotionally.[50]

During this period of living with a fatal illness, family relationships can become extremely vulnerable to stress. The stress of a fatally ill member may be superimposed on a family with problems to begin with. The stress of fatal illness on the family has been studied extensively with the family of a child with leukemia. It appears that in many situations the parents initially shared their feelings of loss and concern but that sharing decreased over time.[25] In many cases the mother physically and psychologically abandoned the rest of the family to focus on the ill child in an attempt to do everything possible to ease his remaining days.[39] The other children might have been supported by the father but usually they were left psychologically on their own. The father often resorted to busying himself in activities away from the family, maybe because he could not define his role as father to a sick child. His abandonment often took the form of excessive hours at work or working two jobs.[4] It may be that the father believed he could not "break down" and mourn as his wife was doing because someone had to be strong.

After many months or years of this polarization, the family ties became weak. After the child died, the family largely dissolved into separate people sharing a roof with little interpersonal contact. The mother frequently believed that the purpose to which she had devoted much of her life was now over and she was often restless and depressed. Both parents reported much pent-up anger towards each other. Estimates of divorce between parents of children with leukemia after the child's death run as high as 80 percent.[54,58]

While preventing family dissolution is difficult, some actions of the nurse might help. First, the nurse can point out the dangers to the family from the stress of having a fatally ill member and encourage them to discuss them and work to prevent family breakdown.

Second, if family life could go on as normally as possible, members would not be forced into their own separate worlds. Parents with an ill child might be helped by pointing out to them that their child will feel most secure and loved when he is prompted to continue in his usual activities and contributions to the family and held to the same limits on his behavior as before. It is important that this be done from the beginning. Attempts to treat him as special will decrease his security and cause him guilt over his special treatment and justified resentment from his siblings. He may also develop into a master at using his condition to manipulate others which does not bring him happiness either.[25] Parents who have a tendency to want to give the ill child everything he wants before he dies might be helped to realize that it is never possible to give someone all he wants, nor does the attempt necessarily contribute to his happiness.

Third, the family might profit from learning flexibility of roles so that one member alone does not become totally and exclusively involved with the dying member. Thus, in the case of the child with leukemia, the father and mother can arrange turn taking or sharing of responsibility for the dying child and the other siblings. The father must be encouraged not to withdraw but to visualize the needs of the family for his participation.[4] The mother should not give up her life for the child—she needs interests and outlets.[15] Most families might at first assume that the mother should quit work when care demands for the fatally ill child become great but it might be best for both parents to work part time instead.

Fourth, families and patients facing a fatal illness need opportunities and the impetus to frequently talk together and share feelings and concerns. This can get brushed aside as the dying member's care becomes more demanding. Emotional withdrawal of members from each other can result if sharing ceases.

The family will not always be most concerned with the individual with the fatal illness and at times family members may seem to the nurse to be denying the condition altogether. This is probably necessary when living with a long term fatal condition.[38] One cannot grieve continuously for years on end.

The family and the patient do not have an easy task and help from as many appropriate sources as possible is beneficial. The family must continue with anticipatory mourning leading to relinquishing the patient, but they must still maintain an attachment and commitment to the patient. They must try in a sense to master a situation which essentially involves defeat.[29] And, of course, life for the patient and the family does not stand still so they both are struggling to cope with the unusual demands of the dying situation and the resulting changes while continuing to progress in growth and development of their own life perspectives.[29] Often individual family members can benefit from referral to sources of support and the nurse should know what counseling services are available and appropriate.

So far it has been assumed that the patient was told of his diagnosis, but this is not always the case. In some situations the family is informed of the condition and allowed to decide if the patient should be told. This area is one of particular controversy and concern. At first thought, it seems cruel to tell an individual that he is dying. Why not let him enjoy his life without the extra burden of worrying about dying?

However, the problem is not this simple. The individual with a fatal illness almost always determines that he is dying from the behavior of others even when not told. He notices that others avoid eye contact with him. There may be an avoidance of conversation about the future.[57] People may tiptoe around, darken the room, or whisper. His questions may be dismissed.[59] Sometimes a sense of false cheerfulness or an altered emotional climate is obvious.[57] He may overhear snatches of conversation. It is believed that the patient will learn about his fatal condition even if he is as young as four years of age.[45,57] Thus, in most situations, the patient is aware that he is dying but he and the family engage in a pretense of not knowing. This means that the patient cannot talk even to those most important to him about his approaching death. He may be isolated and avoided and yet believe that he must maintain the masquerade.

For these reasons, many individuals maintain that those who are dying should be told that they are dying so they can prepare to face their death and so they can more easily and openly discuss death if they wish. However, it has not been shown that those who have been explicitly told they are dying are any more comfortable with dying than those who have not been told explicitly.[20] Nor does it necessarily follow that they or their families are any more able to talk openly about death. In fact, it could follow that conversation may be more difficult and the patient more avoided.[20] Obviously, whether or not to tell a patient that he is dying is not the crucial issue. He will know he is dying whether he is told or not. Pretending that nothing is seriously wrong, however, seems likely to lead the patient to feel isolated and alienated. There is much more to be learned about this area such as when a person should be told, how, by whom, what he should be told, and who should not be told.[20]

Telling a patient that he is dying, therefore, is not a magical formula which leads to discussion and peaceful acceptance. The real issue is how to tailor help for each individual based on his personal wishes and desires for information and his desires to talk to others.

A stage may have been reached at which it is popular to tell all patients about their conditions in great detail including statistical probabilities on the length of their lives even if they do not want to know, and then fail to provide the help needed to deal with the information after it is given.

Many situations occur in which the patient and the family both know that the patient has a fatal illness and yet no direct discussion of the approaching death occurs. Is it not understandable that in our society many cannot speak of their own death? It is believed that there may be patients who know they are dying but never wish to be told so. In support of this is the fact that some never ask despite repeated hospitalizations, surgeries, and radiation therapy. If the patient never asks, it is believed that he probably should not be forced to face his illness.[56] He may ask questions about his condition but not want to hear an explicit death sentence.[56] There may also be the patient who, for various reasons, will turn to the physician or the nurse as his source of support, and not his family.[3]

Probably the most important factors in this issue are: (1) those around the patient even as young as four years old should be aware of the fact that the patient inevitably knows he is dying even if he has not been explicitly told; (2) the nurse and the family should understand that the patient may at some time wish to talk about death; (3) the patient may first approach the subject by vague, indirect statements and questions to see if it is safe to discuss the topics;[51] and (4) the patient's needs to talk about his approaching death may become more pressing as he picks up clues that his condition is deteriorating and death is approaching. The nurse and the family can discuss how they can talk with the patient about death and how to recognize clues that the patient is ready to discuss death.

When the patient is a child, it may seem extremely difficult to discuss death. Children, like adults, want to know how their treatment is progressing—even when it is not going well. They resent evasiveness most of all. The nurse should be alert for the child who is too afraid to ask and try to help him by anticipating his questions. She can try to always leave room for hope even when the situation seems hopeless. "Things don't look too good right now but we are working to help you by all methods we know." Some believe that children can talk about their own death and accept it much more easily than adults.[37]

It is often assumed that adults who are more religious comprehend, accept, and talk about death in general and their own death in particular better than those with less adherence to religious beliefs. This has not been shown to be necessarily true. The nurse may find it easier to talk with those with religious beliefs similar to hers because they may relate and derive comfort from a common faith. She may wonder how to talk with the nonreligious person and how they view death without overwhelming fear. A nonreligious person may feel that when he dies he can live on in others as memories. Thus the lack of formal religion does not preclude a belief that one extends on in the world after death. The nurse must make attempts to learn how each person views his death and not superimpose her own religious beliefs on a patient or family member.

Due primarily to the writings of Dr. Kübler-Ross, it is currently popular to expect every dying person to eventually accept his death gracefully. The critically ill patient is applauded for fighting for his life. Doesn't the dying patient have a right to fight for life and never give up until the end also? The nurse must guard against expecting acceptance to the point that she refuses to allow patients to express other reactions which are less comfortable to deal with. Current theories suggest that acceptance may not be the goal for every patient or even most patients. Depression and withdrawal seem more likely for most and hostility and anger for a lesser number as previously described.

The nurse may find herself in situations where the patient's desires to discuss his death with her cause conflicts with the family. This commonly happens when the patient is a child or teenager.

> Ted was a 15-year-old boy newly diagnosed with Hodgkin's disease. He was cheerful, talkative, and constantly active. His parents were having great difficulty accepting the condition of their bright eldest son. A student nurse who worked in pediatrics on weekends became a good friend of Ted's. One Saturday night Ted talked extensively about his feelings about his condition and how he wished he could help his parents. The student listened carefully and encouraged him to talk. Ted became very depressed and cried periodically during the conversation. When his parents visited on Sunday they found Ted decidedly pensive. He began to tell them about his talk with the student nurse and how much she was helping him to understand himself and how he wished they would talk with her some time. The parents became quite angry and told the head nurse to keep the student away from their son because she was "upsetting him" and "dredging up things that shouldn't be discussed." The head nurse complied and warned the student to avoid Ted from then on.

The nurse in a situation such as this is caught in the middle. The child is usually less stressed by his condition than his parents and finds talking about it easier than they do. Parents may be so preoccupied with their own distress that they are unable to offer much support to their child. The parents may be jealous of the nurse if she succeeds in a role they feel belongs to them. Occasionally the child ends up engaging in denial behavior to make things easier for the parents. Parents may not understand that people who are dying are helped sometimes by opportunities to discuss their feelings—even children. One study found that children who had a chance to discuss their diagnosis and treatment had lower death anxiety which is contrary to the popular notion that talking about death would lead to higher anxiety.[57] To most parents it seems most logical to follow the culturally accepted pattern of a conspiracy of silence about death. Some parents have not been open and honest with their children in the past or oriented towards giving serious consideration to their feelings. This will not magically change because the child is seriously ill.

The student nurse in the situation with Ted talked with the physician who was able to assume her role with Ted and pick up where she and Ted had left off without further offending the parents who were not yet ready to support their son.

It is not unusual for adult patients also to discuss with the nurse what they cannot bear to discuss with their families. Conversely, families may discuss with the nurse what they cannot talk about with the patient. The nurse should support these attempts for both sides to express their feelings.

Sometimes the nurse can get so involved in the psychological aspects of caring for the dying patient and his family that she forgets more obvious aspects of physical care. The dying patient needs competent and safe physical care because his physical needs will usually be challenging. The nurse who cares for the total patient should be thoroughly familiar with the patient's condition and be expert in the associated care and teaching. Pain relief is very important because dying patients may fear pain more than death.[22] In addition, the presence of physical discomfort may aggravate psychological distress. The fatally ill person is not immune to pain because he has been through so much.[23] There are many nuances to pain medication administration which the nurse should learn. The family and patient both benefit greatly from physical care which helps the patient appear comfortable.

The nurse must also remember that the fatally ill patient who is hospitalized is prone to all the common problems which face all hospitalized patients. The harmful aspects of hospitalization do not cease from existing just because the patient is fatally ill.[3] The adult is possibly suffering from loss of self-esteem, boredom, and anxiety over treatments, and the child is afraid of tests, angry at his mother when she leaves him, and limited in physical activity. Nor do the developmental tasks of the patient cease. For example, the teenager is coping with his changing body and with his disease. The adult woman may be fearful of aging and coping with her condition. The nurse can remember to help the patient with all of these.

The dying patient, whether hospitalized or not, and his family frequently suffer from a lack of information about the treatment that is going on.[60] They need concrete information and they need to feel that they are running the show. The nurse can focus efforts on providing them with the information they need to do so.[40] Knowledge of the condition and treatment helps to provide a feeling of control.[38]

When the patient is a child, the nurse can focus her support of the patient in relation to his age and understanding. Many children may interpret their treatment as punishment and she can assure them that they have done nothing wrong to cause their illness. The nurse can do much to make the child feel in control and informed. Statements should be present oriented and concrete.[35] For example, a child being given a blood transfusion might be told, "This is to make you feel stronger." A trip to the lab may be explained as, "This will tell Dr. Smith if your medicines are working the way they should be."

Some families appreciate being able to help in providing physical care. Sitting by the bedside day after day can be a trying experience. Families who are able to participate in physical care often feel better about their contribution because of their opportunity to do things for the patient. The nurse can assess the family's feelings about giving physical care and proceed to teach them as much as they desire to know.

Some families may wish to keep the patient at home until death if they have help and guidance in planning and providing care. The nurse can refer information about services of value to the family and patient such as transportation services, housekeeping services, and equipment rental.[6] The nurse needs to anticipate problems that could occur and prepare the family for them so that the unknowns in the future are less uncertain.[40] It is also good to provide the family with someone who can come to the home periodically to lend support and a method to contact help at any time. Reports of rewarding experiences families have had caring for fatally ill patients at home are becoming more frequent.

Many families describe as helpful getting to know other families who are struggling with the same problems they are.[4] Groups are becoming more frequent and the nurse can learn of their focus. For example, there are in several cities groups for parents who are losing or have lost a child.

It is most important that the nurse encourage or even insist that the family take periods of escape from the situation. The continual burden of living with a terminally ill patient and the associated emotional stress can be unrelenting without periods of diversion.[6] Also, the family can become angry and frustrated with the patient and at the same time feel intense guilt for their feelings and guilt for seeking escape.[25]

A particular note is necessary related to the children in the family who may be overlooked as the crisis of fatal illness peaks. The children in the family may be experiencing special problems which the nurse and the parents should be alert to.[25] Many times the children feel guilty about the condition which is affecting their parent or sibling. This may seem unrealistic to the parents but they may want to make special efforts to assure the children that none of them in any way has caused the current situation. In addition, the children may be afraid of developing the same problems as the patient and need assurance, if truthful, that they will not. They may quite logically feel jealous of any special attention and concern the patient receives and the corresponding lack of usual attention they are receiving. Just a few minutes individually with each child to discuss his feelings may help. This is often feasible just before bedtime.

Outside of the home the children may be teased by playmates about the appearance of the patient or taunted with "My mother says your mother is going to die." This can be discussed and the parent can express understanding of the situation and suggest ways for the child to respond. Parents may need reminders to spend time listening to their children's concerns and how they are relating to the patient. One fatally ill child was upset by her two brothers continually arguing over which one of them would get her room when she died. The parents were made aware of the situation and told that the reaction by the siblings was very normal. The parents were then able to resolve the matter in a way that did not cause the brothers to feel guilty.

The siblings of a fatally ill child may show their suffering through deteriorating performance at school, hyperactivity, depression, severe separation anxiety, abdominal pains, headaches, and enuresis.[4,16] School nurses can watch for these problems and bring them to the parent's attention.

Parents need to be cautioned that they may begin to unconsciously overprotect their children as a reaction to the threat they are experiencing to the integrity of the family. Once they are aware of this, they can monitor their limits to see if they are becoming overprotective.

One specific problem which can develop is the problem of telling a seriously ill patient about the death of someone else. It is often feared that the news might worsen the condition. Individuals who have studied this in relation to children with burns suggest that it is very risky to withhold the information because repeatedly the patient has found out about the death by accident and this is unnecessarily cruel. They suggest that the family inform the patient as soon as possible of the death and stay with the patient afterwards. In many cases it was discovered that the patient had already decided that his relative or friend was dead, and his ideas were confirmed by the revelation. If the patient is a child, his possible guilt over the death must be dealt with.[46]

During this time as the patient's condition deteriorates, the family and patient will become aware of and grieve for additional losses. The nurse can help them discuss their losses before or as they occur. For example, as the health of a father deteriorated and he became more withdrawn, the wife and teenage children began to grieve for the loss of his companionship.

Some families may find themselves becoming isolated from former relatives, friends, and neighbors. Some of this is probably due to their friends' hesitancy about what to do or say combined with their own fear of death. Another factor is that the family members themselves may be withdrawing from former friends due to feelings of envy and irritability as they cope with their losses.[41] Sometimes relatives and friends express their lack of faith in the diagnosis and the family find themselves surrounded by disbelievers.[19] They may feel they need to continually explain and support the diagnosis.[41] Helping the family to explore this area may be valuable to them. Friends and relatives may plague the family with advice and information they have read or heard on miraculous cures and better treatment. The family can be helped to anticipate this problem and plan how to respond to these well meaning friends.[25]

It may be wise to encourage the family to accept the offers of help that others make.[40] Otherwise they may progressively be depleted of support systems. Families may be helped to realize that offers of help are attempts by friends to share their burdens in the only way they can. The nurse may need to be the patient's advocate to mobilize other resources of help for the patient and family. For example, the family may not have thought about contacting their pastor and they may also appreciate visits by the hospital chaplain.[41]

The school nurse who is working with a patient who attends school should arrange a conference with the child's teachers. The teachers and other school personnel will need guidance and assistance in how to best maintain a normal routine at school for the ill child.[24,25] The child's classmates may want to know why he is frequently absent and why certain physical changes are occurring. The teacher may want to discuss this with the class and help them decide how to help the child. Some modifications may be necessary. For example, as the child becomes weaker, he may need to take a nap at lunch time rather than play with the others.

Similarly, if the adult patient is employed by a company having industrial nurses, coordination may be possible to promote a more normal life at work.

The patient frequently becomes more and more withdrawn as death approaches. This may be a difficult time for the family and they will need the support of the nurse in learning how to cope while keeping their ties to the patient intact.[42] The patient may fear nighttime and going to sleep as death nears and may be helped by a night light and the promise that someone will check often.[10]

As the patient's death draws near, the family experiences many conflicts. If the condition has been prolonged and painful they may welcome signs that the ordeal for the patient is nearly over, yet long for a few more good days at the same time. Many patients now begin or have previously begun a withdrawal psychologically from those they love.[40] Expression of intense fear or anxiety is more likely from the family than the patient at this time.[18] If the patient becomes unconscious, the family may find themselves suspended in limbo wondering how long death can take. They are afraid to leave the patient, yet they find the continual watch at the bedside overwhelmingly difficult. They have many questions, some of which they may not be able to put into words. How will the patient die? Is he experiencing pain now? Is this really the end? Can't anything more be done? How long can this last? Can the patient hear them talking to him? The nurse can anticipate some of these and answer them tactfully for the family. Some family members may wish to continue care routines as their contribution to the patient. Some may find physical care at this stage too difficult and the nurse can assume total care. The nurse should watch out for the health of family members at this time by encouraging meals and rest as appropriate.

Some family members may not be able to stay in the patient's room as he approaches death and may talk to others in the lounge or to hospital personnel at the nurse's station. Sometimes the nurse may feel annoyed at these individuals who seem unconcerned or callous about what is happening. She can remember that they are unable at that time to get close to death which might overwhelm them if they stayed in the room with the patient.

Things said to the family at this time may be particularly remembered so the nurse should avoid cliches which may evoke bitterness despite the fact that the nurse meant to be helpful.[25] For example, "You're so lucky that you have other children."

When the patient does die, the family experiences relief and sadness. At once, they are freed from the prolonged nightmare and yet they have lost a family member. It is necessary to tell them that many people experience a sense of relief when the death finally occurs and that this is normal.[25] They need privacy so that they can fully express their emotions without fear of embarrassing themselves.[25] They need to be told what will happen next. They may want to linger with the deceased's body. Some may never have seen a dead body before and they may be curious and at the same time repulsed.

It is wise for someone to phone and visit the family periodically to assess their grief reaction and offer support.[25] They are likely to again feel guilty when the family settles into a normal routine and life seems more carefree. Additional information on helping the family that is grieving is found in Chapter 9.

A summary of possible nursing actions to use with the fatally ill individual and his family is found in Table 13-1.

**Table 13-1.** Possible nursing actions to help patients and their families adapt to fatal illness

1. Initially work to reduce uncertainty and guilt.
2. Encourage discussion and verbalizations early.
3. Provide written information if needed.
4. Help family to prepare for the questions of others.
5. Provide contact with the family to assess reactions and promote expression of feelings through use of the helping process.
6. Determine the dying trajectory of family members and how it will influence the future.
7. Provide for the maintenance of hope.
8. Accept the tendencies of the patient and family to occasionally and periodically deny the diagnosis.
9. Work to prevent family polarization and diffusion.
10. Use additional sources of support and counseling.
11. Realize that the patient almost always realizes the seriousness of his condition.
12. Prepare for the possibility that the patient may wish to discuss his death with the nurse or his family.
13. Do not expect acceptance from everyone.
14. Remember to assure careful physical care and especially pain relief.
15. Plan for meeting other needs also present.
16. Provide the patient and family with enough information so that they can control the situation.
17. Allow family members to participate in care if desired.
18. Prepare family to care for the patient at home if desired.
19. Consider referring the family to an appropriate group.
20. Encourage family members to periodically escape from the situation.
21. Promote attention to the needs of children in the family.
22. Promote anticipatory mourning for losses.
23. Counteract the tendency of the family to isolate themselves and refuse help.
24. Use referrals to school and industrial nurses if appropriate.
25. Provide intensive help as the patient's condition worsens and when he dies.
26. Provide for help after the family returns home.

## A TOOL FOR ASSESSMENT AND EVALUATION

The tool in Table 13-2 is intended to alert the nurse to dimensions of the patient's and family's behavior which could indicate possible successful or unsuccessful adaptation to fatal illness. Those whose behaviors are predominantly less optimal need intensive intervention. This tool can also be used to evaluate the effectiveness of nursing intervention. If nursing action is effective, the patient or family member should show more optimal behaviors.

## THE NURSE AND FATAL ILLNESS

The nurse is probably as uncomfortable with the subject of death as most people. She may carry an extra burden, however, because, as a member of the health team, she may feel that she should be able to alter or slow the patient's death. Because of these factors, she may avoid dying patients because they remind her of her helplessness in the face of death.[37] Even if the nurse accepts comfort and not cure as the goal for individuals with fatal conditions, she may be frustrated in her attempts to provide comfort.

**Table 13-2.** Tool for assessment of adaptation to fatal illness

| Behavior | Less optimal | More optimal |
| --- | --- | --- |
| Use of denial | So strong that treatment is ignored | Occasional |
| Use of condition by patient | Used to manipulate family | Condition accepted realistically |
| Family's view of patient | Has become special, of utmost importance in the family | Maintains normal position in family but may require more attention |
| Family's sharing of feelings | Decreased | Normal |
| Family polarization | One member totally aligned with patient and not family | Sharing of care of the patient |
| Reactions of children in the family | Jealousy, guilt, and anger which interferes with play, school, etc. | Occasional guilt, anger, jealousy |
| Father's reaction if patient is a child | Increasing attention to activities outside of family | Continues usual activities with family |
| Mother's reaction if patient is a child | Devotes attention exclusively to ill child | Continues usual activities in the family |
| Family and patient's acceptance of diagnosis | Hostility toward referring physician, physician shopping | Efforts turned towards cooperation with treatment |
| Family's relationships with friends, neighbors, and relatives | Withdrawal and intolerance | Slight withdrawal, acceptance of help |
| Behavior of family when with patient | Denial predominant or "premature burial" | Realistic[8,9,12,16,32,50] |

Nurses who choose to work with dying patients may not receive the prestige accorded those who choose to work in critical care settings.[44] In fact, others may question the mental health of a nurse who chooses to work with the terminally ill.

Nurses may experience many troublesome emotions when working with dying patients. Studies have found that nurses, like other health care workers, tend unconsciously to avoid terminally ill patients or to feel hostile towards them. Withdrawal is very likely.[1] Other reactions may be for the nurse to displace her anger against the patient onto the physician. This is especially true if the patient procrastinated in seeking help or the physician had difficulty in reaching the diagnosis of the patient.[43,53] Or she may use humor with her coworkers at the patient's expense.[11] It is likely that she may find pretending she is unaware of the patient's condition and engaging in social chitchat easier than allowing the patient to actually discuss his death.[17] Frequent sedation and delegation of the terminally ill patient to auxiliary personnel are other ways to escape and avoid facing the patient.[6] She may provide barriers to communication by focusing her attention on other things such as an intravenous infusion, or ignoring statements by the patient or family which could be anxiety provoking to explore. She may feel that her priority for use of her time belongs to the living and not the dying.[44]

All of these defenses against death are understandable, but they can be deleterious to the patient and family with a fatal illness and they can be altered if the nurse can seriously examine her attitudes and behaviors towards death and fatal illness. Guidelines for getting in touch with one's attitudes about death are given in Chapter 9.

The nurse caring for the dying patient is usually under considerable stress. Caring for a dying patient and his family may be the most challenging nursing situation possible. The patient and the family can, at times, be rude, demanding, and hostile. At other times she may feel overwhelming sorrow for them and find herself affected by their depression. It is most essential that she has supports independent of the family with whom she can share her own anger, grief, guilt, depression, and exasperation.

Because the nurse is aware of the natural tendency to avoid a dying patient and his family, she can make a conscious effort to increase the time she spends with them. Rather than thinking of the dying patient as evidence of her helplessness, she can concentrate on what she can do for him.[8]

Many nurses worry about what to say if the dying patient begins to talk about his death. It is essential to remember that what one says is less important than how one listens.[34] If the nurse attends to what the patient is trying to say and uses her skills of nondirective communication, she is unlikely to say anything which will harm the patient. One particularly frightening aspect for many nurses is a fear that the patient will ask questions she cannot answer such as, "Am I dying?" or "How long do I have?" It is good to remember that the patient may not really want an answer but instead a chance to discuss the question. Thus, she can say, "Why do you ask?" or "What do you think?" so that they can look at the question in light of what the patient believes.

A child may also ask brutally difficult questions: "Am I going to die?" "Do I have cancer?" He may mean, "Will someone take care of me?" and "Will I be safe?"[16] The nurse can help him express himself in direct and indirect symbolic ways.

Many nurses suppress their own fears about death and dying and claim that they cannot talk with patients because they would be overstepping the physician's role and because they do not know what the patient has been told.[13] One can always find out what the physician has told the patient. The nurse may be better able to work with dying patients than a physician because death may be a defeat for the physician who defines his role as preserving life. The nurse may feel less defeated because she can define her role as helping others cope with whatever happens—even death.

The nurse who has accepted the fact that she can help patients to talk about their approaching death should remember that patients who are less able to express themselves and are hostile or withdrawn need her support as much as those who are more accepting and who can verbalize about death.[44]

In some situations the nurse will find herself deeply involved with the patient and his family. She may cry openly and grieve acutely when the patient dies. In these situations she should realize that her reaction is acceptable and understandable but that she is not able to support the family at this time and should, therefore, find someone who can be with the family. She should avoid putting the family in the position of having to support her. She should not pretend that she is a part of the family at the funeral.[50] Many families appreciate knowing that others are saddened by their loss and care enough about them to visit the funeral home or to phone or drop them a note later or visit their home. The nurse does not need to deny her feelings or attempt to mask them but she should put the needs of the family for support first, and if she cannot provide the support they need, she should arrange for someone else to do so.

The nurse can use experiences she has caring for dying patients and their families to increase her own understanding of her attitudes towards death. She too will eventually die. Acceptance of this fact is the first step in learning to look at death.

The nurse needs to consider how her attitudes about death are reflected in the care she gives others. A positive view of death and acceptance of the inevitability of death can be beneficial for her patients and for the nurse herself.

## AN EXAMPLE OF NURSING INTERVENTION IN FATAL ILLNESS

The following example illustrates how a nurse intervened with a patient facing a potentially fatal illness. The nurse in the example did not have contact with the family.

Ron Justin, a 26-year-old graduate student, came to the university health service after he noticed a large swelling on the side of his neck. John, the nurse practitioner, discovered as he did a history and physical that Ron had a painless enlargement in the area of the cervical lymph nodes. In addition, he found what appeared to be enlarged inguinal and axillary lymph nodes.

John immediately arranged for the health service physician, Dr. White, to see Ron. Dr. White explained to Ron that he needed to be admitted to a hospital soon for a biopsy of one of the nodes. Ron was from another state and decided to have his parents arrange admission for him in a hometown hospital. Ron did not ask any specific questions about the possibilities associated with his condition. The physician explained only that the sure way to know what was causing the enlargements in his neck was by doing a biopsy.

After the physician left, John talked with Ron for a few minutes. Ron stated that he was confident that there was nothing to worry about and yet he seemed anxious. John invited Ron to come in to talk any time he wanted to and advised Ron to keep in touch with him regarding results of his hospitalization.

John had not seen Ron for eight weeks when he came into the health service with a report for Dr. White. He had a few weeks earlier undergone a biopsy which had shown the presence of Hodgkin's disease. A few days later he had undergone a staging surgery to discover the extent of his disease. Unfortunately, the disease was found to be widely disseminated. He had begun to receive a combination of radiation and chemotherapy as treatment. He was being permitted to return to school but was to be followed by the health service between return visits to his oncologist at home.

John encouraged Ron to sit down in his office. John discovered that Ron was in a state of confusion over his condition and his future. Although he knew of his diagnosis and prognosis, he chose to dwell on only the encouraging comments he had heard while hospitalized. Yet at the same time, he was discouraged and uncertain about what to do about school. He had almost finished coursework for a Ph.D. degree in chemistry and had his research project well under way, yet he confessed that he had little interest in schoolwork. He did not want to stay at home with his parents, so returning to school seemed his only option.

John listened carefully as Ron talked and encouraged him to express his feelings. He decided that Ron was vacillating between a tendency to disbelieve the seriousness of his condition on one hand and great anxiety over his condition on the other. John did not try to influence Ron's thinking but rather concentrated on developing a helping relationship. He invited Ron to come back once a week to see him. One goal of this was to help Ron remain cognizant of the seriousness of his situation.

Ron continued to return regularly. Within a few weeks Ron did become more immersed in his coursework. As he was feeling well physically, he rarely mentioned his illness specifically. John had the perception that for a while Ron intended to cope with his knowledge of his condition by becoming so involved in his studies and research that he did not have time to think about his illness. However, there were times when this strategy did not work and Ron became depressed and withdrawn. During these times he thought about quitting school and traveling around the country.

A few months later Ron returned home for another course of treatment. When he returned to school later he had lost several pounds. He was not pleased with being underweight and talked to John about how his weight loss made him look "sickly." In addition to letting Ron express his feelings, John gave him pointers on how he could increase his calorie intake to regain some weight. John provided other information on side effects of treatment and how to minimize them. Ron seemed to believe that if he could regain his weight he would not be constantly faced with a physical reminder of his condition. He was also perplexed over skin coloration changes that had occurred following the recent radiation. Other people on campus often assumed he had been on vacation to some warm climate and he had trouble handling their comments and questions.

John helped Ron discuss how his parents and others who knew him might feel and how they could possibly be uncomfortable in his presence over what to say. Ron was particularly concerned over how to relate to a close girlfriend he had dated for several years. He thought about breaking up with her for her sake and yet he very much needed her to talk to and be with. Ron's parents were being supported by their other children and members of their church.

For the first time, Ron was at a point where he talked with John openly about his concerns for the future, although he never mentioned his actual condition or talked of death. He expressed his desire to take his degree, yet he wondered why he should bother to spend so many of his days studying and working in a dismal lab. He decided at the end of one session with John that maybe he enjoyed visualizing that he could quit and leave school whenever he wanted because the fantasy provided him with an escape from the present.

John and Ron continued to meet regularly for over a year. Ron went through many difficult periods of depression, especially after returning to school following trips home for more therapy or followup. It seemed that at school he could often push from conscious awareness his future concerns but his trips home were vivid reminders of his condition.

Another particularly difficult period followed breaking up with his girlfriend. Ron found that dating her became increasingly painful as he was subtly reminded that something in his life had changed. Interacting with her emphasized his uncertain future. He and his girlfriend were able to part as friends but their contacts became less frequent. John found out that Ron had several close friends at school who were able to provide him with some of the support and interest he had relied on his girlfriend for. Especially at that same time, Ron began to attend a campus ministry program and began to interact with the campus minister. John and the minister met several times to plan together.

As Ron approached the end of his program, a new concern appeared. He had gained some security by going on with his studies as planned. Now that he was about finished, he had to decide what to do next. Unfortunately, his physical condition began to deteriorate at about this time. John saw Ron more frequently as Ron's depression increased over his uncertainty about his future after graduation combined with new signs of his disease. At one point Ron had to be admitted unexpectedly for general supportive care and transfusions. When he returned to school, he was more frightened than ever. While hospitalized at home, he had experienced a transfusion reaction during which he had become delirious. The experience had seemed to him a warning of his approaching death. He now talked to John at length about his fear related to dying and his pessimism about ever being cured of Hodgkin's disease. His hopes for the future now became more specific and time-limited such as getting his degree in June and publishing his research. Ron's vision of his dying trajectory now incorporated the concept of death within a year or two. Ron had been reading several books including ones on life after death and was finding some solace in them. He had decided to return home with his parents after graduation. He talked about doing postdoctoral work at a nearby university but he did not make any concrete plans to do so.

As graduation approached and the spring weather arrived, Ron began to progressively mourn for the losses he was experiencing. Usually he looked forward to the summer and the associated activities. He had been an exceptional tennis player in high school and in college and now knew he would not play in the coming summer. He began dispersing various belongings he had among his friends. He also became worried about his mother who was not taking his illness well and he spent considerable time writing her letters. He reported feeling closer to his parents than he had ever felt before.

Ron became progressively weaker as graduation day approached. John watched his condition closely. Ron was able to attend the commencement program although he had to be taken in a wheelchair. He seemed to experience a lot of satisfaction from displaying his diploma and doctoral hood.

Ron's parents had come for graduation and now packed his belongings and took him home. John was able to meet them and bid Ron farewell. Ron was very tired and lethargic.

John received a letter from Ron within a week. Ron had been admitted to a hospital and was being treated for an overwhelming infection. His letter conveyed an awareness that his death was near combined with hopes that the infection could be overcome so he could get out of the hospital. Two days later Ron's parents phoned John to inform him that Ron had died that day. Ron had given them John's telephone number and asked them to call him when he died. He wanted them to thank John for his help while he was at school. His parents were upset by Ron's death but were thankful that he had died peacefully.

John concluded that through a helping relationship he had enabled an individual with a fatal illness to grow in his understanding and awareness of his own death.

## SUMMARY

The nurse who cares for an individual with a terminal illness and his family can offer specific help which enables the individuals involved to adapt in a manner that promotes personal growth. The nurse must understand what it is like to live with a fatal illness, what effects fatal illness may have on a family, and the process of anticipatory mourning.

The nurse can use the difficult situation of caring for fatally ill patients and their families to refine her own thinking about death and dying.

## REFERENCES

1. Aronson, G. J.: "Treatment of the dying person," in Feifel, H. (ed.): *Meaning of Death.* McGraw-Hill, New York, 1959.
2. Benoliel, J. Q.: "Loss," in Clark, A. L., and Affonso, D. D.: *Childbearing: A Nursing Perspective.* F. A. Davis, Philadelphia, 1976.
3. Benoliel, J. Q.: "The terminally ill child," in Scipien, G. M. et al.: *Comprehensive Pediatric Nursing.* McGraw-Hill, New York, 1975.

4. Binger, C. M., et al.: "Childhood leukemia: Emotional impact on patient and family." New Eng. J. Med. 280:414, 1969.
5. Blauner, R.: "Death and social structure." Psychiat. 29:384, 1966.
6. Bozeman, M. F., et al.: "Psychological impact of cancer and its treatment. The adaptation of mothers to the threatened loss of their children through leukemia. Part I." Cancer 8:10, 1955.
7. Buehler, J.: "What contributes to hope in the cancer patient?" Am. J. Nurs. 75:1353, 1975.
8. Carlson, C. E.: "Grief," in Carlson, C. E., and Blackwell, B. (eds.): Behavioral Concepts and Nursing Intervention. J. B. Lippincott, Philadelphia, 1978.
9. Chodoff, P., et al.: "Stress, defenses and coping behavior: Observations in parents of children with malignant disease." Am. J. Psychiat. 120:743, 1964.
10. Davidson, R. P.: "To give care in terminal illness." Am. J. Nurs. 66:74, 1966.
11. Davitz, L. J., and Davitz, J. R.: "How do nurses feel when patients suffer?" Am. J. Nurs. 75:1505, 1975.
12. Engel, G. L.: "Grief and grieving," Am. J. Nurs. 64:93, 1964.
13. Everett, M. G.: "How health professionals help each other." Am. J. Nurs. 75:1355, 1975.
14. Feifel, H. (ed.): The Meaning of Death. McGraw-Hill, New York, 1959.
15. Foley, G. V., and McCarthy, A. M.: "The child with leukemia in a special hematology clinic." Am. J. Nurs. 76:1115, 1976.
16. Fond, K. I.: "Dealing with death and dying through family centered care." Nurs. Clin. North Am. 7:53, 1972.
17. Francel, C. G.: "Loneliness," in Burd, S. F., and Marshall, M. A. (eds.): Some Clinical Approaches to Psychiatric Nursing. Macmillan, New York, 1963.
18. Francis, G. M., and Munjas, B.: Promoting Psychological Comfort. Wm. C. Brown, Dubuque, 1975.
19. Friedman, S. B., et al.: "Behavioral observations on parents anticipating the death of a child." Ped. 32:618, 1963.
20. Gottheil, E., et al.: "Is it right to joke with a dying man?" Prism 2:16, 1974.
21. Glaser, B., and Strauss, A.: Time for Dying. Aldine, Chicago, 1968.
22. Graner, A.: "The effects of pain on child, parent, and health professional," in Martinson, I. M. (ed.): Home Care for the Dying Child. Appleton-Century-Crofts, New York, 1976.
23. Green, M.: "Care of the dying child." Ped. 40:492, 1967.
24. Greene, P.: "The child with leukemia in the classroom." Am. J. Nurs. 75:86, 1975.
25. Gyulay, J. E.: "The forgotten grievers." Am. J. Nurs. 75:1476, 1975.
26. Gyulay, J. E., and Miles, M. S.: "The family with a terminally ill child," in Hymovich, D. P., and Barnard, M. U. (eds.): Family Health Care. McGraw-Hill, New York, 1973.
27. Harrison, S. I., et al.: "Children's reactions to bereavement." Arch. Gen. Psychiat. 17:593, 1967.
28. Hinton, J. M.: "The physical and mental distress of dying." Quart. J. Med. 32:1, 1963.
29. Hoffman, I., and Futterman, E. H.: "Coping with waiting: Psychiatric intervention and study in the waiting room of a pediatric oncology clinic." Comp. Psychiat. 12:68, 1971.
30. Ingram, C.: "Of service to families with children having cystic fibrosis," in Hall, J. E., and Weaver, B. R. (eds.): Nursing of Families in Crisis. J. B. Lippincott, Philadelphia, 1974.
31. Jaffe, L., and Jaffe, A.: "Terminal candor and the coda syndrome." Am. J. Nurs. 76:1889, 1976.
32. Kennerly, S. L.: "What I've learned about mastectomy." Am. J. Nurs. 77:1430, 1977.
33. Klagsbrun, S. C.: "Don't make nice, make real." Am. J. Nurs. 77:1432, 1977.
34. Kneisl, C. R.: "Thoughtful care for the dying." Am. J. Nurs. 68:550, 1968.
35. Krause, D. M.: "Children's concepts of death," in Martinson, I. M. (ed.): Home Care for the Dying Child. Appleton-Century-Crofts, New York, 1976.
36. Kübler-Ross, E.: On Death and Dying. Macmillan, New York, 1969.
37. Kübler-Ross, E.: On Death and Dying. Presented on National Broadcasting Company Television, November 24, 1974. Narration written by Philip J. Scharper.
38. Leventhal, B. G., and Hersh, S.: "Modern treatment of childhood leukemia: The patient and his family." Child. Today 3:2, 1974.
39. Levitt, C. J., et al.: "Parent support groups for the grieving parent," in Martinson, I. M. (ed.): Home Care for the Dying Child. Appleton-Century-Crofts, New York, 1976.
40. Martinson, I. M. (ed.): Home Care for the Dying Child. Appleton-Century-Crofts, New York, 1976.
41. Martinson, I. M., and Jorgens, C. L.: "Report of a parent support group," in Martinson, I. M. (ed.): Home Care for the Dying Child. Appleton-Century-Crofts, New York, 1976.
42. Martinson, I. M., et al.: "Home care for the dying child." Am. J. Nurs. 77:1815, 1977.
43. Meinhart, N. T.: "The cancer patient: Living in the here and now." Nurs. Outlook 16:64, 1968.
44. Mervyn, F.: "The plight of dying patients in hospitals." Am. J. Nurs. 71:1988, 1971.

45. Morrissey, J. R.: "Death anxiety in children with a fatal illness," in Parad, H. J. (ed.): *Crisis Intervention: Selected Readings.* Family Service Association of America, New York, 1965.
46. Morse, T. S.: "On talking to bereaved burned children." J. Trauma 11:894, 1971.
47. Nesbit, M., and Kersey, J.: "Acute leukemia of childhood," in Martinson, I. M. (ed.): *Home Care for the Dying Child.* Appleton-Century-Crofts, New York, 1976.
48. Parsons, T.: "Death in American society—A brief working paper." Am. Behav. Scient. 6:61, 1963.
49. Pearson, H. A.: "The leukemias," in Nelson, W. E. (ed.): *Textbook of Pediatrics.* W. B. Saunders, Philadelphia, 1969.
50. Petrillo, M., and Sanger, S.: *Emotional Care of Hospitalized Children.* J. B. Lippincott, Philadelphia, 1972.
51. Quint, J. C.: "The threat of death: Some consequences for patients and nurses." Nurs. Forum 8:286, 1969.
52. Schulz, R., and Aderman, D.: "Clinical research on the stages of dying." Omega 5:137, 1974.
53. Sonstegard, L., et al.: "The grieving nurse." Am. J. Nurs. 76:1490, 1976.
54. Strauss, A.: *Chronic Illness and the Quality of Life.* C. V. Mosby, St. Louis, 1975.
55. VandenBergh, R. L.: "To overcome inhibiting emotions." Am. J. Nurs. 66:71, 1966.
56. Verwoerdt, A., and Wilson, R.: "Communication with fatally ill patients: Tacit or explicit?" Am. J. Nurs. 67:2307, 1967.
57. Waechter, E. H.: "Children's awareness of fatal illness." Am. J. Nurs. 71:1168, 1971.
58. Weisensee, M.: "A myriad of relationships," in Martinson, I. M. (ed.): *Home Care for the Dying Child.* Appleton-Century-Crofts, 1976.
59. Weisman, A. D., and Hackett, T. P.: "Predilection to death; death and dying as a psychiatric problem." Psychosom. Med. 23:232, 1961.
60. Woehning, M.: "Children in the family with a dying member," in Martinson, I. M. (ed.): *Home Care for the Dying Child.* Appleton-Century-Crofts, 1976..
61. Wygant, W. E.: "Dying, but not alone." Am. J. Nurs. 67:574, 1967.

# BIBLIOGRAPHY

Assell, R.: "An existential approach to death." Nurs. Forum 8:200, 1969.
Bunch, R., and Zahra, D.: "The unlearned role." Am. J. Nurs. 76:1486, 1976.
Craven, J., and Wald, F. S.: "Hospice care for dying patients." Am. J. Nurs. 75:1816, 1975.
Davis, F.: *Passage Through Crisis.* Bobbs-Merrill, Indianapolis, 1963.
Decker, D. J.: "In the valley of the shadow." Am. J. Nurs. 78:416, 1978.
Easson, M.: *The Dying Child.* Charles C Thomas, Springfield, Ill., 1970.
Etzel, B.: "The role of advocacy in the rite of passage," in Martinson, I. M. (ed.): *Home Care for the Dying Child.* Appleton-Century-Crofts, 1976.
Fox, N. L.: "A good birth, a good life, why not a good death?" Nurs. Dig. 4:24, 1976.
Fox, J. E.: "Reflections on cancer nursing." Am. J. Nurs. 66:1316, 1966.
Friedman, S.: "Care of the family of the child with cancer." Ped. 40:498, 1967.
Giaquinta, B.: "Helping families face the crisis of cancer." Am. J. Nurs. 77:1585, 1977.
Glaser, B., and Strauss, A.: *Awareness of Dying.* Aldine, Chicago, 1965.
Glaser, B., and Strauss, A.: "Social loss of dying patients." Am. J. Nurs. 64:119, 1964.
Goldfogel, L.: "Working with the parent of a dying child." Am. J. Nurs. 75:1675, 1975.
Greene, P.: "Acute leukemia in children." Am. J. Nurs. 75:1709, 1975.
Hershberger, P. A.: "Waiting with a dying man and his family," in Hall, J. E., and Weaver, B. R. (eds.): *Nursing of Families in Crisis.* J. B. Lippincott, Philadelphia, 1974.
International Work Group on Death, Dying and Bereavement. "Assumptions and principles underlying standards for terminal care." Am. J. Nurs. 79:2967, 1979.
Karon, M., and Vernick, J.: "An approach to the emotional support of fatally ill children." Clin. Ped. 7:274, 1968.
Kastenbaum, B. K., and Spector, R. E.: "What should a nurse tell a cancer patient?" Am. J. Nurs. 78:640, 1978.
Kübler-Ross, E.: "Life in transition." Convocation presented at Purdue University, West Lafayette, Ind., April 27, 1978.
Kübler-Ross, E.: "What is it like to be dying?" Am. J. Nurs. 71:54, 1971.
Martinson, P. V.: "The health professional and the dying child: Toward a theoretical framework," in Martinson, I. M. (ed.): *Home Care for the Dying Child.* Appleton-Century-Crofts, New York, 1976.

Miller, M.: "Nursing the nonliving," in Hall, J. E., and Weaver, B. R. (eds.): *Nursing of Families in Crisis.* J. B. Lippincott, Philadelphia, 1974.

Northrup, F.: "The dying child." Am. J. Nurs. 74:1066, 1974.

Paige, R. L., and Looney, J. F.: "Hospice care for the adult." Am. J. Nurs. 77:1812, 1977.

Pillitteri, A.: *Nursing Care of the Growing Family: A Child Health Text.* Little, Brown and Company, Boston, 1977.

Regan, P.: "The dying patient and his family." JAMA 192:666, 1965.

Rose, M. A.: "Problems families face in home care." Am. J. Nurs. 76:416, 1976.

Sauer, S. N.: "The hospital setting for the child with cancer," in Martinson, I. M. (ed.): *Home Care for the Dying Child.* Appleton-Century-Crofts, New York, 1976.

Schowalter, J. E.: "The child's reaction to his own terminal illness," in Schoenberg, B., et al. (eds.): *Psychosocial Aspects of Terminal Care.* Columbia University Press, New York, 1972.

Schumann, D., and Patterson, P.: "Multiple myeloma." Am. J. Nurs. 75:78, 1975.

Sharp, D.: "Lessons from a dying patient." Am. J. Nurs. 68:1517, 1968.

Shneidman, E.: "You and death." Psychol. Today 5:43, 1971.

Sutherland, A. M., and Orbach, C. E.: "Psychological impact of cancer and cancer surgery. Part 2. Depressive reactions associated with surgery." Cancer 6:958, 1953.

Svoboda, E. H.: "Wilm's tumor and neuroblastoma: The child under treatment." Am. J. Nurs. 68:532, 1968.

Ufema, J. K.: "Dare to care for the dying." Am. J. Nurs. 76:88, 1976.

Vernick, J., and Lunceford, J. L.: "Milieu design for adolescents with leukemia." Am. J. Nurs. 67:559, 1967.

Wade, N.: "Crib death." Science 184:447, 1974.

Weiss, R. S.: "The fund of sociability." Trans-action 6:39, 1969.

Wentzel, K. B.: "The dying are the living." Am. J. Nurs. 76:956, 1976.

Whitman, H. H., and Lukes, S. J.: "Behavior modification for terminally ill patients." Am. J. Nurs. 75:98, 1975.

# CHAPTER 14

# PARENTHOOD

Nurses frequently have contact with individuals in numerous health care situations who are coping with the physically and emotionally taxing task of being a parent. Opportunities abound to promote effective parenting. All too frequently the nurse is confronted with situations wherein she suspects actual or potential problems with the parent-child relationship. More severe disorders of parenting such as the failure-to-thrive syndrome and the child abuse syndrome are receiving considerable emphasis. Although intervening in parenthood is not widely considered as a realm of nursing practice, the nurse who understands the concept of parenthood as it relates to adults and children in her care and learns ways to evaluate parent-child relationships and intervene appropriately can help ensure that parenthood reaches a favorable conclusion so that the optimal development of the child and of the parents is reached. The nurse not uncommonly is or becomes a parent herself and she can benefit personally from an exploration of parenthood.

## REVIEW OF THEORY

Parenthood in American society is commonly thought of as a process which involves:

1. Marriage of a male and female adult.
2. Biologic production of one or more children.
3. Physical activities involved in caring for the child (such as bathing, feeding, etc.).
4. Psychosocial activities designed to socialize the child and guide him toward maturity (such as disciplining, teaching, etc.).
5. Release of the offspring as independent adults.

These ingredients need not always be present for parenthood to exist. Parents are not always married, nor are they always adults, nor are there necessarily two of them. Some couples of the same sex consider themselves parents. In some instances there may be an institution that considers itself to be a parent. The child involved is not always a biologic offspring of the parents. He may be, among other things, adopted, a foster child, or a grandchild. Parents do not always engage in the physical or psychological activities of rearing the child. They may hire someone else to do this or they may be unable because of disability or unavailability. And offspring may not necessarily be released at a certain prescribed time as adults and may never leave home, or may leave earlier or later than expected. Parenthood, therefore, is a concept which embraces many arrangements and situations within which children are reared.

Parenthood is frequently described in the literature as the final step into adulthood of an individual.[56] Parenthood typically demands the ability to put the needs of another person on the same level as or above the needs of self in a way that may not have been experienced before. It is believed that earlier in history adjustment to marriage and parenthood was an almost simultaneous process but, with the advent of more effective birth control measures and changing attitudes toward the timing of the first pregnancy, a wider separation has occurred between marriage and the first pregnancy in many cases.[85] Parents report that parenthood changed their lives much more than marriage,[56,58] although they had been led to believe that adjusting to marriage was the only significant task ahead of them in their adult life. Unfortunately, adjustment to marriage seems to receive considerably more attention than adjustment to parenthood in publications, courses, and services offered.

The reasons why individuals become parents are multiple and range from selfish to altruistic. Pronatalism is believed to be rampant in our society so that men and women may feel that parenthood is expected and drift into having children as a logical course without much consideration of their actual interest and ability. Parents have been known to produce children to carry on the family line, provide income tax deductions, increase the family labor pool, fulfill religious beliefs, provide security for their later years, provide an opportunity for vicarious experience, cement a marriage, prove their virility, gain an opportunity to be a mother or father, provide heirs for their possessions, compensate for loneliness, provide a link with eternity, prove their adulthood, share their love, and so forth. The reasons any one person has for desiring children are probably numerous and mostly unconscious. Of course, parenthood is not always the result of a conscious decision and all too frequently is unplanned.

Just as the reasons for having children vary, so do the situations into which children are born. While it is popular to think of the young, healthy, financially stable couple anxiously awaiting the arrival of their first little bundle, this is not often the case. Parents vary in terms of their mental and physical health, age, financial resources, abilities, marital status, and stability.

## Motherhood

It is generally considered in our society that parenthood is not an identical experience for women and men. Women develop feelings about mothering and child rearing as young girls receiving care and nurturance from their parents and playing with friends. As a woman passes through childhood and adolescence, she clarifies her feelings about the roles of women and men, and the requirements and importance of motherhood. These feelings will all affect her readiness to become a mother and her reactions to the mothering role.

As the woman matures, her relationships with men and her husband are believed to influence further her self-concept as a woman. When the woman becomes pregnant, the timing of the pregnancy and the course of the pregnancy begin to have an effect on how she perceives the developing fetus and form a basis for the beginning of the mother-child relationship. According to some sources, at least 80 percent of all pregnancies are rejected early in the pregnancy. By three months, this has decreased to only 15 percent of mothers rejecting the pregnancy and it is believed to decrease even further when fetal movements begin.[15] Early rejection of a pregnancy does not seem to correlate with negative feelings later towards the infant.[98]

Events occurring in the period surrounding birth are believed to influence the later relationship of the mother with her newborn.[62] Long and painful labors are believed to cause a strain in the relationship. Normal reactions after the birth of the baby seem to be initially a feeling of emptiness or loss and a feeling of strangeness toward the infant. This is followed at some point by a feeling of love towards the baby. Some mothers are distressed over the initial lack of maternal feelings for their infants and need reassurance that it will develop.

The establishment of an emotional bond between the mother and her infant is referred to as attachment. Attachment is considered to be crucial for the optimal physical and emotional development of the child and is demonstrated by behaviors such as how the mother holds, feeds, and looks at the infant.[1,49] The process of attachment is not believed to be totally dependent on the mother but is thought to be a reciprocal process in which the infant searches for and accepts the actions of the mother, which augments further her desire to care for the infant.[53] Early and prolonged separation of the mother and infant is believed to possibly alter the attachment process.

Much research is now being done to determine if there is a critical period after delivery when the attachment process must occur. Studies have shown that if the process is interfered with, later problems are more likely to occur, such as child abuse and behavioral problems in the child.[49] The importance of maternal attachment can be seen when one considers the fact that the human infant is born in a rather helpless state and is not able to obtain his own food supply. For this and other reasons he is dependent on the mother or someone else for nurture. The baby needs his mother more than she needs him, however, so that attachment of the mother to her infant is probably crucial to insure that the infant's needs will be met.[53] Current discussions in the literature seem to imply that attachment is either "high" or "low," and that the best possible situation is high attachment. It would seem reasonable to expect that attachment between a mother and her infant probably exists on a continuum with a frequency like the normal curve with most mothers falling somewhere in the middle. The dangers of low attachment behavior seem to be apparent and real in relation to disturbed mother-child relationships. It is interesting to speculate whether there is a danger in extremely high attachment to an infant. Will the highly attached mother have difficulty with tasks such as separating herself from the infant, promoting his independence, and setting limits?

Just as the child's behavior influences attachment, he continues to influence the evolving maternal-child relationship as he develops. Infants are not all alike as anyone who has spent time in a newborn nursery will attest. Thomas, Chess, and others have described several dimensions of behavior which they found in infants.[93,94] The particular infant's pattern of behavior was shown to persist almost unchanged over several years. One child might be placid, basically cheerful, adaptable, and easily amused. Another might be hyperactive, predominantly uncheerful, slow to adapt, and difficult to please. One can speculate that the first child is easy to nurture and a pleasant relationship between parent and child could be predicted while the second child would be best with a mother who is a saint—and there are not many of those around! More information on behavioral differences in children will be given later. The area of the child's effects on the parents has often been overlooked but is now being more thoroughly explored. It is becoming more recognized that the infant's responses or lack of responses greatly influence how he is cared for and the maternal attachment which develops.[6,83]

Of course, the mother's life is not static as she rears her child. There may be changes in her health, goals, marriage, attitudes, responsibilities, and perceptions of her child, any of which might affect her relationship with the child. Thus it is easy to see why no two parent-child relationships are ever alike.

## Fatherhood

Very little information is available about how men experience parenthood.[37] Men are nonexistent in most discussions of child rearing or are casually mentioned as the one who gives his wife "unlimited emotional support."

It is likely that boys develop their attitudes toward male and female roles and fatherhood beginning early in childhood as do their female counterparts. Girls usually can readily see what mothers do when they grow up by watching and imitating their mothers, but boys may have to cope with more uncertainty about what fathers do and learn by abstraction. Fatherhood seems to be much less of a preoccupation with males than does motherhood with females. It is common for girls and women to list motherhood as a high priority goal for their lives, but boys and men give much lower priority to fatherhood as a goal. Perhaps an overemphasis on motherhood has led to a de-emphasis on fatherhood in our culture.[37]

The feelings of men during their mate's pregnancy are infrequently described and studied or are described jokingly. Recently a process of attachment in the father called *engrossment,* which is similar to attachment in the mother after the birth of the child, has been described. Fathers experienced absorption, preoccupation, and interest in their newborn infants which was manifested through a desire to hold the baby, look at the baby, and a reported increase in self-esteem within a few days after birth.[30]

Probably the role of father is subject to more variation today than is the role of mother. Currently fathers must wonder what their role is.[57] Is a father an equal partner in the care and upbringing of his children or "mother's little helper?" Is his only significance in financially supporting the family or does he provide an equal and explicit input into the personality of the developing child? Is he warm and tender or stern and authoritarian, essential or easily replaced?

A man may experience fatherhood at a time in his life when he is preoccupied with concerns outside of the home. He may desire that his wife keep things at home including the children under control and bother him as little as possible. As he reaches a level of security and maturity he may become more interested in his family only to discover that his children have grown up while he was otherwise distracted. The attention and concern he is now ready to give may be rejected by his teenage children or lavished on his grandchildren much to the amazement of his wife and his children.[88]

While it is common to consider fatherhood and motherhood separately, it should be remembered that the parents usually develop into parenthood as a couple. The two person group is considered by some to be the best form of human relationship. The addition of the first child requires a realignment of the existing two person group into a three person group and a complex of new roles and responsibilities. The three person group poses a potential threat to personal relations because it can easily become a pair and an isolate.[99]

It is not difficult to see this occurring in couples with their firstborn child. The mother and the child may become the pair and the father a semi-isolate. If the couple try to function somewhat as a pair, society may condemn them as poor parents who are not properly devoted to their child.[56] If the father has been cast in a peripheral role, the addition of each child may serve to reinforce his role as outsider. The mother may give her "all" to the children and, indeed, this is considered very normal and expected in middle class society. Obviously, children can be divisive in a marriage.

Family size may be somewhat indicated by family relationships. Where husbands and wives share child care activities, fewer children are usually desired than where the husband has little involvement.[80] Family size is, of course, also dependent on religious beliefs and the use or effectiveness of contraception.

It has been shown that parenthood does not affect the partners equally. Women tend to show a decrease in personal development and self-esteem during child rearing years while men do not.[85] It is a sobering thought to realize that the person considered most influential in developing the child's personality and self-esteem—the mother—is also the one losing ground in these areas during parenthood.

## Stresses That Can Affect Parents

An adequate discussion of parenthood would not be complete without highlighting some sources of stress that most parents face as they raise their children. A primary stress lies in the fact that parenthood is an extremely challenging task for which parents are usually only casually prepared. Most individuals becoming parents today have had very little experience living with or caring for young children.[43] Parents tend to do what their parents did, or in some situations try not to do what their parents did, in the hopes that the knowledge passed on from generation to generation will be sufficient.[4] Of course, much of what is passed on from parents to children is unrecognized so that most parenting activities could be considered primitive responses based on unconscious learning.

Although much information exists on child development and effective parenting, it is generally disseminated unevenly into the general population[13] or not at all. There does seem to be intense interest among some segments of the population in learning about parenting as shown by the popularity of books, articles, and discussion groups for parents. Unfortunately, those who need this type of information the most are often the least likely to receive it. The advice available to parents can vary from one extreme to another with or without clinical basis. And whose advice should one take—a child psychiatrist's, an educator's, a physician's, a psychologist's, or a minister's? Much of what one reads about children with problems and their parents is based on *"ex post facto"* research which may not be reliable. Parents are sometimes advised in lay publications to discuss parenting with their family physician. An examination of medical school curricula rarely shows any identifiable content on advising parents. Medical journals, even in pediatrics, are not replete with this information either. Where can parents turn for advice?

Another stress which is frequently unrecognized is that rearing children calls for a wide variety of behaviors on the parent's part and these behaviors must evolve as the child matures. For example, a 2-year-old, a 6-year-old, and a 14-year-old need much different types of limits. Stress occurs when parents are unable to recognize that their behavior must change as their child matures. It is possible that some parents are not capable of much change. In addition, parents may have difficulty recognizing that methods of functioning which were effective with one particular child may be ineffective with another child. Many parents tend to keep trying what worked before rather than trying something different.

The concept that parents must change in their behavior along with their child and that they must adapt their behavior to each child may help explain to some parents problems that they are having with their children. This usually occurs when the child needs another type of response from that which the parents have become accustomed to giving. There usually follows a period of disequilibrium until the parents find a new response that works both for them and the child. This explains why parents may be readily "expert" at coping with children of a certain age but have tremendous difficulties with children of another age. For example, the mother who is very restrictive may have "well-behaved" young children but unless she learns to be less restrictive, her children may be very rebellious or overly submissive as teenagers.

Most parents enter parenthood with tremendously unrealistic expectations.[16,64] They are going to be wise, patient, and devoted—not at all like those people they see with their children in the grocery store. It is inevitable that they have set a romanticized standard against which they can only fail. Their expectations of their children are also unrealistic. Their daughters will be dutiful, popular, loving, and show the world their parents' virtue. Their sons will be able to achieve and accomplish what they were not able to. Again feelings of frustration and failure are inevitable when reality clashes with expectations. Because the parents' self-esteem is linked with the accomplishments of the child, disappointment is taken personally.

A further stress is that most parents are totally unprepared for the amount of effort, physical and emotional, that raising children requires. Specifically, parents are not prepared for the amount of change that will occur in their lives when they have children. No wonder thinly veiled resentment seems to be a partner of parenthood. Imagine the new father assuring himself, "The baby can't walk or talk. It's only 8 pounds. How big of a deal can this be?" In one study, 83 percent of couples interviewed stated that the birth of their baby was an extensive or severe crisis. The fact that the pregnancy was planned and desired did not seem to make parenthood any less of a crisis.[56]

Another source of stress for parents is our varied and complex society. Parents can easily see wide differences in how children are being raised. These differences can encourage parents to stick rigidly to their convictions, to fluctuate with the season, or to worry excessively over what they are doing. When the Smiths next door put their 14-year-old daughter on the "pill," a search of convictions and values is likely to haunt the neighbors. Earlier in our history, it may have been easier to parent as there were fewer schools of thought on parenting in what was once a more homogeneous and less mobile society.

Women are especially prone to stress during parenthood.[64] Because public opinion emphasizes that the mother is of primary importance in child rearing, she must bear the primary responsibility for how her children develop.[8] Due to our Freudian heritage, the mother is subject to much free floating parental anxiety. She may at some point begin to realize that mothering is fundamentally a lonely task.[85] Frustrations can occur as home becomes where the children play, father relaxes, and mother works.

Few women are adequately prepared to be mothers. Pregnancy does not allow the women to make a gradual transition into the role of mother.[85] She becomes a mother overnight. If the mother throws herself into the lives of her children and husband, she is destined to bask only in reflected glory.[88] If she tried to pursue her own independent interests outside of marriage and family as men do, she may be chastised by society as a neglectful mother. If she plunges herself into volunteer work and "self-development" activities, she finds that she has not gained legitimate work experience or salary benefits. No wonder the average "homemaker" is described as neurotic by some. If the mother has been raised to consider motherhood as her only role and purpose in life, she may wonder why she is not happier and more successful than she is.[25] Mothers with young children are probably more isolated now than at any other time in history, which can lead to a condition which Bronfenbrenner has referred to as "momism."[12] There is reduced chance that today's isolated suburban mother will see role modeling examples of other mothers raising their children.[43]

Both mothers and fathers today face the stress of having fewer family supports available than previous generations.[85] New parents are likely to be removed both geographically and philosophically from their parents. The young mother is more likely to look for advice on problems of child rearing to her neighbors or her physician, rather than asking her mother. Note that in our society a woman does not go to her mother's home to have her baby, she goes to a hospital.

Our society has also plotted against parents in the current confusion over techniques versus relationships in child rearing. A look at current magazines would lead one to believe that if she had natural childbirth, breast fed her baby, and later sent him to a Montessori preschool, she could not fail as a parent. It is, of course, possible to do all of that and fail, or do none of it and succeed as a parent. Missing from the magazines and books are discussions about the goals of child rearing and the parents' role in teaching their children desirable character traits, for example. It is no wonder that a woman may confuse being a good mother with keeping her home and her children cleaner and neater than anyone else.

The cult of parenthood is surrounded by many pervasive myths which may contribute to parental stress, resentment, disappointment, and dissatisfaction. Consider the following:

1. Your greatest pleasures and fulfillment in life will be through your children.
2. Your life will be empty and barren unless you have children.
3. Your children will bring you and your spouse closer.
4. The American middle class nuclear family is the ideal family style.
5. As long as you really *love* your children, you can be a good parent.
6. Parents should sacrifice their desires and goals for the sake of their children.
7. Parents and children should spend all available time together.
8. Large families are happier than small families.
9. The only child is lonely and maladjusted.
10. Your children will take care of you in your old age.
11. Once your children have matured and left home, you will not have to worry about them any more.
12. You own your children and you are responsible for their behavior.
13. Your children will be grateful for what you do for them.

Children will seldom provide all that they are expected to provide and parents may conclude that the fault is theirs. Parents must learn to look elsewhere for fulfillment, security, and happiness besides to their children.

There is some confusion in society today over the goals of child rearing. It is difficult to remain focused on the long range goal of parenthood which is to produce an individual who will be able to function independently in society, control his behavior, work productively, and love others. Parents may tend to focus on short term goals such as controlling behavior which may not necessarily contribute to the achievement of the overall goals. For example, some methods parents may use to make a child behave may be instilling in the child a need to have others control his behavior for him, while other methods may develop in the child the ability to control his own behavior.

## Parents Likely to Experience Unusual Stresses

There have been a number of situations described in the literature as likely to produce excessive stresses for parents over and beyond the usual stresses of parenthood. These parents are potentially at high risk.

Teenage parents are frequently mentioned in the literature as prone to excessive stress as parents. Marital stress may be one problem for them as they have a three to four times higher divorce rate than those who marry later.[52] Teenage workers usually earn salaries at the bottom of the wage scale so that financial resources may be limited. Education or occupational training may need to be sacrificed. Medical problems may occur for teenage parents which are not as much of a problem for older parents. Pregnancy during adolescence is a higher risk than is a later pregnancy. The rate of premature births is markedly increased.[17]

Teenagers who become parents may not have had a chance to adequately cope with the developmental task of adolescence which is establishing their identity. They are prematurely thrust into coping with the developmental task of adulthood which involves generativity or the creating and nurturing of new life. Somewhere, maybe lost in the transition, is the developmental stage of young adulthood which focuses on developing intimacy in relationships.[67] Thus the teenager who becomes a parent is engulfed with three sets of developmental tasks simultaneously. It is most likely that he will not be able to cope equally with all of them and there may be little psychic energy left to help a child cope with his developmental tasks.[73] Another problem is that some tasks a child faces may mimic or conflict with those of his parents.[42] A preschooler attempting to assert his independence and autonomy may be quite a problem when his adolescent parent is still striving to assert his independence from his parents. The negativism of a two-year-old may be difficult to accept when the teenage parent is himself learning to control his moods.

Many teenage parents are single women. It is estimated that over 200,000 junior and senior high school age females deliver babies each year and 85 percent of them are choosing to keep their babies. The very young single mother is the most likely to keep her child. Single mothers have a tendency to avoid prenatal care and this can lead to health problems.[17] They face all the problems previously described for teenage parents and they face them alone. Some authorities propose that out-of-wedlock pregnancy is not usually an accident but is unconsciously planned by the mother. An unconscious desire to perplex her parents seems more prominent than a desire for or interest in having a baby.[102] It is an understatement that pregnancy out of wedlock is usually a crisis although the extent of crisis is believed to vary in sociocultural groups.

The single female parent is often viewed with suspicion in the community. Unconscious or conscious attitudes may reflect on her, such as feelings that she may be out to steal away other husbands or that she is inferior because she was unable to get or keep a man. Even information she sees in the media dwells excessively on the fact that her home is without a father rather than with a mother. Because of her inability to earn what a man would earn, usually she must cope with marginal income, housing, schools, and surroundings.[11] In addition, she often faces the pervasive expectations of others that she should quickly marry or remarry.

Nonadolescent single parents do not seem to be confronted with as many problems as teenage single parents. Their greater maturity and health status may lead to less stress. Single male parents usually have an advantage over single female parents because of higher income.[81] Single parents who are older are still without the support of a spouse and, faced with the unrelenting demands of child care, may need a reliable network for supports to help them. It is estimated that one out of every seven children in the United States is being raised by a single parent.[66]

Adoptive parents are described in the literature as under some stresses that biologic parents may not experience.[2,33,48,87,104] If infertility was a problem and if the parents were very distressed by being infertile, they may have feelings of inadequacy and failure.[32] Adoptive parents are frequently sensitive to the fact that parenthood by adoption is still considered in American society as a last resort if you cannot have "your own." Few individuals grow up planning to adopt. It is possible for adoptive parents to feel overly sensitive about their children's performance and behavior because they may believe that neighbors, teachers, or relatives expect adopted children to be different from biologic children. They may unconsciously worry about the child's biologic heritage.

Parents who choose to adopt may also experience apprehension and embarrassment over adoption procedures such as home inspections, the questioning of neighbors, financial investigations, proof of infertility, legal hassles, lengthy personal interviews which frequently call for complete disclosure of personal affairs, surveillance after placement, and appearance in court.

There is some suggestion that adoptive parents may be more overprotective than biologic parents because the adopted child was difficult to obtain and would be difficult to replace. Adoptive parents also experience some slights by others that may be upsetting. For example, adoptive parents are not likely to receive as much attention upon the placement of their child as that bestowed on biologic parents upon the birth of a child. The placement may not bring flowers, cards, visitors, and free gifts from merchants. The new father may not be granted time off from work and insurance policies must often be changed to include adopted children by special amendments. These slights or differences may remind the parents that what they have done is not quite sanctioned by society as equal to biologic parenthood. As the child matures, new challenges regularly appear such as questions from peers.

Parents of a child with physical or mental defects are described in the literature as likely to experience unusual stresses.[31] Although parents may wonder during pregnancy if their child will be normal, few really anticipate that their baby could be abnormal. The child who is defective is a threat to the parents' self-esteem because the presence of a defect reflects that they too must be defective. Possible negative responses to the birth of a defective child which may occur are shock, denial, guilt and shame, bitterness, envy, and rejection. It is obvious that none of these reactions provides a desirable basis for a beginning parent-child relationship. Acceptance of the child and his condition can occur only after a period of disorganization which leaves the child in limbo and the acceptance of the child is more often a goal than a reality.[96] The stresses on parents may be increased if the child requires extensive health care and other special services. It is noteworthy that men can usually accept a defective female child more easily than a defective male child. Acceptance by both parents is conditioned to some extent by socioeconomic standing, length of marriage, and the presence of other children.

Giving birth to a premature child can lead to parental stress. Parents of a premature infant may experience a crisis when the birth occurs.[17] Feelings of shock, disbelief, grief, guilt, shame, and anger over the birth of their baby are common. The baby, who is often seriously ill and requires intensive medical care, may be in danger of not surviving and the parents may attempt to hold back from an emotional involvement. It has been suggested that there may be problems with maternal attachment later when the infant is seriously ill enough to require restrictions of parental visiting.[49]

The premature infant is not capable of the same level of response to his parents as the full term newborn, which may lead the parents to feel unsuccessful and rejected.[54] In addition his appearance may be somewhat abnormal or repulsive to the parent.[14] It has been shown that prematures are statistically more likely to be later diagnosed as having failure-to-thrive syndrome and as child abuse cases. There may also be some basis for suspecting that mothers who deliver their infants prematurely vary from mothers who do not in terms of emotional health and adjustment.[10]

Foster parents are not without special stresses.[27,61] There are over 250,000 children living with foster families in the United States at any one time. Children in foster homes may be challenging to raise because of the unmet needs and emotional difficulties they may bring to the foster care situation. In addition, there are new elements in the foster care situation which must be adjusted to such as new siblings, teachers, neighbors, and foster parents. Foster parents may be raising their biologic children as well as foster children and they may wonder about effects of the interaction of their children with the foster children. Foster parents may be held in high esteem in the neighborhood or regarded as individuals who are responsible for bringing "undesirable influences" into the community.

Foster parents may struggle to remain objective about the biologic parents of their foster children, but may be tempted to compete with the biologic parents for the affection of the children. They may suffer repeated emotional distress as children they have cared for and learned to love are removed from their homes.

It has been shown that the incidence of behavioral problems increases in foster children with the increase in the length of foster care and with lack of contact with biologic parents. One-half of all children in foster homes will spend the major part of their youth in foster care. For these reasons, foster parents need supports and resources over and beyond those of other parents.

Parents with critically ill children, whether the children are acutely or chronically ill, are faced with unusual demands.[68] Financial burdens may be overwhelming. The time involved in the care of the child may leave little time for much else. The child may develop emotional disturbances or learn to use his illness to control his parents. The mother may find herself allying with the ill child and the rest of the family excluding her gradually. Well siblings may be jealous of the ill child and suffer from a lack of attention to their needs.

Whether the family experiences a crisis or not is dependent on the resources of the family and the previous experiences they had had. The type of illness the child has is not usually as important to the functioning of the family as the meaning the illness has to the family.

Even if the child recovers from the illness or his life is no longer in danger, the child who has been critically ill may become a victim of the "vulnerable child syndrome" as described by Green and Solnit.[29] It is hypothesized that the syndrome results from a persistent grief reaction even though the child is no longer in danger of an early death. This is likely to happen if the child was not expected to live. The parents' treatment of the child may appear to indicate that they still consider him to be a special child who is destined to die in his youth. The child senses his parents' unconscious predictions of doom and accepts them. The child may develop school phobias, behavior problems, difficulties with toilet training and weaning, sleep problems, overconcern with bodily functions, and school underachievement. In addition to seriously ill children, premature infants, infants with congenital defects, children born to parents who had experienced many miscarriages or stillbirths, children born following a difficult pregnancy where the fetus was in danger, and children born in families with hereditary medical disorders are all prone to the vulnerable child syndrome.

It should be mentioned that in this discussion of the problems of parents who are under unusual stress, the negative aspects have been exclusively dwelt on. No one seems to ever look for positive aspects. It could be argued that, for each of the parents mentioned, there are advantages to parenting. For example, teenage parents may have an advantage over older parents in terms of increased physical energy and their ability to devote themselves to altruistic goals. Much needs to be done in terms of looking more for parental strengths and focusing less on weaknesses.

## Other Determinants of Parenting Behavior

Parental behavior is determined largely by unconscious learning as mentioned and by cultural factors such as socioeconomic status. The investigations by individuals predominantly from the middle class of the parenting behavior of the lower socioeconomic class are most prominent in the literature and the reports are replete with terminology such as "limited" and "deficient." Little study has been done which looks for positive factors.[97] From what has been written there does seem to be an increased potential for disturbed relationships between lower socioeconomic parents and their children which appears to perpetuate itself from one generation to the next. Particularly detrimental seems to be the presence of prolonged and prevalent male unemployment which is correlated with many pathologic conditions in the family.[34]

Less has been written about the parental behavior of middle class parents which is all too frequently presented as the ideal, and even less is known about the parental behavior of upper class parents. There is no doubt, however, that class standing must exert an influence on parenting which writers are only vaguely aware of. Much of what one thinks is the proper and right way to rear one's child comes from an immersion in the attitudes and values of one's social class and culture rather than from any source of wisdom.

Another determinant of parental behavior is the environment in which the family exists.[69] One can imagine the differences in child rearing practices in one situation where many individuals live together in a small space versus a situation where a few people occupy a larger space. Other conditions of the environment which might affect parental and child behavior include climate, hazards, resources, and possessions. The fact that features in the environment can alter family functioning is all too often overlooked. It may be quite different raising a child in an environment with space and abundant resources available than raising a child in a crowded environment with few resources available. It cannot be altogether easily determined that one environment is better than another. It is possible that environmental adversity or stress is beneficial. Thus one can never fully comprehend a parent-child situation until one fully considers the situation in which the interaction occurs and the constraints or variables operant because of it.

## Severe Parenting Disorders

It appears that there are some situations which arise out of the grave inability of parents to provide appropriate care to their children for some reason. In some instances, this may take the form of excessive physical abuse which may range from infliction of mild injury to manslaughter. This is referred to as the child abuse syndrome. One of the discouraging findings is that children who were abused tend to grow up to be abusing parents themselves.[5]

Another disorder believed due to an inability to provide appropriate physical and psychological care which results in a physically and developmentally delayed infant is called the failure-to-thrive syndrome. Infants who have failed to thrive will often show dramatic weight gain when hospitalized but will fail to continue to gain when returned to their home situations. Both of these syndromes will be explored more later. The role the child plays in each of these situations is not yet clear.

## THE FAMILY TIME LINE

By viewing the family development on a time line with six stages, new insights can be gained about periods in the life of a family. This concept of a family time line is based somewhat on the family life cycle as described by Duvall.[23] The age of the oldest child indicates the stage of the family on the time line because the interests and activities of the family usually slowly shift from one stage to another at the initiative of the oldest child's interests and activities.

The interaction between the family and the environment in each stage could be as characterized in Table 14-1. The young couple usually must experience some degree of separation from the environment in order to form a bond together and to decide who they are as a couple. The family with young children usually faces an isolation from the environment which may be necessary in order to meet the burdensome demands of raising young children. The family with school-aged children faces an increasing awareness of the environment as their children advance into the world away from home. The family with teenage children must compete with the environment as home becomes less attractive to the child and his thinking is increasingly influenced by others outside of the family. The family with dispersing children retracts as children diffuse into the environment. The mature couple must reintegrate their lives again with the environment as a couple.

Sources of family stress are most likely when the family moves from one stage to another or when they are unable to interact with the environment appropriately. Although families will vary in terms of size, goals, and socioeconomic characteristics, families in a particular stage will evidence characteristics in common with other families in the same stage.

The family time line in a typical American family is changing, particularly because parents are having fewer children and having them closer together. This decreases the length of time spent overall in child rearing activities. When this is combined with the lengthening life span for both men and women, the amount of time any one individual

**Table 14-1.** Interaction between family and environment

| Stage | Interaction |
| --- | --- |
| The young couple | Separation from the environment |
| The family with young children | Isolation from the environment |
| The family with school-aged children | Awareness of the environment |
| The family with teenage children | Competition with the environment |
| The family with dispersing children | Diffusion into the environment |
| The mature couple | Reintegration with the environment |

spends as a parent is becoming less. Figure 14-1 represents an example of a family time line for a nuclear family with two children.

Several interesting factors can be emphasized about the time line in Figure 14-1.

1. Considering the entire life span, each parent will spend only about 25 percent of his lifetime actively in child rearing. Seventy-five percent will be spent otherwise.
2. The couple in the example will spend only about 33 percent of their married life engaged in the activities of actively raising children. They will spend 66 percent of their married life as a young or mature couple without children in the home.

Of course, considered here has been all too exclusively the elusive and rare "typical family." It is a beneficial exercise to consider the appearance of the family time line, the stages which would result, and the interaction with the environment for the following situations:

1. The couple whose oldest child is mentally retarded.
2. The single parent.
3. The couple who marry after the birth of their first child.
4. The couple who have their first child at 16.
5. The couple who have their first child at 35.
6. The family with two children 19 years apart.
7. The couple who have a late child when in their 40s.
8. The couple without children.
9. The couple who adopt a 6-year-old as their first child.
10. The couple with a child who never leaves home.
11. The couple who marry after both have children from a previous marriage.

This exercise should allow one to predict possible sources of stress which would be unique to each of these cases. Other relevant information on family development can be found in the study by Duvall.[23]

Looking at the family time line indicates some of the activity and growth going on within a family at any given time but it must be emphasized that the entire attention of a parent during the child rearing years is not focused exclusively on his family or on the task of

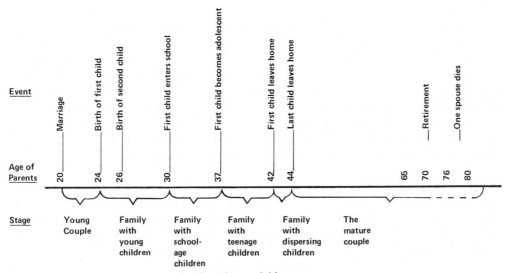

**Figure 14-1.** A family time line for a family with two children.

guiding his children through their growth and developmental tasks. The role of parent is not necessarily the individual's only or primary preoccupation. The parent is also coping with his own developmental needs as he matures such as seeking identity, security, and facing change and crises which are outside of those involving his family and children.[88]

In addition to facing his own developmental tasks, a parent can relive each stage that his children are going through and experience the child's developmental tasks again as if they were his. Hopefully, he resolves the tasks of each stage more completely than as a child. In fact, this is one of the potential rewards of parenthood—reaching a higher level of maturity.[64]

There are other rewards of parenthood.[58] For most parents, the production of children provides a greater sense of continuity with the future. Parents know they cannot live forever, and it may be comforting to know that their children will most likely live on after they die. For many parents, watching a child grow and develop can provide satisfaction in spite of the frustrations along the way. Accomplishments of the child can be flattering to parental egos. Having a child provides an opportunity for sharing an intimate relationship with another human and may enrich the parent's personality in the process. Some parents may enjoy the feeling that they are providing their children with more than they had, although children rarely seem to grasp or be interested in this point. For some parents, becoming a parent can lead to a new relationship with and appreciation for their own parents. Very few parents upon finding themselves overburdened and underappreciated at some point in their child rearing years have not wondered with a new found amazement and respect, "How did Mom and Dad ever get through this?"

## NURSING INTERVENTION IN PARENTHOOD

### Primary Prevention of Disturbed Parent-Child Relationships

Primary preventive efforts would involve actions designed to promote successful parenting.

Efforts aimed at preparing individuals for parenthood may be effective at reducing problems in the future.[24,56] Primary efforts are being made in school systems in some areas of the United States to introduce content on family life, child development, and parenthood into curricula.[18,19,44,63,84,90] Although programs vary, most of them include theory and practice related to the responsibilities of parenthood, the growth and development of children, problems commonly encountered in working with young children, ways to communicate with children, and how to plan appropriate learning experiences. It is uncertain at this time, but courses like these may help to increase the preparedness of parents in the future. Of course, these programs are reaching only a small percentage of the school-aged population.

Nurses may have an opportunity to support the inclusion of family life, education for parenthood, or child development courses for both males and females in school curricula and to help plan content and experiences. Courses such as these are subject to budget cuts and are controversial to the extent that some individuals feel more attention should be given to more traditional school subjects. The nurse may need to help make others aware of the importance of courses which deal with family life. In some school systems, driver's training gets far more attention than parenthood training.[52] Unfortunately, in some school systems, family life courses are only for those not destined for college because college bound students are encouraged both by high school and college counselors to take course offerings in other subjects. Fortunately, family life courses are becoming more plentiful and popular in some college programs.

There is a trend which nurses could support to include more content on parenthood in prenatal classes or to offer separate classes for new parents on parenthood.[65] Content which could be covered includes characteristics of normal infants, changes in the life style of the couple which will occur, providing nutrition, care, and proper stimulation for the baby, and an opportunity for soon-to-be or new parents to discuss their concerns about becoming a parent. Fatherhood may need particular emphasis and discussion.[39,74] The parent who is realistically prepared may cope better.[101] The population these courses might attract is most likely to be similar to the population which has the time and resources to attend prenatal classes.

Some health care projects for lower income families have also embarked on offering classes on parenthood to mothers.[3] Usually the classes are held in the daytime with child care services provided for the children. Content covered is similar to that discussed above with emphasis on an awareness of the mother's role in the promotion of the growth and development of her young child.

Some day care centers for low income parents have programs which provide day care services and involve the parents in activities at the day care center which will enable them to observe the growth and development of their children and learn effective ways of care, teaching, and discipline. Some centers are training lay members of the community to work with families in their area to improve the quality of family life.[76] Efforts like these have a potential for helping to increase the knowledge and competence of parents but they are now few in number and not widely available. The professional nurse could have much to offer in the development and implementation of such programs in the media, community centers, churches, mental health centers, inpatient and outpatient child care services, private and public nursery, elementary, and high schools, day care centers, and community service organizations.

It appears from the literature that nursing frequently stops one step short of programs which help prepare patients for parenthood. For example, there is a considerable amount of information published on helping unwed adolescent mothers care for themselves during pregnancy and prepare emotionally and physically for labor and delivery, but there is almost nothing in the nursing literature on helping them deal with parenthood after they have their babies. And this lack of attention to parenthood is repeated again and again in many areas. In situations where nurses have contact with prospective or actual parents, programs are usually possible which focus on the primary prevention of parent-child disturbances.

One source has described the creation of "parent training packages" which could be sent to parents through the mail.[92] The packages described are being tailored for parents with children who have handicaps but the idea of packets might be useful for many parents. There is also a newsletter available in one community which can be subscribed to by new parents which arrives each month to prepare them for the baby's expected development during the coming month and tips on feeding and care. As the child grows, the newsletter covers such topics as sibling rivalry, temper tantrums, and environmental safety.

Underlying many of the efforts previously described is the subtle objective of deromanticizing parenthood. If individuals developed a more realistic view of what parenthood is and is not, parenthood might be a more pleasant experience for many. The nurse can seek out opportunities to promote realism about parenthood in contacts with potential parents.

Efforts to reduce the pervasive pronatalism in our culture might reduce the pressures individuals feel unconsciously to reproduce without thought. The availability of family planning services is a primary preventive measure so that caretakers have children if and when they want them.

Some problems of altered caretaker-child relationships might be avoided if families likely to experience stress could be identified and followed in some manner.

Foster parents may need help in dealing with specific problems their foster children may bring to them and support as they cope with the day-to-day demands of both their biologic and foster children.[27,61]

Adoptive parents can sometimes benefit from group meetings of other adoptive parents where situations which arise in raising adopted children are discussed.[2]

Parents who have given birth to defective or premature infants need support and assistance in coping with their reactions and in forming affectional bonds with the child.[54] They need sufficient experience with the child to develop attachment and competence in their role as caretakers. They can be helped by a nurse who increases their feelings of adequacy.

The vulnerable child syndrome might be prevented by avoiding overly stressing the seriousness of a child's condition while attachment is occurring. If the child has recovered, one should avoid stressing how close the child came to dying and instead emphasize that the child is now well. The parents should be cautioned against treating their child as special because of the possibility of harmful effects on the child's development. Continuing to follow the child needlessly in clinics and community health nursing visits also emphasizes to the child and his caretaker that he is vulnerable. The parents need to know that their child is not unusually susceptible to other problems.[29,49] Health care personnel could do much more to facilitate continued family functioning during medical treatment of children.[55]

If the child is handicapped, the nurse can teach the mother ways to parent her handicapped child.[26,92] For example, the caretaker of a mentally retarded child may need information on how to teach a child who is slower to learn, has memory lapses, is less interested in the environment, has unevenness in his abilities, and has a shorter attention span. She may need information about some behaviors which she is probably unprepared for such as pica, repetitive behavior habits such as head banging, and hyperactivity. The nurse can coach her in using behavior modification techniques and other learning theories to teach habit training and self-care.

The young teenage mother needs help in coping with a school system which seems embarrassed by her presence, a health care system which was not designed with her in mind, and a need for effective supports.[73] Group parenting is an alternative.

Nursing actions to promote effective parenting are summarized in Table 14-2.

**Table 14-2.** Possible nursing actions to promote effective parenting

1. Initiate or support programs to prepare individuals for parenthood.
2. Promote programs which might help individuals who are already parents.
3. Work to reduce the myths surrounding parenthood and pronatalism.
4. Promote the availability of birth control.
5. Identify parents at risk and provide assistance.

## Secondary Prevention of Disturbed Parent-Child Relationships

What can the nurse do when she encounters a situation where the relationship between a caretaker and child is less than optimal? The nurse can look upon the needs of the caretaker as acceptance, emotional support, information, and guidance.[26] In all situations it seems important that the nurse's initial efforts be directed towards developing a helping relationship with the caretaker in order to provide acceptance and support. This is the most important intervention the nurse can perform. The need of the caretaker for support is greater than her need for information in the early stages of intervention. Also, advice about child rearing is likely to be unheeded if the caretaker does not yet trust the advice giver. Excessive advice might increase the caretaker's sense of inferiority and uselessness.

Many mothers are overwhelmed by their offspring and feel that they are the only people who must be puzzled over raising their children. Statements by the nurse which help the mother to feel accepted include, "Many mothers have told me that they feel that way" or "I can understand how you might feel." The nurse can help the mother to realize that her ambivalence toward her parental role is normal and to recognize that conflicts she is experiencing can be explored and coped with. It is crucial to focus on the caretaker so that her feelings of self-worth can be increased and reinforced. When the mother has had ample opportunities to express her feelings and receive understanding, she may be ready to turn her attention to solving the problems she has as a mother. Statements which encourage the caretaker to problem solve are, "What have you thought you might do about this?" or "How do you think you could handle that next time?" The parent can apply this method later on her own.

The nurse may need to give the caretaker information about the normal development and behavior of children. Many caretakers who have had little contact with young children have misconceptions about how a baby or child can be expected to behave in certain situations. Mostly their expectations are unrealistically high.[22]

The nurse can teach the caretaker normal development and help the mother become aware of the growth and developmental achievements the child is making so that she becomes more interested in and sensitive to the child. Many parents are amazed to learn how much individual children vary in temperament and are relieved to learn that they have not created every characteristic which their child has. The nurse can then help the caretaker learn ways to live with the particular temperament of the child.

The nurse may be able to help the caretaker learn to become more discriminating in picking up cues from her child. This intervention may help the caretaker see the child's behavior as less ambiguous.[53] The mother's sense of competence may increase when her actions more accurately and predictably produce results. The nurse can interpret the child to the caretaker so she can be helped to see the reasons why her child engages in certain behavior. This may help especially if the caretaker has a very negative view of the child. The mother may have many questions about sibling rivalry, discipline, and toilet training, for example. The nurse can provide guidance and acceptance of the mother's feelings as well.

Many inexperienced mothers are unaware of the need most children have for some routine in their lives and the mother may need help in establishing a schedule. A frantic child who previously had little order in his life may become more pleasant when he has regular meals, nap times, and bedtimes. The mother will benefit from the more planned work periods which she can arrange around the child's schedule. Sometimes the caretaker may have a routine but it may need rearranging. Every baby will not need his bath in the morning even though it was done in the morning at the hospital when he was a newborn. Giving the bath in the evening when Daddy is home to entertain the other children might work better.

Another intervention which the nurse can focus on involves helping the mother find more pleasure in her relationship with her child.[53] This may include teaching her how to enjoy play with her child.

The nurse may be able to correct negative reactions to a child by pointing out to the caretaker accomplishments and assets of her child which she was not aware of and by explaining normal behavior which the parent may interpret incorrectly.

Periods of time away from the child can help some caretakers to rejuvenate their sense of self. The caretaker may need "permission" from the nurse to have time to herself. Although employment was never suggested as desirable or as possibly beneficial to the mother and the child by the sources reviewed, it is reasonable to believe that part time or full time employment might help some caretakers to be better parents. Employment could provide the parent with a chance to spend some time away from her child and extra financial resources. Studies reviewed by Howell reveal that maternal employment is frequently related to an increased self-esteem for the woman involved and various beneficial effects for her children such as increased creativity, independence, and higher self-esteem.[40] After all, parents have a need to be valued and respected as persons in their own right apart from the role of being a parent, and employment may enhance this. At least, current sources suggest that if the mother wishes to work, there is no evidence to suggest that she should be persuaded not to because of possible harmful effects on her children, her own self-esteem, or her marriage.[40]

It is particularly helpful for the nurse to comment on the parent's strengths and abilities in ways which are sincere and honest such as, "I think it is amazing that you have time to manage all of this."

At this point, the nurse would be well advised to concentrate on the caretaker's strengths and use them to the most advantage. For example, if the caretaker is a person who likes to read, she may be interested in a well written and entertaining book about parents such as McBride's *The Growth and Development of Mothers*.[64] If the caretaker is socially outgoing she may be well suited to attend a "mother's morning out" type group where she would have a chance to meet other mothers.

An important and often overlooked role involves helping caretakers discover and use sources of information and support such as churches, neighbors, spouses, school, community programs, and relatives. Some caretakers may need encouragement to ask others for information or help. Other caretakers may have found sources of support and information in the past but may not have thought of using them in the present situation.

If the caretaker is faced with multiple stresses other than child rearing such as financial and marital problems, the nurse can direct her in finding resources for resolving as many as possible so that her energies are freer to cope with her child. If the caretaker is struggling to meet her own developmental tasks, the nurse can focus her intervention on helping her with these. Some mothers can profit by temporary homemaker services which might help them survive a period of turmoil and crisis.

Different mothers may need help with different problems. For one mother, setting limits may be difficult and the nurse can help her learn to be consistent and more confident in her authority. Another mother may be overly directive and may need the support of the nurse in letting her child become more independent.[70,71] Most mothers need to talk to someone about accepting rejection from children and about tolerating the criticism and rejection of older children. Another mother may need support in the face of a critical parent or in-law who is harrassing her. Some mothers need to learn how to successfully separate from their children. Other problems may be encountered when two parents differ over how situations should be handled.

Many of the problems perplexing the parents will be normal problems that are destined to be encountered in raising children, but that does not make them any easier to deal with. Perennial problems which may be presented to the nurse include jealousy, sibling rivalry, temper tantrums, stealing, TV, fighting, sexual curiosity, enuresis, sex education, and chores. The nurse can serve a vital function just by using communication skills which help the parent clarify in her own mind what the problem is and using her knowledge of the problem solving process to find solutions.

It is especially important for the nurse to provide anticipatory guidance to the caretaker.[62] This can prepare the caretaker for what is ahead so that she begins to feel more competent and in control of the future. Measures can be used which focus on increasing the caretaker's adaptive capacities such as role playing difficult situations and various solutions.

It is important that the nurse attempt to provide intervention as early as possible for a family before attitudes and relationships become so confused that major efforts at intervention are needed. For this reason, major concerns should be focused on situations where new parents are found because early case finding presumably provides the best hope for promotion of change.

A complete discussion of methods of dealing with children which the nurse might find helpful in teaching to parents is beyond the scope of this chapter but some recommendations can be made. Nurses who frequently work with children and parents may find these resources valuable: general: Angela McBride, *The Growth and Development of Mothers;*[64] communicating with children: Haim Ginott, *Between Parent and Child,* New York: Macmillan, 1965; understanding child behavior and discipline: Rudolph Driekurs and Vicki Stoltz, *Children: the Challenge,* New York: Hawthorne Books, 1964; Raymond J. Corsini and Genevieve Painter, *The Practical Parent,* New York: Harper and Row, 1975.

Information can be suggested to parents which avoids a cookbook approach but instead educates them about why the child behaves as he does and how the parents can respond. For caretakers who are interested in reading, the use of a resource book can have several advantages. They may become more consistent in relating to their child, which is beneficial to them and the child. They may have more confidence because they are implementing what they read in print, and their increased confidence may be communicated to the child. Not all parents will be interested in reading books but the nurse who is familiar with the information can convey it to parents by teaching or remodeling. This will expand the caretaker's repertoire of child rearing techniques. Experiments the nurse suggests with different ways of handling a situation may help the caretaker to see that changes in parents' behavior may lead to changes in a child's behavior. Caretakers may begin to see that the way their parents handled their childhood is not necessarily the only way or the best.

A parent may feel relief when she can see that her sense of self-esteem need not be completely dependent on the accomplishments of her children. The nurse can help the caretaker see her parenting role as only one facet of her life. If she has accomplishments and abilities which she has developed outside of raising children, she may be more able to let her children be themselves rather than overcontrol them to meet her needs for recognition.

A parent may appreciate discussing the myths he believed on entering parenthood. He may realize that he has not necessarily failed as a parent because parenthood has not turned out to be the joyful experience he was led to think it would be.

The nurse can help a parent to gain perspectives about his family's stage of development by constructing a time line. A time line may also emphasize what is ahead, and preparing for the future can be discussed. In particular a parent may not be aware of the long period of his life which will likely be spent without children present in the home.

Possible nursing actions for improving parent-child relationships are summarized in Table 14-3.

**Table 14-3.** Possible nursing actions to improve parent-child interactions

1. Develop a helping relationship with the caretaker.
2. Teach the parent to problem solve.
3. Provide information on normal development and variability in children's behaviors.
4. Interpret the child to the caretaker to increase her sensitivity.
5. Help the parent establish routines or rearrange nonfunctional ones.
6. Search for ways to increase the caretaker's pleasure in the relationship.
7. Attempt to change negative views of the child.
8. Give the parent permission to have a life apart from his child.
9. Utilize parents' strengths.
10. Encourage use of other resources.
11. Work to remedy concurrent personal or family problems.
12. Provide specific help for specific problems.
13. Provide anticipatory guidance to increase the caretaker's sense of competence and control.
14. Intervene as early as possible.
15. Use resources on child rearing directly or indirectly.
16. Put parenthood in its proper perspective as only one component of an individual's life.
17. Help the caretaker develop realistic views about the benefits of parenthood.
18. Use a family time line to gain insight and prepare for the future.

## Tertiary Prevention of Disturbed Parent-Child Relationships

Tertiary prevention involves intervening in situations where long standing or severe disruption has occurred in the caretaker-child relationship so that the child's development has been altered either physically or emotionally and the functioning of the parents is inadequate and they are not providing sufficient or appropriate physical or psychological care.

Most of what has been described previously in the section on secondary prevention is of use to the nurse in working with parents where severe parenting disturbances exist. If one assumes that parenting is a learned behavior, then it could be concluded that caretakers who are functioning inadequately can be rehabilitated by learning new behaviors. Behavior change is usually considered a slow and difficult process so that nursing intervention in these situations will be prolonged and extensive.

Again it should be emphasized that the most important aspect of the nursing intervention is the formation of a helping relationship with the caretaker. Some sources suggest that the caretaker needs to be "mothered" or "reparented" by the nurse.[20,86] This could build up resources of self-esteem and security which she may never have had as a child. Sometimes a parent may fear close relationships and be resistant to the nurse's approach. If the nurse can persist in being warm, accepting, and nonjudgmental, she may eventually succeed.[82] It is very important in severely disrupted situations that someone focus almost exclusively on the caretaker.[5] It is understandable that most of the individuals interacting to help the family may tend to be primarily concerned about the child. To place the focus on the child further depletes the mother's ego and can increase her mistrust. The nurse is usually in a position where she can focus primarily on the caretaker.

Focusing on the mother is not always easy to do, especially if the nurse is concerned about the physical safety of the child. It is crucial for the nurse to remember that most caretakers, no matter how inadequately they are performing, do love their children.[7,20] Rehabilitating the caretaker, if possible, will usually provide a better solution in the future than placing the children in another care situation although the risks involved are greater.[45] For example, it has been found that infants who need increased stimulation are more likely to improve when the mother is supported and taught how to help her infant than when someone works with the infant outside of the home.

Some parents can benefit from having contact with parent's groups. One such group is Parents Anonymous which exists for supporting all caretakers who are experiencing difficulty raising their children. One service of the group which many have found beneficial is the provision of a telephone support service which caretakers can use for help at any time. Similarly, some cities are experimenting with 24-hour-a-day child care centers where caretakers can leave their children when they need relief.[20] Other parents may have other resources where they can turn in times of stress but they may need "permission" from the nurse to seek help. Some areas are experimenting with the use of lay visitors to support the caretaker who is under stress.[7,76]

The nurse herself may be able to serve as a subtle role model in her behavior toward the child[86] or the nurse may be able to arrange for the caretaker to have contact with other effective mothers so that the caretaker can pattern her behavior after theirs.[38] This is especially appropriate with the woman who saw negative role models as she grew up. Positive reinforcement should be given when the parent is engaging in appropriate behavior.

It seems particularly necessary to avoid appearing to be an authority or a stern parent figure. This means that interaction must be informal and casual with teaching done by suggestion.[82]

After the caretaker begins to feel more accepted and secure, the nurse can begin teaching and general supportive measures as described previously.

The nurse's responsibilities for the child involve seeing that he has any needed services—some of which she may be able to provide herself. The best help for the child is to improve the functioning of his parents, but temporary removal from the home may be warranted in certain circumstances. As an alternative, experiences outside of the home on a daily basis might be feasible.[79]

If the nurse discovers that a vulnerable child syndrome exists in the family, she can do much to help.[29] The parents are unaware that the problems they are experiencing with the child are because of their unconscious fear that the child may die. The nurse can ask if the child was ever seriously ill and let the caretaker thoroughly relive the situation involved. The caretaker will usually relate the story with considerable emotion and appear relieved to have discussed the fears she has been building up. The nurse can then help the caretaker to realize that she may still be reacting to the child as particularly vulnerable and that her treatment of the child as somehow special can be causing the behavioral problems the child is experiencing. This must be done with tact and sensitivity and cannot be accomplished quickly. Once the parents have seen the connection between the earlier situation and their problems with the child, the nurse can help them begin to rectify current problems. They will usually need help with setting limits, becoming less protective, and encouraging the child's independence. They also need to refrain from dwelling on how they almost lost the child. The caretaker needs assurance that the child has recovered and is not particularly prone to other illnesses or calamities.

The nurse should, of course, be cognizant of the development and personality of the child to see how he related to his caretaker and plan intervention for the child as appropriate.

Most situations which require tertiary prevention involve extensive and pervasive family disorganization and social deprivation.[72] There may be many problems of more priority to the family than those the nurse is concerned about. The nurse can mobilize efforts at resolving these problems. The family may evidence apathy and resignation which are very difficult for the nurse to change if even possible. The length of time involved in tertiary intervention can be extensive. Zacha describes work with a mother which lasted for several years and involved visits of more than once a week during some periods.[103] Reports of successful interventions with multiproblem families are not prevalent.

This information on tertiary prevention is presented in Table 14-4.

**Table 14-4.** Possible nursing actions to alter severely disrupted parent-child relationships

1. Focus primarily on forming a helping relationship with the principal caretaker.
2. Provide role models of effective parenting.
3. Use measures described under secondary prevention.
4. Intervene with the child as needed.
5. Help parent recognize vulnerable child syndrome if necessary.
6. Provide generalized measures to reduce family disorganization.

## THE NURSE AND PARENTHOOD

The professional nurse usually has a good basic background in psychology and sociology which may be helpful to her as a parent in understanding the development of her children and the functioning of her family. The processes which a nurse uses in her practice such as communication and problem solving are very useful in child rearing. The nurse's knowledge of nutrition and health promotion may enable her to intelligently care for her children.

But the special knowledge of a nurse may make her prone to worry about her role in her children's development and their health status too. And of course, she may suffer more if something does happen because she may feel that, as a nurse, she should have been able to prevent the problem or discover the problem earlier. Nurses must learn that they are as vulnerable as any parent to the stresses that face all parents but they also are well equipped to cope with parenthood and to share their knowledge with others.

The nurse must deal with her own feelings such as anger and disgust which may develop when she has contact with parents who have harmed or neglected their children and who may reject her help.[5] The nurse will need a support system of her own to discharge her feelings through. The nurse will be most effective with the caretaker if she does not add to their stresses by communicating displeasure and distrust of them.[38]

The nurse who works with extensively disrupted families will need support if she experiences discouragement. It may be helpful for the nurse to remind herself that she is not there to change the family but to work with the family within their life style and frame of reference. Some change in the caretaker-child relationship which she is able to promulgate may ensure that the child involved will be able to establish somewhat more optimal parent-child relationships when he becomes an adult than those he experienced as a child. Thus, slowly, will changes occur.

## A TOOL FOR ASSESSMENT AND EVALUATION

Because parenthood is often a central part of an individual's life experiences and because the relationships between parents and their children are instrumental in determining to a large extent the development of the child, the nurse needs to develop competence in assessing parenthood.

It is suggested that the nurse initially draw a family time line specifically designed for the family she works with. By studying this, the nurse can determine the family's position on the time line in relation to potential crisis periods and what concerns the family has experienced or is likely to experience. The nurse can reflect upon the interactions of the family with their particular environment and how it influences parent-child behavior.

Assessment of the socioeconomic frame of reference of the family may help the nurse in understanding values and conflicts they are experiencing. There may also be additional stresses with which the family is coping at any one time and these should be noted. Lastly, the nurse can assess the specific interactions between all family members. A framework for assessing the interactions between the caretaker and children of various ages will be detailed because this type of assessment can give the nurse a large amount of useful data.

### Assessing Parent-Child Relationships

The goal of the nurse's assessment is not to sort out "good" parents from "bad" parents but to determine if there are areas of the interaction between parents and their children where intervention might be helpful. No parent-child relationship is ever perfect. Some information can be obtained by interview techniques and some by observation. It is important to survey the relationship between each caretaker and each child separately and not survey only the interactions between the parents and the children as an aggregate. To do so might cause the nurse to miss subtle details.

To begin with, it should be stated that assessing the relationships in a child's environment is very risky and difficult for various reasons. First of all, assessment must be based on several periods of observation because any one situation may not be typical of the normal way people relate to the child but may reflect a temporary or unusual situation. Equally important, however, is the problem of observer bias. Each nurse has her own opinions of what is appropriate and what is not appropriate. Most nurses are by habit and nature oriented to the behaviors expected of middle class parents and the corresponding reactions of the child. Thus a nurse may classify all behavior by individuals not in the middle class as somewhat abnormal. This is, of course, not accurate. Unfortunately, much of what is written about looking at parents and their children reflects this middle class bias. The behaviors of caretakers differ with many factors including socioeconomic class. The typical behaviors of the middle class mother are not necessarily better than those of the mother in the lower socioeconomic class, but the nurse is more likely to identify with them and believe them to be appropriate.

Another bias is that, as members of the middle class, we are all too prone to consider almost exclusively the mother-child interaction and to a small incidental extent the father-child interaction. In order to accurately assess the child's environment, the nurse must turn her attention to the totality of experiences that surround the child. A child who gets little love or attention from his biologic mother and has no father present may be getting very adequate parenting by another individual in the environment. The nurse must determine who the principal caretaker is rather than assuming it is the biologic mother. In fact, it is possible for a child to grow up to be mentally and physically healthy without one clearly identifiable primary caretaker.

The nurse is looking for situations where the parent or caretaker is experiencing feelings of frustration and failure predominantly and the child is in danger of possible inappropriate emotional or social development because of the parent-child interaction.

The information given can be used by the nurse to evaluate the effectiveness of her intervention. The interaction should appear more like the characteristics described as more optimal if she is intervening appropriately.

## Assessment of the Mother's Potential for Parenthood

Because it is believed that the rudiments of motherliness develop early in an individual's life when she herself is an infant or a child, some assessments about her behavior as a child may have relevance to her future behavior as a mother. Some authors have attempted to classify females as highly or minimally maternal. It should be stated that there are probably many degrees of maternal behavior just as there are many degrees of maternal attachment, and most women are probably in the middle ranges rather than at the extremes. It is of interest to note that recent studies of the behavior of young girls show that "tomboys" are probably much more common than had been previously thought. In fact, there is some suggestion that most girls are "tomboys" as they grow up and that the very feminine little girl is the exception to the rule. Other behaviors shown later when the woman is pregnant are believed to be predictive of her future interaction with her child. Table 14-5 summarizes the information which was found in the literature. The relevance of these factors is unknown so the information is presented more as speculation than fact.

**Table 14-5.** Factors assumed to be predictive of the mother's potential for a successful mother-child relationship

| Behavior | More optimal | Less optimal |
| --- | --- | --- |
| Play as a young girl | Interested in dolls, playing house, babysitting | Tomboy |
| Relationship with mother | Positive identification | Rejection |
| Length of monthly menstrual flow | Long period of flow | Short period |
| Perceptions of fetus | Developing baby | Animal or tumor |
| Sexual preference | Desires either boy or girl | Definitely one preference |
| Fantasies of coming baby | Small, helpless infant | Older competent child |
| Attitude towards pregnancy | Positive | Negative |
| Feelings toward female role | Positive | Negative[15,49,50] |

## Assessment of Caretaker-Infant Interaction During the First Contact

Considerable significance is given to what the mother says and does upon first seeing and holding her baby. Table 14-6 details the variation in responses which may occur. Studies seem to indicate that there is an increased incidence of child abuse and other problems when the mother's responses were like those described as less optimal.[21]

**Table 14-6.** Responses of the mother on first contact with her newborn infant believed to be predictive of the beginning mother-infant relationship

| Behavior | More optimal | Less optimal |
|---|---|---|
| Comments about baby | Describes baby in positive terms—beautiful, cute | Describes baby in negative terms—ugly, frog |
| Interest in baby | Intense preoccupation | Disinterest |
| Handling | Holds baby close and so that their eyes meet "en face" | Holds baby away or so eyes do not meet |
| Positioning | Holds baby over heart | Baby not held in physical contact with body |
| Responses | Takes cues from baby | Not responsive |
| Vocalizations | Soft cooing sounds | Normal tone and inflection[9,49,50,60] |

## Assessment of Characteristics of the Infant

It should be restated at this point that the child and his unique behavioral characteristics probably influence the caretaker-child interaction at least as much as does the parenting style of the caretaker. For this reason, it would be beneficial for the nurse to describe the child using Thomas and Chess's nine dimensions of personality which were found to be discernible shortly after birth and which appear to persist somewhat during childhood.[93,94] These dimensions are identified in Table 14-7. Each child will vary in terms of his position on each category and on many of them he will fall in the middle.

Thomas and Chess were able to identify characteristics which they felt identified some children as "easy" to raise and others as "difficult." It would seem logical to believe that certain characteristics which might annoy one caretaker might be valued by another. For example, one caretaker may admire lively, noisy, physically active children and be annoyed by a child who sits motionlessly and quietly much of the time. Another caretaker may find that a very active child makes her "nervous" and enjoy a child who is placid and serene. It all depends on her perspective. And since caretakers' perceptions and reactions to children vary, the nurse needs to assess the caretaker's perceptions and compare them to hers. They may vary considerably and this should be noted. Because caretakers cannot order what kind of child they want, the potential for problems is higher when a child does not for some reason fit into the desires and expectations of his caretaker. Similarly, problems are predictable when the nurse's assessment differs markedly from the mother's, which may indicate that the mother is not accurately perceiving her child.

**Table 14-7.** Behavioral characteristics of infants which can be assessed shortly after birth

| Characteristics | Behavioral continuum | |
|---|---|---|
| Activity level: motor function | High: continually active, can hardly be still | Low: passive, slow, quiet |
| Rhythmicity: regularity of sleeping, hunger, eating, bodily functions, rest | Regular: consistent pattern present | Irregular: no recognizable pattern |
| Approach or withdrawal: initial reaction to new food, person, toy, situation | Approach: reacts positively, adjusts quickly to change | Withdrawal: reacts negatively, slow to adjust to change |
| Adaptability: how easily child's responses can be modified over time | Adaptive: will change responses with experience, flexible | Nonadaptive: responses change little, rigid |
| Intensity of reaction: degree of reaction to new stimuli, change, restriction, hunger | Intense: delight or distress is exaggerated | Mild: little reaction |
| Threshold of responsiveness: degree of stimulation necessary to provoke a response | Low: responds to small degrees of stimulation | High: responds only to large amounts of stimulation |
| Quality of Mood: | Negative: unfriendly, unhappy, whines, cries | Positive: friendly, joyful, smiles, laughs |
| Distractibility: degree to which one can influence child to change present activity for another | Distractible: will easily turn attention to next activity | Nondistractible: refuses to be lured by another activity |
| Attention span and persistence: length of time a particular activity will be pursued | Long: engages in activity for a prolonged time | Short: quickly changes activity |
| Response when presented with obstacles | Persistent: ignores or attempts to overcome obstacles in order to continue activity | Nonpersistent: changes behavior[93,94] |

## Assessment of Caretaker-Infant Behavior After Initial Contact

During the first few months after birth, certain behaviors indicate how the mother-infant interaction is proceeding. Table 14-8 represents some possible observations which were reported in the literature as indicating the functioning of the relationship. The point must be emphasized that one must differentiate between a lack of knowledge and experience in taking care of a baby and a lack of attachment to the baby. For example, a mother who demonstrates responses consistent with those less than optimal may need teaching on how to feed and hold the baby and may in reality have an optimal relationship with her baby.

The young infant may give clues about the caretaker-child relationship. Table 14-9 lists some behaviors which have been suggested as observable in young infants which are significant.

**Table 14-8.** Responses of mothers with young infants possibly predictive of the quality of the caretaker-infant relationship

| Behavior | More optimal | Less optimal |
| --- | --- | --- |
| Bottle feeding | Holds bottle so that nipple is filled with milk | Holds bottle carelessly so baby sucks air |
| Interest in baby | Preoccupation | Disinterest |
| Physical contact | Fondles baby, holds close, supports head | Avoids touch, holds baby awkwardly, lets head dangle |
| Verbal behavior | Talks to baby while giving care | Cares for baby in silence |
| Reaction to baby's crying | Appears anxious, attempts to soothe | Appears indifferent, always lets baby "cry it out" |
| Vigilance | Protects baby when in precarious situations | Lack of protective functioning |
| Reaction to separation | Hesitant to separate, worries about baby when apart | Separates readily, appears relieved, rarely thinks about baby when apart |
| Description of baby | Describes baby in positive terms, calls by name or nickname | Describes baby in negative terms, "bad," "difficult," "spoiled" |
| Ability to elicit smile from baby | Skillfully coaxes baby to smile | Unable to get baby to smile |
| Ability to describe new behaviors of baby | Aware of developmental changes | Unaware of changes |
| Ability to interpret baby | Can differentiate types of cries and implications | Unaware of baby's needs |
| Reaction to painful procedure done to baby (injection) | Reacts as though she herself were hurt | Expression unchanged |
| Reaction when baby complimented, "This is a beautiful baby" | Smiles, looks at baby, agrees | Expression unchanged, does not look at baby or disagrees |
| Reaction to child's attempts for physical contact | Accepts contact | Rejects contact |
| Use of punishment | Infrequent | Frequent use of harsh physical punishment |
| Play | Imitates baby, plays games, provides baby with appropriate toys | Toys unavailable, does not play with baby |
| Individualization of infant | Can describe baby's differences from other children, uniqueness | Describes baby as the same as all children |
| Reaction to baby's noises, body products, odors | Realistic acceptance | Repulsed |
| Beliefs about condition of baby | Appropriate | Believes baby has a defect |
| Beliefs about baby | Does not attribute negative emotions to baby | Believes infant dislikes her or attempts to expose faults[9,36,47,51,53,91] |

## Assessment of the Caretaker-Child Relationships of Young and School-aged Children

Table 14-10 details some parameters which have been suggested for assessing the relationships of caretakers with children over one year of age.

There are some observations about the behaviors of the child which have been sug-

**Table 14-9.** Responses of young infants believed to be predictive of the quality of the caretaker-infant relationship

| Behavior | More optimal | Less optimal |
|---|---|---|
| Focus of interest | More interested in mother | More interested in objects in the environment |
| Behavior after separation from caretaker | Attempts to approach caretaker | Not affected by separation |
| Responsiveness | Normal for age | Hypotonic or unresponsive |
| Developmental status | Normal for age | Delayed |
| Physical growth | Normal for age | Underweight |
| Autoerotic activity | Normal for age | Increased |
| Emotional responses | Normal for age | Restricted |
| Play activity | Normal for age | Unable to play |
| Exploration of environment | Uses mother as a base | Does not periodically return to mother[53] |

gested as helpful in looking at the caretaker-child relationship. These are presented in Table 14-11.

It is apparent that what we know about assessing caretaker-child relationships is rather subjective and judgmental. The reliability of such observations must not be overestimated. The nurse will have to rely on information as presented with caution. Note also that maternal behavior predominates in reported assessment characteristics. Appropriate paternal behavior appears to be an almost unrecognized area. However, some criteria have been suggested for assessing the father's responses to pregnancy of the mother and to the new baby. These are considered in Table 14-12.

**Table 14-10.** Characteristics of the relationship and behaviors of caretakers of children older than one year of age believed to be predictive of the quality of the caretaker-child relationship

| Behavior | More optimal | Less optimal |
|---|---|---|
| Warmth of the relationship | Warmth and affection predominate | Distance and coldness predominate |
| Parent's affective responses to child | Appropriate, i.e., caretaker smiles when child is happy | Inappropriate, i.e., caretaker laughs when child hurts himself |
| Consistency of reactions | Usually consistent | Inconsistent |
| Attitude toward misbehavior | Sees misbehavior from the child's point of view | Believes child purposefully misbehaves to discredit her |
| Ability to limit culturally unacceptable behavior by child | Limited effectively | Unable to limit |
| Communication pattern | Two way dialogue | Predominantly one way, commands, demands |
| Allowance of exploration by child | Encouraged | Discouraged |
| View of the future for the child | Hopeful | Has a negative view of the future for the child |
| Enjoyment in parenting | Feelings of pleasure predominate | Describes little or no pleasure |
| Acceptance of the child's personality | Views child as a unique and separate individual | Tries to change child's personality; views child as representative of someone else |
| Fault finding | Occasional | Continuous |
| Ability to enforce compliance | Usually successful | Unable, i.e., "he wouldn't take his medicine"[41,35,91] |

**Table 14-11.** Responses of children over one year of age which are suggested as predictive of the quality of the caretaker-child relationship

| Behavior | More optimal | Less optimal |
|---|---|---|
| Ability to relate to others | Normal | Decreased |
| School performance | Consistent with ability | Not equal to ability |
| Play | Plays freely | Restricted in play activities, bizarre use of toys |
| Roles played in the family | Roles change with the growth of the child and facilitate family functioning (clown, helper) | Roles are fixed and have a limiting effect on the child and family (scapegoat, troublemaker) |
| Sexual curiosity | Normal for age | Increased |
| Impulse control | Normal for age | Less than appropriate for age |
| Perceptions of the environment | Appropriate | Distorted |
| Range of emotional expression | Normal for age | Restricted |
| Mood | Normal | Pervasive depression, unhappiness, withdrawal |
| Health | Appropriate | Presence of headaches, stomach aches, speech problems, etc.[79,29,100] |

## Assessment of Child Abuse

Young children who have many injuries which are not logically explained may have been abused by their caretakers. When abuse has occurred the caretakers often gave vague, contradictory, or unrealistic descriptions of how the child was injured, were hostile, or showed little interest or concern about the child by avoidance of the treatment situation.[5,75] Many consider parents who abuse their children to be average parents who are inadequately coping with above average stresses,[89] but others feel abusing parents had a disturbed childhood themselves and demonstrate personality characteristics such as immaturity, impulsivity, and paranoia towards others.[86] It is possible that both descriptions of abusing parents could be accurate at different times for different parents.

Potential abusers may share some characteristics in common which the nurse might be able to assess.[21,38,45,47,51,78] It has been noted that parents who may abuse their children seem particularly sensitive to crying by their child and believe that their child cries excessively. They may feel depressed when he cries and have difficulty managing the child

**Table 14-12.** Responses of fathers to young infants believed to be predictive of the future father-child relationship

| Behavior | More optimal | Less optimal |
|---|---|---|
| Response during pregnancy | Anticipates assuming a new role | Foresees no change in role |
| Reaction to birth of child | Changes feelings about himself, life style, wife | No change in feelings |
| Perception of infant | As separate individual | Does not see as unique individual |
| Physical response | Touches and holds infant | Does not approach physically |
| Emotional response | Describes feelings of love and tenderness towards baby | Not present[57] |

when crying. They may give the nurse the impression that they expect the child to mother them. In some situations, an older child may have learned to "mother" the mother to avoid being hurt. Some potentially abusive parents will state that they dislike being alone with the child and this is believed to be because they fear what they may do to the child. They may express that they feel they have many critics and that they dislike having people watch them interact with their child. Questioning may reveal that they have rigid and unrealistic ideas on discipline which demand behavior from the child before it is possible. Many were themselves abused as children. Some potentially abusive parents seek help by seemingly inappropriate visits to health care settings in the hopes that someone will be able to help them and discover their fear that they will hurt their child before actual abuse occurs. Chronic deliberate child abuse is not synonymous with accidental injury inflicted on a child by a caretaker who has lost his temper.

Certain children seem more likely to provoke child abuse than others. Those who were premature, defective, unwanted, or ill have been noted as more frequently abused than others.[45,89] It has been noted that abused children have later been abused when placed in a foster home where abuse had not occurred previously.[28] This might suggest that the child is definitely a factor in precipitating abuse. In many situations, only one child in the family is abused. Children who have been abused, in addition to signs of physical damage, may manifest increased autoerotic behavior, restricted or exaggerated emotional outbursts, lack of crying, fear of others, lethargy, and will not usually turn to their caretakers for comfort.[5,45]

## Assessment of the Failure-to-Thrive Syndrome

Children who are neglected usually have parents who appear to have characteristics much like those who abuse their children except that the element of physical abuse is absent. Neglect has been described as passive child abuse and may be one end of the parental dysfunction continuum with child abuse at the other end.[46] The parents may appear disinterested and unsatisfied by their children. A frequent picture is a lonely mother under stress in an unhappy marriage who has an unwanted baby after a difficult pregnancy or delivery.[82]

The infant who is failing to thrive displays marked malnourishment and growth failure with delays in social and motor development. Specifically, he may have poor muscle tone, lethargy, increased autoerotic behavior, an inability to cuddle, and delayed or absent vocalizations. He may not show the expected fear of strangers or protest when left alone.[82] Many children have been described as displaying a peculiar intense eye contact which appears to almost represent a plea for human contact.[77] Some infants may resist physical contact[95] while others may fail to demonstrate the expected resistance of an infant to bodily manipulation.[77] Some infants refuse to feed while held but will take their bottles if the bottle is propped and the infant is placed in his bed.

The infant who is a true victim of the failure-to-thrive syndrome will show steady weight gain when hospitalized. Failure to maintain improvement when he returns to his usual home situation is a significant observation. Physical illnesses may mimic a failure-to-thrive syndrome and must be ruled out. There are probably degrees of severity of the maternal deprivation which causes failure-to-thrive syndrome.[59] The nurse must be alert to only slight evidences.

## AN EXAMPLE OF NURSING INTERVENTION IN PARENTHOOD

The following example of nursing intervention describes the actions of two nurses working in a children's unit. This example was chosen because it illustrates that even brief encounters with parents in episodic settings can be used to promote healthy parent-child relationships and support distraught parents.

Six-year-old Bobby Hadley and his mother were occupying a private room. Bobby had been admitted late the night before for an appendectomy. His appendix had been found during surgery to be ruptured and gangrenous. The team leader, Kathy, encountered Ms. Hadley and Bobby while making rounds after report. Bobby was in a crib and appeared flushed and irritable. He had an intravenous infusion, a urinary catheter, and a nasal gastric tube for suction. Ms. Hadley, who appeared to be in her early 40s, was hovering over Bobby, saying over and over, "I know my baby is so sick." Ms. Hadley had spent the night and had slept in her clothes since the trip to the hospital had been unexpected and she had not had time to pack a suitcase.

Upon seeing the team leader, Ms. Hadley commented that she was sure Bobby's temperature was elevated again and wanted some medication for him. She talked anxiously and her voice had a tone of great urgency. Kathy assured the mother than she would check into Bobby's temperature and need for medication.

Kathy's next contact with Bobby and his mother occurred a few minutes later when she returned to their room to give Bobby a suppository for his elevated temperature. The mother helped with the procedure and stated repeatedly and emphatically, "Mommy won't let her hurt my baby." Kathy was impressed by the mother's high level of anxiety as evidenced by her behavior and the way she was relating to her son. After comforting Bobby, who screamed with terror during the procedure, she talked with Ms. Hadley briefly. Kathy discovered that Ms. Hadley had been awake most of the night watching over Bobby and was exhausted from the experiences of the previous day and the almost sleepless night. She was very concerned that the surgeon who had operated on Bobby had not come to see him after surgery or yet that morning. Ms. Hadley told Kathy with a lot of emotion that Bobby had been sick for a few days before the surgery and she thought he had influenza as several neighborhood children did and had not taken him to the doctor immediately. Kathy made a mental note that the mother had a lot of concerns she seemed to want to talk about but Kathy thought that they would be best discussed somewhere away from Bobby since the general tone of Ms. Hadley's comments projected fears over her son's illness which were probably being communicated to Bobby. Kathy decided to plan a time to talk with Ms. Hadley away from Bobby's room.

Kathy had a few other glimpses of the activity in Bobby's room during the morning. Ms. Hadley maintained a constant vigil over Bobby's bed and directed all activity by Joan, the nurse who was assigned to him. On one occasion, she had the nurse put Bobby back to bed almost immediately after he was up in a chair because "He looks so weak. He's too tired to sit up."

Kathy and Joan spent a few minutes comparing notes about Ms. Hadley's behavior and they wrote down the following hypotheses which they believed to be relevant in this situation.

1. Ms. Hadley wishes to help Bobby recover and her present behavior represents the best response she is capable of making at this time.
2. Ms. Hadley is many miles from home and her husband in a strange environment and without her usual sources of support.
3. Ms. Hadley feels guilty over not taking Bobby to the doctor sooner and this is manifested in anxiety over his condition.
4. Ms. Hadley believes that a ruptured appendix is associated with a very serious illness.

## Kathy and Joan decided on the following actions.

1. Ms. Hadley needs a chance to express her concerns away from Bobby's room.
2. The nurses caring for Bobby are usually focusing on Bobby and his care out of necessity but Kathy should focus on Ms. Hadley separately.
3. Ms. Hadley may need some information about the illness Bobby has had and his expected convalescence.
4. Ms. Hadley's concern for Bobby is a strength to be utilized in the intervention, but she needs some help in channeling her concern for Bobby into activities that are more purposeful.

## The following action was planned.

1. Kathy would invite Ms. Hadley to lunch in the hospital cafeteria with the assurance that Joan would take care of Bobby while the mother was gone.
2. Kathy would give Ms. Hadley a chance to talk about what she had gone through. Kathy would try to convey understanding and support and help Ms. Hadley deal with her guilt if possible.
3. After lunch, Joan would encourage Ms. Hadley to take a nap while Bobby took his.
4. Joan and the other staff would make a conscious attempt to communicate with Bobby in a calm manner which respected his age and competencies in the hopes that Ms. Hadley might begin to adopt their approach.
5. Joan would try to suggest specific activities that Ms. Hadley might do for Bobby in place of her anxious hovering and overstimulation.
6. Information about Bobby's condition would be brought in whenever the mother was receptive.
7. Kathy and Joan would evaluate their progress at the end of the afternoon and prepare notes for the evening staff.

Ms. Hadley accepted Kathy's invitation to lunch and appeared to be relieved to leave the children's unit with Bobby under the watchful eye of Joan. On the way to the cafeteria Kathy asked the mother about her experiences of the day before. Ms. Hadley explained Bobby's illness, the rushed admission, and the surgery. She again expressed distress that he had been ill for several days and she had not realized the seriousness. Kathy commented throughout the conversation with statements such as, "It must be difficult to know a child is sick, but to wonder how serious the illness is" and "You must have been really frightened when the doctor told you to bring him to the emergency room." Kathy found out that Ms. Hadley had not eaten any supper the night before or any breakfast that morning. She was also worried about how her husband was managing at home with their 13-year-old daughter to care for. Ms. Hadley seemed more relaxed as she ate. On the way back to the children's unit, Ms. Hadley asked Kathy if Bobby had peritonitis. Kathy was able to cover several things which she had wanted to tell Ms. Hadley. Ms. Hadley was obviously surprised to learn that most appendectomies in children involve a ruptured appendix. Kathy was able to mention that she thought the fact that the surgeon had not placed Bobby in the intensive care unit was a good sign that he expected a positive recovery. Ms. Hadley commented thoughtfully that she had not considered that.

After returning to the children's unit, Joan noticed that Ms. Hadley definitely appeared less agitated. Bobby's nasal-gastric tube had been taken out and he looked less restrained.

Joan handed Ms. Hadley some children's books and suggested that she read some stories to Bobby before his nap. She pulled up a chair for her to sit in which was near by. She stressed that Ms. Hadley could probably make the stories more interesting to Bobby than she could. Ms. Hadley read until Bobby was asleep but she declined taking a nap and sat watchfully beside Bobby. Joan and Kathy concluded that some progress was being made and communicated their plan to the evening shift.

The next morning, Kathy and Joan learned that the evening and night staff had carried on the plan. Ms. Hadley had left to eat dinner, with a nurse watching Bobby, had called her husband, and had slept most of the night. During the morning Joan provided Ms. Hadley with activities such as giving Bobby his bath and taping up pictures he had chosen around his room. Joan again stressed that Ms. Hadley was special to Bobby. Ms. Hadley was much less likely to hover over Bobby's bed and she appeared less harried. Kathy commented on Bobby's stabilizing temperature and his progress. Ms. Hadley still seemed watchful for things to go wrong, however. Although Joan and Kathy tried to consistently talk to Bobby in an optimistic and mature manner, Ms. Hadley continued to communicate with him as though he were helpless and unable to comprehend his situation. She did not refer to him as "baby" at all during the second day.

In order to promote adult contact, Kathy suggested to another mother that she invite Ms. Hadley to the parent's lounge during the afternoon nap time. Kathy dropped in to visit and found them comparing their children's illnesses and physicians. Ms. Hadley seemed to gain some perspective about the fact that her child was not as seriously ill as other children in the unit and commented later on how lucky Bobby was only to have had an appendectomy.

As Ms. Hadley relaxed, Bobby became less irritable. Kathy and Joan concluded that they had brought some relief of anxiety to Ms. Hadley in small periods of contact during two days of focusing on her and her needs as an individual and as a parent by providing chances for her to ventilate her feelings, acknowledging her difficult yet special role as a mother, rechanneling her good intentions into more constructive activities, providing her with information which lessened her fears over her child's condition, and providing an impetus for her to have periods of escape from her son's bedside. The hoped for support they had provided to Ms. Hadley to deal with her own stresses had allowed her to eventually channel her energies into activities related to her role as Bobby's parent.

## SUMMARY

The nurse in many settings will have contact with teenagers and adults who are parents. The nurse often can promote healthy parent-child relationships. She is frequently in a good position to assess and intervene in situations where something is amiss in relation to the significant relationships that a child is experiencing. It is hoped that the nurse can learn to recognize potential situations which can lead to altered relationships, assess the interactions which are occurring, and intervene to prevent problems or to promote improvement in the relationships which surround the child. Through this action, the nurse may help some children to one day become mentally and physically healthy parents themselves. In addition, the nurse may likely be a parent herself. She can use her specialized knowledge of parenthood and her nursing skills to good advantage.

# REFERENCES

1. Ainsworth, M.: "Attachment and separation of children under pediatric care." Paper presented at the 11th Annual Conference, Association for the Care of Children in Hospitals, Denver, 1976.
2. Bache-Wiig, B. J.: "Adoption insights: A course for adoptive parents." Child. Today 4:22, 1975
3. Badger, E. D.: "A mother's training program: The road to a purposeful existence." Children 18:168, 1971.
4. Balter, L.: "Psychological consultation for preschool parent groups: An educational-psychological intervention to promote mental health." Child. Today 5:19, 1976.
5. Bassett, L. B.: "How to help abused children and their parents." RN 37:44, 1974.
6. Bell, R. Q.: "Contributions of human infants to caregiving and social interaction," in Lewis, M., and Rosenblum, L. (eds.): *The Effect of the Infant on Its Caregiver.* John Wiley and Sons, New York, 1974.
7. Besharov, D. J.: "Building a community response to child abuse and maltreatment." Child. Today 4:2, 1975.
8. Birdwhistell, R. L.: "The idealized model of the American family." Soc. Casework 51:195, 1970.
9. Bishop, B.: "A guide to assessing parenting capabilities." Am. J. Nurs. 76:1784, 1976.
10. Blau, A., et al.: "The psychogenic etiology of premature births: A preliminary report." Psychosom. Med. 25:201, 1963.
11. Brandwein, R. A., et al.: "Women and children last: The social situation of divorced mothers and their families." J. Marriage Family 36:489, 1974.
12. Bronfenbrenner, U.: "Nobody home: The erosion of the American family." Psychol. Today 10:40, 1977.
13. Bronfenbrenner, U.: "Socialization and social class through time and space," in Maccoby, E. E., Newcomb, T. M., and Hartley, E. L. (eds.): *Readings in Social Psychology.* Wolt, Rinehart and Winston, New York, 1958.
14. Brown, J., and Hepler, R.: "Stimulation: A corollary to physical care." Am. J. Nurs. 76:578, 1976.
15. Caplan, G.: *Concepts of Mental Health and Consultation.* Children's Bureau, Washington, D.C., 1959.
16. Clark, A. L.: "Stresses and conflicts: Their relevance to the expanding family," in *Parent-Child Relationships: Role of the Nurse.* Rutgers University, New Brunswick, N.J., 1968.
17. Clark, A. L., and Affonso, D. D.: *Childbearing: A Nursing Perspective.* F. A. Davis, Philadelphia, 1976.
18. Clayton, M., and Dow, P.: "Exploring childhood." Child. Today 2:8, 1973.
19. Cohen, D. J.: "Meeting adolescents' needs." Child. Today 2:28, 1973.
20. Davoren, E.: "Working with abusive parents—A social worker's view." Child. Today 4:2, 1975.
21. Dean, J.: "Prediction and prevention." Paper presented at the 11th Annual Conference, Association for the Care of Children in Hospitals, Denver, 1976.
22. Dixon, G.: "Helping infants, toddlers and parents to thrive in the hospital and in the community." Paper presented at the 10th Annual Conference, Association for the Care of Children in Hospitals, Boston, 1975.
23. Duvall, E. M.: *Marriage and Family Development.* J. B. Lippincott, Philadelphia, 1977.
24. Dyer, E. D.: "Parenthood as crisis: A re-study," in Parad, H. J. (ed.): *Crisis Intervention: Selected Readings.* Family Service Association of America, New York, 1965.
25. Friedan, B.: *The Feminine Mystique.* Dell Publishing, New York, 1963.
26. Garrett, B. L.: "Foster family services for mentally retarded children." Children 17:228, 1970.
27. Garrett, B. L.: "The rights of foster parents." Children 17:113, 1970.
28. Gil, D. G.: *Violence Against Children.* Harvard University Press, Cambridge, Mass., 1970.
29. Green, M., and Solnit, A. J.: "Reactions to the threatened loss of a child: A vulnerable child syndrome." Ped. 34:58, 1964.
30. Greenberg, M., and Morris, N.: "Engrossment: The newborn's impact upon the father." Am. J. Orthopsychiat. 44:520, 1974.
31. Grossman, G. K.: *Brothers and Sisters of Retarded Children: An Exploratory Study.* Syracuse University Press, Syracuse, N.Y., 1972.
32. Gustin, K.: "The adopting family," in Hymovich, D. P., and Barnard, M. U. (eds.): *Family Health Care.* McGraw-Hill, New York, 1973.
33. Hammons, C.: "The adoptive family." Am. J. Nurs. 76:251, 1976.
34. Handel, G.: "Sociological aspects of parenthood," in Hymovich, D. P., and Barnard, M. U. (eds.): *Family Health Care.* McGraw-Hill, New York, 1973.
35. Hartmann, K., and Bush, M.: "Action-oriented family therapy." Am. J. Nurs. 75:1184, 1975.
36. Helfer, R., and Kempe, H. C. (eds.): *The Battered Child.* University of Chicago Press, Chicago, 1968.

37. Hines, J. D.: "Father—The forgotten man." Nurs. Forum 10:176, 1971.
38. Hopkins, J.: "The nurse and the abused child." Nurs. Clin. North Am. 5:589, 1970.
39. Hott, J. R.: "The crisis of expectant fatherhood." Am. J. Nurs. 76:1436, 1976.
40. Howell, M. C.: "Effects of maternal employment on the child (II)." Ped. 52:327, 1973.
41. Hurwitz, J. I., et al.: "Designing an instrument to assess parental coping mechanisms," in Parad, H. J. (ed.): *Crisis Intervention: Selected Readings.* Family Service Association of America, New York, 1965.
42. Hymovich, D. P.: "The family with a young child," in Hymovich, D. P., and Barnard, M. U. (eds.): *Family Health Care.* McGraw-Hill, New York, 1973.
43. Jongeward, D., and Scott, D.: *Women as Winners.* Addison-Wesley, Reading, Mass., 1976.
44. Jones, P. S.: "Parenthood education in a city high school." Child. Today 4:7, 1975.
45. Kalisch, B. J.: "Nursing actions in behalf of the battered child." Nurs. Forum 12:365, 1973.
46. Kaplan, H. S.: "Problems of parenting: Child abuse," in Waechter, E. H., and Blake, F. G.: *Nursing Care of Children.* J. B. Lippincott, Philadelphia, 1976.
47. Kempe, H. C., and Helfer, R. (ed.): *Helping the Battered Child and His Family.* J. B. Lippincott, Philadelphia, 1972.
48. Kirk, H. D.: *Shared Fate.* Free Press, New York, 1964.
49. Klaus, M. H., and Kennell, J. H.: "Mothers separated from their newborn infants." Ped. Clin. North Am. 17:1015, 1970.
50. Klaus, M. H., et al.: "Human maternal behavior at the first contact with her young." Ped. 46:187, 1970.
51. Korsch, B.: "Practical techniques of observing, interviewing and advising parents in pediatrics as demonstrated in an attitude study project." Ped. 18:467, 1956.
52. Kruger, W. S.: "Education for parenthood and the schools." Child. Today. 2:4, 1973.
53. Lamper, C.: "Faciliating attachment through well-baby care," in Hall, J. E., and Weaver, B. R. (eds.): *Nursing of Families in Crisis.* J. B. Lippincott, Philadelphia, 1974.
54. Lancaster, J., and Roberts, F. B.: "Impact of intensive care on the maternal-infant relationship," in Korones, S. B.: *High Risk Newborn Infants: The Basis for Intensive Nursing Care.* C. V. Mosby, St. Louis, 1972.
55. Lawson, B.: "Chronic illness in the school-aged child: Effects on the total child." Matern. Child Nurs. J. 2:49, 1977.
56. LeMasters, E. E.: "Parenthood as crisis," in Parad, H. J. (ed.): *Crisis Intervention: Selected Readings.* Family Service Association of America, New York, 1965.
57. Leonard, S. W.: "How first-time fathers feel toward their newborns." Matern. Child Nurs. J. 1:361, 1976.
58. Lidz, T.: *The Person: His Development Throughout the Life Cycle.* Basic Books, New York, 1968.
59. Lipp, J. P., and Specht, E. E.: "Growth, development, and care during the first year," in Waechter, E. H., and Blake, F. G.: *Nursing Care of Children.* J. B. Lippincott, Philadelphia, 1976.
60. Luddington-Hoe, S. M.: "Postpartum: Development of maternicity." Am. J. Nurs. 77:1171, 1977.
61. Macintyre, J. M.: "Adolescence, identity, and foster family care." Children 17:213, 1970.
62. Maebius, N. K.: "The nurse and the expanding family: A mother's viewpoint," in Hymovich, D. P., and Barnard, M. U. (eds.): *Family Health Care.* McGraw-Hill, New York, 1973.
63. Marland, S. P.: "Education for parenthood." Child. Today 2:3, 1973.
64. McBride, A. B.: *The Growth and Development of Mothers.* Harper and Row, New York, 1973.
65. McCabe, S. N.: "Anticipatory guidance of families with infants," in Hymovich, D. P., and Barnard, M. U. (eds.): *Family Health Care.* McGraw-Hill, New York, 1973.
66. McRae, M.: "An approach to the single parent dilemma." Matern. Child Nurs. J. 2:164, 1977.
67. Middleman, R.: "A service pattern for helping unmarried pregnant teenagers." Children 17:108, 1970.
68. Millar, T. P.: "The hospital and the preschool child." Children 17:171, 1970.
69. Minturn, L., and Lambert, W.: "Motherhood and child rearing," in Bell, N. W., and Vogel, E. F. (eds.): *The Family.* Free Press, London, 1968.
70. Missildine, W. H.: "Case history interview: Perfectionistic overcoercion." Feelings and Their Medical Significance (Ross Laboratories) 12:1, 1970.
71. Missildine, W. H.: *Your Inner Child of the Past.* Simon and Schuster, New York, 1963.
72. Morris, M. G., Gould, R. W., and Matthews, P. J.: "Toward prevention of child abuse." Children 11:58, 1964.
73. Nelson, S. A.: "School age parents." Child. Today 2:31, 1973.
74. Obrzut, L. A.: "Expectant father's perception of fathering." Am. J. Nurs. 76:1440, 1976.
75. Olson, R. J.: "Index of suspicion: Screening for child abuse." Am. J. Nurs. 76:108, 1976.
76. Pavenstedt, E.: "The meanings of motherhood in a deprived environment," in Pavenstedt, E., and Bernard, V. W. (eds.): *Crisis of Family Disorganization.* Behavioral Publications, New York, 1971.

77. Pillitteri, A.: *Nursing Care of the Growing Family: A Child Health Text.* Little, Brown and Company, Boston, 1977.
78. Pollock, C. B.: "Early case finding as a means of prevention of child abuse," in Helfer, R., and Kempe, C. H. (eds.): *The Battered Child.* University of Chicago Press, Chicago, 1968.
79. Pothier, P. C.: *Mental Health Counseling With Children.* Little, Brown and Company, Boston, 1976.
80. Rainwater, L.: *Family Design: Marital Sexuality, Family Size and Contraception.* Aldine, Chicago, 1965.
81. Reeder, S., et al.: *Maternity Nursing.* J. B. Lippincott, Philadelphia, 1976.
82. Rhymes, J. P.: "Working with mothers and babies who fail to thrive." Am. J. Nurs. 66:1972, 1966.
83. Robson, K. S., and Moss, H. A.: "Patterns as determinants of maternal attachment." J. Ped. 77:976, 1970.
84. Rosoff, S. R.: "Education for parenthood: An overview." Child. Today 2:1, 1973.
85. Rossi, A. S.: "Transition to parenthood." J. Marriage Family 30:26, 1968.
86. Savino, A. B., and Sanders, R. W.: "Working with abusive parents: Group therapy and home visits." Am. J. Nurs. 73:482, 1973.
87. Schecter, M.: "About adoptive parents," in Anthony, J., and Benedek, T. (eds.): *Parenthood.* Little, Brown and Company, Boston, 1970.
88. Sheehy, G.: *Passages.* E. P. Dutton, New York, 1974.
89. Smith, S. M.: "The battered child syndrome—Some research findings." Nurs. Mirror 140:48, 1975.
90. Stollack, G. E.: "Learning to communicate with children." Child. Today 4:12, 1975.
91. Stone, F.: "A critical review of a current program of research into mother-child relationships," in Caplan, G. (ed.): *Emotional Problems of Early Childhood.* Basic Books, New York, 1955.
92. Stowitschek, J. J., and Hofmeister, A.: "Parent training packages." Child. Today 4:23, 1975.
93. Thomas, A., et al.: "The origin of personality." Scient. Am. 233:102, 1970.
94. Thomas, A., et al: *Behavioral Individuality in Early Childhood.* New York University Press, New York, 1963.
95. Triplett, J.: "The role of experience in child development," in Scipien, G. M., et al.: *Comprehensive Pediatric Nursing.* McGraw-Hill, New York, 1975.
96. Tudor, M. J.: "Family habituation: A child with a birth defect," in Hymovich, D. P., and Barnard, M. U. (eds.): *Family Health Care.* McGraw-Hill, New York, 1973.
97. Ventura, J., and Dykstal, V.: "Perspectives of health care for a low income family." J. Assoc. Care Child. Hosp. 5:4, 1976.
98. Wallin, P., and Riley, R.: "Reactions of mothers to pregnancy and adjustment of offspring in infancy." Am. J. Orthopsychiat. 20:616, 1950.
99. Wilson, G., and Ryland, G.: *Social Work Group Practice.* Houghton Mifflin, New York, 1949.
100. Work, H. H.: "The resistive child." Feelings and Their Medical Significance (Ross Laboratories) 7:1, 1965.
101. Wuerger, M. K.: "Stepping into parenthood." Am. J. Nurs. 76:1283, 1976.
102. Young, L.: *Out of Wedlock.* McGraw-Hill, New York, 1954.
103. Zacha, M. C.: "Nursing goals in working with families under multiple stress." Nurs. Clin. North Am. 4:69, 1969.
104. Zimmerman, B. M.: "The exceptional stresses of adoptive parenthood." Matern. Child Nurs. J. 2:191, 1977.

# BIBLIOGRAPHY

Baumrind, D.: "Some thoughts about childrearing," in Bronfenbrenner, U., and Mahoney, M. A. (eds.): *Influences on Human Development.* Dryden Press, Hinsdale, Ill., 1975.

Brazelton, T. B.: "The early mother-infant adjustment." Ped. 32:931, 1963.

Brazelton, T. B.: "Listening to toddlers." J. Assoc. Care Child. Hosp. 4:17, 1976.

Bronfenbrenner, U.: *Is Early Intervention Effective?* Department of Health, Education and Welfare, Office of Child Development, Washington, D.C., 1974.

Brown, M. S., and Hurlock, J. T.: "Mothering the mother." Am. J. Nurs. 77:438, 1977.

Erdman, D.: "Parent-to-parent support: The best for those with sick newborns." Matern. Child Nurs. J. 2:291, 1977.

Holaday, B. J.: "Achievement behavior in chronically ill children." Nurs. Res. 23:25, 1974.

Josselyn, I. M.: "Cultural forces: Motherliness and fatherliness." Am. J. Orthopsychiat. 26:264, 1956.

Kagan, J.: "Exploring childhood: A theoretical foundation." Child. Today 2:13, 1973.

Kilker, R., and Wilkerson, B. L.: "Anticipatory guidance of the expectant family," in Hymovich, D. P., and Barnard, M. U. (eds.): *Family Health Care.* McGraw-Hill, New York, 1973.

Laymann, E. M.: "Discussion: Symposium: Father influence in the family." Merrill-Palmer Quart. 7:107, 1961.

Mattson, A.: "Long term physical illness in childhood: A challenge to psychosocial adaptation." Ped. 50:801, 1972.

Minuchin, S., et al.: *Families of the Slums: An Exploration of Their Structure and Treatment.* Basic Books, New York, 1967.

Morris, M. G.: "Maternal claiming—identification processes: Their meaning for mother-infant mental health," in Clark, A. L. (ed.): *Parent Child Relationships: The Role of the Nurse.* Rutgers University, New Brunswick, N.J., 1968.

Pavenstedt, E.: "To help infants weather disorganized family life," in Reinhardt, A. M., and Quinn, M. D. (eds.): *Family-Centered Community Nursing: A Sociocultural Framework.* C. V. Mosby, St. Louis, 1973.

Rubin, R.: "The family-child relationship and nursing care." Nurs. Outlook 12:36, 1964.

Viren, M.: "Economics and the family," in Hymovich, D. P., and Barnard, M. U. (eds.): *Family Health Care.* McGraw-Hill, New York, 1973.

Wonnell, E.: "The education of the expectant father for childbirth." Nurs. Clin. North Am. 6:591, 1971.

Zigler, E. F.: "A national priority: Raising the quality of children's lives." Children 17:166, 1970.

# *INDEX*

**425**